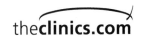

CHILD AND ADOLESCENT PSYCHIATRIC CLINICS OF NORTH AMERICA

Neuropsychiatric Genetic Syndromes

GUEST EDITOR
Doron Gothelf, MD

CONSULTING EDITOR
Andrés Martin, MD, MPH

July 2007 • Volume 16 • Number 3

SAUNDERS

An Imprint of Elsevier, Inc.
PHILADELPHIA   LONDON   TORONTO   MONTREAL   SYDNEY   TOKYO

W.B. SAUNDERS COMPANY
A Division of Elsevier Inc.

Elsevier Inc. • 1600 John F. Kennedy Boulevard • Suite 1800 • Philadelphia, Pennsylvania 19103-2899

http://www.childpsych.theclinics.com

CHILD AND ADOLESCENT PSYCHIATRIC CLINICS	**Volume 16, Number 3**
OF NORTH AMERICA	**ISSN 1056–4993**
July 2007	**ISBN-13: 978-1-4160-5044-5**
Editor: Sarah E. Barth	**ISBN-10: 1-4160-5044-2**

The ideas and opinions expressed in *Child and Adolescent Psychiatric Clinics of North America* do not necessarily reflect those of the Publisher. The Publisher does not assume any responsibility for any injury and/or damage to persons or property arising out of or related to any use of the material contained in this periodical. The reader is advised to check the appropriate medical literature and the product information currently provided by the manufacturer of each drug to be administered to verify the dosage, the method and duration of administration, or contraindications. It is the responsibility of the treating physician or other health care professional, relying on independent experience and knowledge of the patient, to determine drug dosages and the best treatment for the patient. Mention of any product in this issue should not be construed as endorsement by the contributors, editors, or the Publisher of the product or manufacturers' claims.

Child and Adolescent Psychiatric Clinics of North America (ISSN 1056-4993) is published quarterly by Elsevier Inc., 360 Park Avenue South, New York, NY 10010-1710. Months of issue are January, April, July, and October. Business and Editorial Offices: 1600 John F. Kennedy Boulevard, Suite 1800, Philadelphia, PA 19103-2899. Customer Service Offices: 6277 Sea Harbor Drive, Orlando, FL 32887-4800. Periodicals postage paid at New York, NY and additional mailing offices. Subscription prices are $200.00 per year (US individuals), $302.00 per year (US institutions), $103.00 per year (US students), $227.00 per year (Canadian individuals), $356.00 per year (Canadian institutions), $124.00 per year (Canadian students), $200.00 per year (international individuals), $356.00 per year (international institutions), and $124.00 per year (international students). International air speed delivery is included in all *Clinics* subscription prices. All prices are subject to change without notice. **POSTMASTER:** Send address changes to *Child and Adolescent Psychiatric Clinics of North America*, Elsevier Periodicals Customer Service, 6277 Sea Harbor Drive, Orlando, FL 32887-4800. **Customer Service: 1-800-654-2452 (US). From outside of the US, call 1-407-345-4000.**

Child and Adolescent Psychiatric Clinics of North America is covered in *Index Medicus, ISI, SSCI, Research Alert, Social Search, Current Contents,* and *EMBASE/Excerpta Medica.*

Printed in the United States of America.

CONSULTING EDITOR

ANDRÉS MARTIN, MD, MPH, Professor of Child Psychiatry, Yale Child Study Center, Yale University School of Medicine, New Haven; and Medical Director, Children's Psychiatric Inpatient Service, Yale New Haven Children's Hospital, New Haven, Connecticut

FOUNDING CONSULTING EDITOR

MELVIN LEWIS, MBBS, FRCPsych, DCH

GUEST EDITOR

DORON GOTHELF, MD, Department of Child Psychiatry, The Behavioral Neurogenetics Center, Schneider Children's Medical Center of Israel, Petah Tiqwa; and Tel Aviv University, Tel Aviv, Israel

CONTRIBUTORS

FORTU BENARROCH, MD, Child and Adolescent Psychiatrist, Hadassah-Hebrew University Medical Center, Jerusalem; and Multidisciplinary Clinic for Prader-Willi Syndrome at the Neuropediatric Unit, Shaare Zedek Medical Center, Jerusalem, Israel

ELISABETH M. DYKENS, PhD, Professor, Department of Psychology and Human Development, Peabody College, Vanderbilt University; Associate Director, Vanderbilt Kennedy Center for Research on Human Development; and Director, Vanderbilt Kennedy University Center of Excellence on Developmental Disabilities, Nashville, Tennessee

STEPHAN ELIEZ, MD, Professor, Service-Médico-Pédagogique, Department of Psychiatry, University of Geneva; and Department of Genetic Medicine and Development, University of Geneva School of Medicine, Geneva, Switzerland

CARL FEINSTEIN, MD, Professor, Psychiatry and Behavioral Science-Child Psychiatry, Stanford University School of Medicine, Stanford; Lucile Packard Children's Hospital, Palo Alto, California

JOAQUIN FUENTES, MD, Head, Service of Child & Adolescence Psychiatry, Policlinica Gipuzkoa; and Scientific Advisor, GAUTENA Autism Society, San Sebastin, Spain

LARRY GENSTIL, PhD, Behavioral Psychologist, Shaare Zedek Medical Center, Jerusalem; and Multidisciplinary Clinic for Prader-Willi Syndrome at the Neuropediatric Unit, Shaare Zedek Medical Center, Jerusalem, Israel

BRURIA BEN ZEEV GHIDONI, MD, Associate Professor, Sackler School of Medicine, Tel-Aviv University, Tel-Aviv; Head, Pediatric Neurology Unit, Safra Pediatric Hospital, Sheba Medical Center, Ramat-Gan, Israel

DORON GOTHELF, MD, Department of Child Psychiatry, Behavioral Neurogenetics Center, Schneider Children's Medical Center of Israel, Petah Tiqwa; and Tel Aviv University, Tel Aviv, Israel

VARDA GROSS-TSUR, MD, Professor, Pediatric Neurologist, Shaare Zedek Medical Center, Jerusalem; Multidisciplinary Clinic for Prader-Willi Syndrome at the Neuropediatric Unit, Shaare Zedek Medical Center, Jerusalem, Israel

SCOTT S. HALL, PhD, Center for Interdisciplinary Brain Sciences Research, Stanford University School of Medicine, Stanford University, Stanford, California

HARRY J. HIRSCH, MD, Pediatric Endocrinologist, Shaare Zedek Medical Center, Jerusalem; and Multidisciplinary Clinic for Prader-Willi Syndrome at the Neuropediatric Unit, Shaare Zedek Medical Center, Jerusalem, Israel

ROBERT M. HODAPP, PhD, Professor, Department of Special Education, Peabody College, Vanderbilt University; Director of Research, Vanderbilt Kennedy Center for Excellence Developmental Disabilities, Nashville, Tennessee

SHELLI R. KESLER, PhD, Senior Research Assistant, Department of Psychiatry and Behavioral Sciences, Stanford University, Stanford, California

YAEL E. LANDAU, MA, Developmental Psychologist, Shaare Zedek Medical Center, Jerusalem; and Multidisciplinary Clinic for Prader-Willi Syndrome at the Neuropediatric Unit, Shaare Zedek Medical Center, Jerusalem, Israel

PAUL J. LOMBROSO, MD, Elizabeth Mear and House Jameson Professor, Child Study Center, Yale University School of Medicine, New Haven, Connecticut

M. CONCEPCIÓN MARTÍN-ARRIBAS, RN, PhD, Section Head, Research Institute of Rare Disorders, (National) Institute of Health Carlos III, Madrid, Spain

ANDREAS MEYER-LINDENBERG, MD, PhD, MSc, Investigator, Unit for Systems Neuroscience in Psychiatry; Neuroimaging Core Facility; Clinical Brain Disorders Branch; Genes, Cognition and Psychosis Program, National Institute of Mental Health, NIH, DHHS, Bethesda, Maryland

ALLAN L. REISS, MD, Center for Interdisciplinary Brain Sciences Research, Stanford University School of Medicine, Stanford University, Stanford, California

MARIE SCHAER, MD, Service-Médico-Pédagogique, Department of Psychiatry, University of Geneva, Geneva; and Signal Processing Institute, Swiss Federal Institute of Technology, Lausanne, Switzerland

TONY J. SIMON, PhD, Associate Professor of Psychiatry and Behavioral Sciences, University of California, Davis, M.I.N.D. Institute, Sacramento, California

SONIA SINGH, Undergraduate, Stanford University School of Medicine, Stanford; Lucile Packard Children's Hospital, Palo Alto, California

DEEPA V. VENKITARAMANI, PhD, Post-Doctoral Fellow, Child Study Center, Yale University School of Medicine, New Haven, Connecticut

CAROLINE F. ZINK, PhD, Post-Doctoral Fellow, Unit for Systems Neuroscience in Psychiatry; Clinical Brain Disorders Branch; Genes, Cognition and Psychosis Program, National Institute of Mental Health, NIH, DHHS, Bethesda, Maryland

Cover artwork Courtesy of Socorro Rivera G., Mexico City, Mexico

CONTRIBUTORS

CONTENTS

> The past decade has seen tremendous advances in our understanding of the molecular and genetic basis of many neuropsychiatric disorders. Although the genetic aberrations that lead to these syndromes have been identified in many cases, not much is known about specific gene products and their function. This article reviews the molecular basis of well-known neurogenetic disorders. The syndromes discussed here follow a Mendelian pattern of inheritance and are predominantly single-gene disorders; however, most childhood and adolescent psychiatric disorders are polygenic in nature. This genetic complexity and heterogeneity has made it difficult to identify the genes involved in their etiology. Identification of genetic and environmental risk factors involved in the etiology of complex disorders, such as autism, will help in the discovery of medications that can ameliorate the symptoms.

> For almost two decades, a considerable amount of work has been devoted to the accurate delineation of normal and abnormal brain

development using cerebral MRI. In the broad field of neuroimaging research, specific genetic conditions associated with impaired cognitive performances or with psychiatric symptoms have received increased attention because of their potential for revealing insight on the biologic correlates of behavior. First delineated by volumetric measurements of cerebral lobes or regions of interest, new image processing techniques are currently defining cerebral phenotypes associated with neurogenetic disorders with increasing precision. In this article the authors review the contribution of structural brain imaging in advancing our understanding of the pathogenic processes underlying altered brain development in Down, fragile X, and velocardiofacial (22q11DS) syndromes.

Many neuropsychiatric disorders of childhood and adolescence have a strong genetic component, and all present challenging questions about the neural abnormalities that underlie complex and unique behavioral and cognitive phenotypes. A useful research strategy in this setting is imaging genetics, a relatively new approach that combines genetic assessment with multimodal neuroimaging to discover neural systems linked to genetic abnormalities or variation. In this article, the authors review this strategy as applied to two areas. First, the authors present results on dissecting neural mechanisms underlying the complex neuropsychiatric phenotype of Williams syndrome. Second, they examine neural systems that are linked to candidate gene genetic variation that mediate risk for psychiatric disorders in a gene by environmental interaction. These data provide convergent evidence for neural circuitry mediating emotional regulation and social cognition under genetic control in humans.

This article presents the cognitive profile observed in children with one of several common genetic syndromes associated with "nonverbal learning disorders." It introduces the concept of a cognitive endophenotype to help explain the similar pattern of impairments across the syndromes. It explores the explanation of diverse impairments in higher-order visual, spatial, temporal, numerical, and executive cognitive competencies deriving from origins in more basic attentional and spatial cognitive dysfunctions. The importance of a developmental approach to understanding dysfunction is stressed.

As the numbers of syndrome-specific behavioral articles continue
to grow, it seems a good time to pause and take stock of patterns
that are emerging across these many studies. This article takes note
of these patterns and summarizes the authors' reading of the behavioral phenotype waters. The authors propose that there are (at
least) three overarching themes that relate to individual differences
within syndromes. These include the roles of (1) development
across the lifespan, (2) gender differences, and (3) other subject
and environmental factors. The authors end with a cautionary note
about measures and the need to supplement (alongside weaknesses and psychiatric vulnerabilities) the strengths and positive
affect and attributes of individuals who have genetic syndromes.

Many of the known genetically based neurodevelopmental disorders are associated with a distinctive behavioral phenotype. As
these behavioral phenotypes have been elucidated by clinical research, distinctive profiles of social traits have emerged as prominent syndromic features. This article reviews social phenotypic
findings for fragile X syndrome, Down syndrome, Prader-Willi
syndrome, Smith-Magenis syndrome, Turner syndrome, Williams
syndrome, and velocardiofacial syndrome. An analysis of these
social profiles raises several questions regarding the relationship
between identified social impairments and autism and the relationship between social impairments in neurodevelopmental disorders
and those found in normative child populations. The unique
profile of certain of the known behavioral phenotypes also serves
to distinguish several dimensions of sociability that are not readily
observed in typical populations.

Neurogenetic disorders share many characteristics with other rare
disorders and raise complex bioethical issues for clinical practice
and research. Because patients frequently present with cognitive
or communicative impairments, special measures to guarantee consent and assent are required. Many neurogenetic disorders present
with autistic behavior or borderline sociocommunicative aspects.
The likelihood that early educational intervention benefits the
adaptive skills of these persons leads to screening programs that
pose bioethical challenges. The biggest conflicts come from the lack
of research in clinical care and the limited application of biomedical
ethics in the personal support services arena. Alternatives include
the development of personal services portfolios, establishing and
supporting bioethical committees, reviewing and improving ethical
aspects in research initiatives in this population, and empowering

clients (and their legally authorized representatives) for participation and representation.

II. Select Syndromes

Fragile X Syndrome: Assessment and Treatment Implications
Allan L. Reiss and Scott S. Hall

Fragile X syndrome (FraX) is the most common known cause of inherited mental impairment. FMR1 gene mutations, the cause of FraX, lead to reduced expression of FMR1 protein and an increased risk for a particular profile of cognitive, behavioral, and emotional dysfunction. The study of individuals with FraX provides a unique window of understanding into important disorders such as autism, social phobia, cognitive disability, and depression. This review highlights the typical phenotypic features of individuals with FraX, discussing the apparent strengths and weaknesses in intellectual functioning, as evidenced from longitudinal follow-up studies. It also discusses recent neuroanatomic findings that may pave the way for more focused disease-specific pharmacologic and behavioral interventions. This article describes the results of an open-label trial of the antiglucocorticoid medication, mifepristone, that the authors have recently conducted in boys and men with FraX, as well as other medication trials designed to target symptoms associated with FraX. It also describes some recent behavioral interventions that were conducted in the authors' laboratory.

Velocardiofacial Syndrome
Doron Gothelf

Velocardiofacial syndrome (VCFS) is the most common known microdeletion in humans. It is also the most common known genetic risk factor for schizophrenia. The aim of this article is to describe the clinical characteristics of the syndrome, with emphasis on the myriad psychiatric disorders and abnormal behaviors from a developmental perspective. In addition, the possible pathways that lead to the psychotic symptoms and cognitive deficits are discussed. Guidelines are suggested to alert clinicians to the possibility of the presence of VCFS, and the cumulative clinical experience and limited research on psychiatric treatments for VCFS are presented. There is an urgent need to conduct treatment trials in this high-risk population.

Prader-Willi Syndrome: Medical Prevention and Behavioral Challenges
Fortu Benarroch, Harry J. Hirsch, Larry Genstil,
Yael E. Landau, and Varda Gross-Tsur

In this article the authors discuss the genetic, medical, and endocrinologic issues of Prader-Willi syndrome and their treatment. The authors also present the typical cognitive profile characterized by specific strengths and areas of disability. The behavioral phenotype of Prader-Willi syndrome affects four domains: food-seeking related behaviors; traits that indicate lack of flexibility; oppositional behaviors, and interpersonal problems. The management of the maladaptive behaviors is challenging and requires lifelong restrictive supervision (to prevent morbid obesity), addressing psychiatric comorbidity, psychopharmacologic management exacerbated by metabolic abnormalities, ongoing medical care, and, in many cases, institutional treatment. The multiple facets of the clinical problems demand a multidisciplinary approach with anticipatory medical and psychiatric care, oriented to enhancing the quality of life of individuals who have Prader-Willi syndrome.

Turner syndrome is a neurogenetic disorder characterized by partial or complete monosomy-X. It is associated with certain physical and medical features, including estrogen deficiency, short stature, and increased risk for several diseases, with cardiac conditions being among the most serious. The cognitive-behavioral phenotype associated with the syndrome includes strengths in verbal domains with impairments in visuospatial, executive function, and emotion processing. Less is known regarding psychosocial and psychiatric functioning in Turner syndrome, but essential aspects of psychotherapeutic treatment plans are suggested. Future investigations should include continued genetic studies and determination of candidate genes for physical and cognitive features. Multimodal, interdisciplinary studies are essential for identifying optimal, syndrome-specific interventions for improving the lives of individuals who have Turner syndrome.

Rett syndrome (RS) is an X-linked neurodevelopmental disorder and the second most common cause of genetic mental retardation in females. Different mutations in MECP2 are found in up to 95% of typical cases of RS. This mainly neuronal expressed gene functions as a major transcription repressor. Extensive studies on girls who have RS and mouse models are aimed at finding main gene targets for MeCP2 protein and defining neuropathologic changes caused by its defects. Studies comparing autistic features in RS with idiopathic autism and mentally retarded patients are presented. Decreased dendritic arborization is common to RS and autism, leading to further research on similarities in pathogenesis, including MeCP2 protein levels in autistic brains and MeCP2 effects on genes connected to autism, like DLX5 and genes on 15q11-13 region. This area also is involved in Angelman syndrome, which has many similarities to RS. Despite these connections, MECP2 mutations in nonspecific autistic and mentally retarded populations are rare.

FORTHCOMING ISSUES

RECENT ISSUES

CHILD AND
ADOLESCENT
PSYCHIATRIC CLINICS
OF NORTH AMERICA

ELSEVIER
SAUNDERS

Child Adolesc Psychiatric Clin N Am
16 (2007) xiii

A Memoriam and Rededication

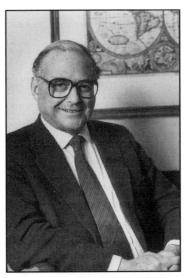

Melvin Lewis, MBBS, FRCPsych, DCH
(1926–2007)

It is with profound sadness that I share with our readers the passing of Melvin Lewis shortly before this issue went to press. As a small token of gratitude and appreciation for his many contributions over the years, the *Clinics'* front matter will now permanently list him as its Founding Consulting Editor (1992–2005).

I cherish the opportunities I had to share my feelings for Mel when he was still alive. A variation of the words that I wrote about him in the January 2006 issue remain fitting, if regrettably now in the past tense:

Mel was the ultimate gentleman, the kindest and most generous of individuals. His grace, poise, and beautiful British accent made one think of royalty, and his signature modesty could not hide innate nobility. Queen Elizabeth II may never have knighted him. But *we* had, his colleagues and disciples all. This issue, and this series henceforth are dedicated to him

—to Sir, with love.

AM

1056-4993/07/$ - see front matter © 2007 Published by Elsevier Inc.
doi:10.1016/j.chc.2007.05.001

childpsych.theclinics.com

ELSEVIER
SAUNDERS

Child Adolesc Psychiatric Clin N Am
16 (2007) xv–xvi

CHILD AND
ADOLESCENT
PSYCHIATRIC CLINICS
OF NORTH AMERICA

Foreword

Stranded

> ...while others did what they could, longing for
> tools still unimagined, medicines still unfound,
> wisdoms still unguessed at.

–Mary Oliver, University Hospital, Boston (1983)

The disorders covered in this issue of the *Child and Adolescent Psychiatric Clinics of North America* may strike the reader as trivial—anomalous clinical situations seen infrequently, when seen at all. But only from the strict standpoint of their prevalence would that assessment be accurate. To dismiss them because they are uncommon would be to miss their relevance to the practice of child and adolescent psychiatry. For starters, one cannot find what one does not look for; as we were taught in *The House of God*, you can't find a fever if you don't take a temperature. And so, if we are unfamiliar with a condition, we will miss it, especially in those cases with incomplete manifestations or with more subtle physical anomalies. Even fragile X syndrome (FXS), the most common inherited form of mental retardation—which with a prevalence of 1 per 4000 boys is in fact not that rare—undoubtedly continues to slip by undetected.

These conditions are also exceptional in how much we know about their underlying mechanisms of disease. The processes of imprinting and methylation that were initially described for Prader-Willi syndrome (PWS), of trinucleotide repeats and anticipation for FXS, of single gene mutations for Rett syndrome, or of restricted chromosomal region anomalies for velocardiofacial syndrome (VCFS) have each proven to be important etiological templates for various forms of developmental psychopathology. We know enough by now to realize that finding single-gene explanations for the most common forms of childhood psychiatric disorders is highly improbable, and it may be precisely because of this realization that we should pay heed to the unique vantage point that these "model" disorders can offer. Specifically, these conditions have provided a powerful heuristic through which to better understand aspects that range from social, cognitive and learning styles, through brain circuitry and neuroimaging, to etiologically-targeted interventions. The twelve contributions comprising this issue provide concrete examples for all of these.

1056-4993/07/$ - see front matter © 2007 Published by Elsevier Inc.
doi:10.1016/j.chc.2007.03.009

We are far from the day when genetic testing will effectively guide our clinical diagnoses and therapeutic approaches. Still, the syndromes covered in these pages provide a glimpse of what our specialty may look like in the decades to come. We already have some examples of how understanding a disorder's etiology can lead to targeted treatments capable of curing, or better yet preventing, specific forms of psychopathology—phenylketonurea readily comes to mind. Glimpsing back into our history books, we may do well to remember that only one hundred years ago tertiary syphilis was still the leading cause of psychiatric institutionalization. It is unlikely that dietary modification or a silver bullet akin to penicillin will save the day in the years ahead, but these hopes may not be completely unwarranted either; pharmacogenetics has already started to make inroads in the selection of our medication choices, and, as this volume makes clear, the refinements in understanding the clinical implications of select genetic mechanisms would have been unthinkable just a few years ago.

These disorders also carry with them a message of professional humility, reminding us that understanding the mechanisms of a particular disease is but a new starting point. It is nowhere near a final destination. The knowledge that we have gained through these disorders only reinforces our commitment as physicians to care for the patients and families affected by them. In this spirit, it is fitting that one of the articles in the issue is specifically devoted to ethical considerations.

I have long admired Doron Gothelf and his uncanny ability to balance ethical standards, superlative clinical and teaching skills, administrative prowess, and scientific rigor with a vision so sharply focused on the genetic neuropsychiatric syndromes of childhood. I am grateful to him for having put all of these talents to work in the making of this important issue. Together with his extraordinary cast of contributing authors, Doron has made it clear that these disorders are not stranded on the shores of our specialty. To the contrary, the lessons that we have to learn from affected patients— from their symptoms and their phenotypes to their strands of DNA—have relevance for all of our discipline.

Andrés Martin, MD, MPH
Yale Child Study Center
Yale University School of Medicine
230 South Frontage Road
New Haven, CT 06520-7900, USA

E-mail address: andres.martin@yale.edu

ELSEVIER
SAUNDERS

Child Adolesc Psychiatric Clin N Am
16 (2007) xvii–xx

CHILD AND
ADOLESCENT
PSYCHIATRIC CLINICS
OF NORTH AMERICA

Preface

A 15-year-old male is referred for a neuropsychiatric evaluation because of academic and behavioral problems in school. Psychiatric evaluation reveals that the adolescent presents with psychotic symptoms and an indiscriminate, overfriendly approach to strangers. Upon neuropsychological evaluation, he exhibits deficits in working memory and in object recognition processes. Functional magnetic resonance (fMRI) evaluation reveals increased activation in the cingulate gyrus and dorsolateral prefrontal cortex during performance of a Go/NoGo task. There is also decreased activation in the region of the intraparietal sulcus when performing a two-dimensional puzzle task. Based on the multimodal assessments, the child psychiatrist suspects that variants of several genes including *COMT*, *PRODH*, elastin and LIM domain kinase 1 (*LIMK1*), are mediating the patient's neuropsychiatric and neurocognitive deficits. Consequently, a blood sample is drawn and a molecular work-up reveals that the patient's genetic profile is consistent with the suspected high- risk genetic variants. Variations in the *COMT* and *PRODH* gene explain the prefrontal cognitive deficits and psychotic symptoms, whereas variations in the *LIMK1* explain the dorsal visual processing stream deficits and the overfriendly approach of the patient. The child psychiatrist presents the results of the clinical evaluation and laboratory tests to the patient and his family, and suggests medications that will regulate the activity of the *COMT* enzyme and that will normalize the expression of the *LIMK1* gene. The described scenario would have been regarded as fantasy or science fiction by child psychiatrists only a decade ago. However, with the rapid technologic advances in the field of neuroscience, the revolution in evaluation and treatment of psychiatric disorders is already on the way. As will be shown in this special issue, neurogenetic syndromes have a pre-eminent role in leading this revolution.

This issue of the *Child and Adolescent Psychiatric Clinics of North America* is devoted to neuropsychiatric genetic syndromes with a known genetic etiology, a field also known as behavioral neurogenetics. Behavioral

Dr. Gothelf is funded by the Basil O'Connor Starter Scholar Research Award of the March of Dimes and by the NARSAD Young Investigator Award.

1056-4993/07/$ - see front matter © 2007 Published by Elsevier Inc.
doi:10.1016/j.chc.2007.03.008

neurogenetics is, in some ways, a potential alternative to the descriptive, non-etiologic approach for studying psychiatric disorders epitomized in the Diagnostic and Statistical Manual (DSM). Behavioral neurogeneticists claim that DSM-defined psychiatric disorders are too heterogeneous and consequently do not easily render themselves to scientific investigation of etiologic and pathophysiologic mechanisms. They are looking for etiologically defined and relatively homogeneous genetic syndromes. These syndromes have neural mechanisms underlying maladaptive cognition, psychiatric symptoms, and abnormal behaviors that can be systematically investigated.

The first part of the issue is composed of a series of articles dealing with the general aspects of neuropsychiatric syndromes. As reviewed by Venkitaramani and Lombroso, much has been learned about the molecular bases of neurogenetic syndromes. Fifteen years ago, as with all psychiatric disorders, the etiology of these syndromes was unknown. With the advance of molecular biology and the development of animal models of neurogenetic syndromes, much has been learned regarding the role of key genes on brain development and function. The articles by Schaer and Eliez, and by Meyer-Lindenberg and Zinc, go on to describe the research literature on brain development and function in individuals who have genetic syndromes using structural and functional magnetic resonance imaging. Of special promise are new image processing techniques that will allow for the definition of anatomic phenotypes with increasing precision. Meyer-Lindenberg and Zinc describe how fMRI studies enable an understanding of the abnormal neural systems mediating the unique visuospatial deficits and social phenotype of Williams syndrome. They also describe a new approach—Imaging Genetics, which combines genetic assessment with multimodal neuroimaging to discover neural systems linked to specific allelic variations.

The article by Simon describes specific cognitive endophenotypes involving spatial, temporal, and attentional domains. Interestingly, deficits in these areas are common to several neurogenetic syndromes presented in this issue, including velocardiofacial, Williams, Turner and fragile X syndromes. These syndromes are also associated with a nonverbal learning disability. Future studies will further elucidate the road from gene to brain development to cognitive endophenotype in these conditions and show how these different pathways converge to yield similar cognitive deficits.

The article by Dykens and Hodapp indicates that research in behavioral neurogenetics has increased exponentially, with some syndromes such as Williams and velocardiofacial showing a fivefold increase in the number of articles published during the last decade. The authors remind us of the definition of behavioral phenotype: "the probability that persons with a genetic syndrome will show certain behavioral or developmental sequelae relative to those without the syndrome." They also urge that in our quest to find the molecular and neural mechanisms mediating the phenotype of genetic syndromes, we not neglect examining more basic, yet important, subject characteristics, such as age, development, gender, or environmental variables.

The article by Feinstein and Singh provides an updated review on the social phenotype of various genetic syndromes. Social deficits are common in all children who have developmental disabilities, including children who have neurogenetic syndromes. Still, it remains highly controversial whether these deficits truly represent a forme frustre of the autistic phenotype.

The article by Fuentes and Martín-Arribas discusses the ethical dilemmas related to clinical practice and research in individuals who have neurogenetic syndromes. Since these patients often suffer from cognitive and communicative impairments, special precautions to guarantee proper consent and assent procedures are crucial. The ultimate goal of researchers in the field is to improve the lives of individuals who have neurogenetic syndromes, but the translation of basic scientific knowledge into concrete treatments will still take time. Meanwhile, much can be done to assist this population, including making patients and their families more aware of the portfolio of services they are entitled to.

The second part of this issue includes articles on specific neuropsychiatric genetic syndromes. These articles emphasize the unique phenotype of each syndrome and what is known about their specific genetic and neural mechanisms, as well as the risk factors mediating their cognitive and psychiatric phenotypes. The articles also highlight the urgent need to develop more effective treatments for the psychiatric symptoms of this population. The article by Reiss and Hall on fragile X syndrome describes a novel approach as to how such behavioral interventions and pharmacologic treatments could be designed. The behavioral intervention could be based on rigorous analysis of the abnormal behaviors. The pharmacologic treatments could be pathophysiologically based, targeting defined disease pathways. Examples include treatment approaches that try to improve fragile X psychiatric symptoms through agents that counteract the downstream effect of fragile X mental retardation protein deficiency.

The article by Gothelf describes the association between velocardiofacial syndrome and schizophrenia-like psychotic disorder. Velocardiofacial syndrome is the most commonly known genetic risk factor for schizophrenia. Recent findings from longitudinal studies show that the evolution of schizophrenia, in individuals who have velocardiofacial syndrome, is a protracted developmental process and several risk factors for the evolution of psychosis in the syndrome have been identified. These include genes (eg, the *COMT* gene), cognitive deficits (eg, decline in verbal abilities), and psychiatric symptoms (eg, obsessive-compulsive symptoms).

The articles of Benarroch and colleagues on Prader-Willi syndrome, and of Kesler on Turner syndrome highlight the pivotal role of endocrinologic factors (eg, growth hormone and sex hormones) on the behavioral and cognitive phenotype of individuals who have these conditions. They also highlight the importance of a comprehensive multidisciplinary approach to treating individuals who have neurogenetic syndromes. Such treatment should be holistic, integrating mind and body facets of the phenotype.

The final article in the volume, by Ben-Zeev, supports the view that we are on the verge of a revolution in our nosological classification of psychiatric disorders. Only a few years ago, Rett syndrome was classified as an idiopathic disorder, a variation of autistic disorder, in the pervasive developmental disorder section of the DSM. Recently it was discovered that the syndrome is caused by a mutation in the *MECP2* gene. Our vision is that, with the knowledge gained from etiologically homogeneous models such as those of these select neurogenetic syndromes, our psychiatric nosology will be likely based more and more on known biological processes, instead of relying solely on clinical evaluations and descriptive assessments.

I wish to thank Dr. Andrés Martin for his thoughtful scientific and editorial advice and guidance, and to Sarah Barth for editorial work. I feel a special debt of gratitude to the late Dr. Donald J. Cohen, my mentor and teacher on the principles of developmental psychopathology. My work is directed in Donald's spirit of uncovering the mechanisms underlying psychiatric disorders in children. Finally, I wish to thank our brave patients and their incredible families for teaching us all we know about genetic syndromes—and about the greatness of the human spirit.

Doron Gothelf, MD
The Behavioral Neurogenetics Center
Feinberg Child Study Center
Schneider Children's Medical Center of Israel
Sackler Faculty of Medicine
Tel Aviv University
14 Kaplan Street
Petah Tiqwa, Israel

E-mail address: gothelf@post.tau.ac.il

ELSEVIER
SAUNDERS

Child Adolesc Psychiatric Clin N Am
16 (2007) 541–556

CHILD AND
ADOLESCENT
PSYCHIATRIC CLINICS
OF NORTH AMERICA

Molecular Basis of Genetic Neuropsychiatric Disorders

Deepa V. Venkitaramani, PhD, Paul J. Lombroso, MD*

*Child Study Center, SHM I-270, Yale University School of Medicine,
230 South Frontage Road, New Haven, CT 06520, USA*

The genetic basis of several childhood neuropsychiatric disorders has been clarified over the last decade and provides a springboard for the development of intervention strategies [1,2]. Aberrant brain development during the fetal and childhood period has been implicated in several neurodevelopmental and psychiatric disorders. The chromosomal location has been mapped for numerous autosomal-dominant, autosomal-recessive, and X-linked disorders; in some cases, specific genes have been implicated in the pathophysiology of the disease [3,4]. The functional relevance of the genes in question is being studied. This article presents an overview of the molecular pathways implicated in neuropsychiatric disorders, with a discussion of some of the mutations that occur in signaling molecules critically involved in learning.

Fragile X syndrome

Our understanding of the molecular basis of fragile X mental retardation syndrome (FXS) has advanced tremendously over the past decade [5]. FXS is a recessive X-linked mental retardation disorder, and the phenotype associated with the syndrome cosegregates with a "fragile" site on the X-chromosome. A break point appears to be present on one of the X-chromosomes in cells grown in medium lacking folic acid [6]. Because of the mutation that is present, this chromosomal region does not stain normally in karyotypic analyses, and this chromosomal abnormality suggested to investigators that a gene involved in the disorder might lie near the disrupted site.

* Corresponding author.
E-mail address: paul.lombroso@yale.edu (P.J. Lombroso).

1056-4993/07/$ - see front matter © 2007 Elsevier Inc. All rights reserved.
doi:10.1016/j.chc.2007.03.003   *childpsych.theclinics.com*

Certain unusual aspects were observed in the phenotypic expression of the disorder before the gene of interest was actually cloned. About 20% of men carrying the mutant version of the gene did not manifest any cognitive deficits. This was intriguing, because if the gene involved lies on the X-chromosome, why were these men with an apparent fragile site unaffected? These individuals are called "normal transmitting males" and pass the mutated copy of the gene to their daughters who also may show few symptoms; however, it was observed that their grandson carried a much higher risk for manifesting the full-blown syndrome. The progressive increase in the severity of a disorder over several generations is called "anticipation."

The molecular basis of anticipation is now clear. A novel type of mutation in the 5′ untranslated sequence of the *FMR1* gene, called a triplet repeat expansion, was identified as the cause for FXS [7]. The size of the expansion increases over generations, and, thus, the mutation and the disorder become more severe over time. Triplet repeats are made up of three consecutive nucleotides repeated several times as a tandem unit. The three nucleotides repeated in FXS are cytosine-guanine-guanine (CGG). In normal individuals, this triplet sequence is repeated between 6 and 50 times in the *FMR1* gene, with 29 being the most commonly occurring repeat number [7]. The number of triplet repeats is increased in affected individuals to between 200 and 1000 repeats. Mothers of affected individuals carry between 50 and 200 repeats, which lies between the number seen in normal individuals and the number seen in affected individuals; this intermediate number of repeats is termed a "premutation" [7]. Individuals with premutations in the *FMR1* gene may show mild cognitive deficits and behavioral abnormalities [8]. Women who are heterozygous for the mutation perform poorly in visuospatial and other memory subtests [9,10]. Furthermore, female premutation carriers show decreased total brain volumes and increased metabolic labeling within the hippocampus and cerebellum, as determined by MRI and positron emission tomography scans [11]. Mothers with the premutation are at a higher risk for producing offspring with expanded triplet repeats, and, hence, lead to the observed increased severity of the phenotype. Although it remains unclear as to why there is an initial expansion to a premutation, the molecular basis of anticipation can be explained by the increase in triplet repeats over the course of several generations.

Although it was originally believed that premutation carriers were mostly asymptomatic, two different phenotypes recently were described in these carriers. Early ovarian failure was reported in 16% to 24% of female carriers, whereas male premutation carriers older than 50 years develop fragile X–associated tremor and ataxia syndrome [12–15]. The molecular basis of these two disorders remains unclear, because it does not correlate directly with the size of triplet repeats or the extent of nonfunctional fragile X mental retardation protein (FMRP).

Cytosine-Guanine dinucleotide connected by phosphodiester bond (CpG) islands are stretches of DNA sequences larger than 200 base pairs, with greater than 50% cytosine and guanine nucleotide content and a high preponderance of CpG sequences. Usually, these sequences are found within the promoter sequences at the 5′ untranslated region of many genes [16]. The triplet repeat in FXS is CGG; it may be repeated many hundreds of times in affected individuals. Thus, patients who have FXS have a large increase in these CpG sequences. The cytosines in the CpG islands can be methylated, and this can regulate the expression of the gene negatively. Thus, the dramatic expansion of CGG repeats in FXS leads to an increase in methylated CpG islands [17]. The degree of methylation within this region is correlated directly to the extent of loss of functional FMRP [18].

What is the normal physiologic function of FMRP in neurons, and how does the lack of this protein lead to clinical symptoms? Shortly after the isolation of the gene in 1991, researchers noticed that the protein contained three conserved domains. These motifs have high homology to amino acid sequences known to be RNA-binding motifs. RNA-binding proteins play a role in regulating the processing, trafficking, or translation of mRNA transcripts within cells [19–21]. A mutation within the RNA-binding domain of these proteins can disrupt the normal binding to mRNAs, and, hence, affect the ability of the cells to produce mature messages or to translate those messages into protein.

The importance of the RNA-binding domain in FMRP was confirmed by the identification of a patient who had FXS and a point mutation that altered a conserved amino acid in one of the RNA-binding domains. This individual lacked the usual expansion of trinucleotide repeat [21–23]. The RNA-binding domain of FMRP is essential for protein function, and mutations within this region may affect the ability of FMRP to bind RNA and process them correctly. Although most cases of FXS are caused by the expansion of CGG repeats, the discovery of this case and others like it suggested that any mutation that interferes with the function of FMRP could lead to a similar clinical syndrome. It is a good example of allelic heterogeneity, where different types of mutations in a gene lead to the expression of the same phenotypes in affected individuals.

Characterization of the intracellular localization of the FMRP also has advanced our understanding of its function. Initially, the fragile X protein was found to associate with polyribosomes, the cellular organelles composed of ribosomal RNAs and various RNA-binding proteins that function as an assembly line in the translation of mRNA transcripts into proteins [24]. The pattern of FMRP expression in various regions of the brain during development also has been studied in detail. The highest expression of the protein is observed in the basal forebrain and hippocampus [25]. Both of these brain regions are involved in the acquisition of short-term memory and sequential processing of information, and they are affected in some neurodegenerative disorders, such as Alzheimer's disease. Clinical neuroimaging studies have detected age-related changes in the brain volume of patients who have FXS, particularly in the cerebellar vermis, fourth ventricle, and hippocampus [26–28]. Finally, the development of animal models, such as the knockout mouse, has been useful to understand some of the molecular processes that are disrupted. FMRP knockout mice show many of the clinical symptoms noted in patients who have FXS [29].

Our understanding of the normal function of FMRP has been helped from two other lines of investigation: the site of protein translation and the mechanism by which mRNAs are transported. The first line of study was to identify the location of protein translation in neurons. According to older dogma, messages transcribed in the nucleus are transported rapidly to the cytoplasm where ribosomes are assembled onto the messages, and the translated proteins are deposited into the cytosol or into the endoplasmic reticulum for posttranslational modification. This mechanism is true for most messages; however, recent work suggested that a subpopulation of neuronal mRNAs is transported along dendrites to locations adjacent to spines. These messages that are shipped out await the arrival of signals, upon which they are translated locally near the sites of synaptic inputs to produce the proteins necessary for biochemical changes at the spine and the synaptic remodeling that must occur.

This new model of local protein synthesis has helped to solve a major hurdle in our understanding of the development of synaptic plasticity. A typical neuron can have up to 10,000 spines. The extracellular signal probably arrives at a few hundreds of these spines. According to the previous model, this signal traveled to the nucleus, where it initiated gene transcription and subsequent translation in the perinuclear region. This brings up the obvious question of how these new synthesized proteins are transported to only a subset of spines that is activated by the original incoming signal. Based on the new model, the messages themselves are transported to the dendritic spines, ready to be translated when the signal arrives. Evidence for dendritic protein synthesis has accumulated over the past few years, with the finding of components of the translation machinery throughout dendrites and within the spines themselves [30]. The various components identified to date include mRNAs, ribosomes, and proteins that function as translation factors necessary for the synthesis of proteins [31].

Local protein synthesis does not preclude that the original signal also might be sent to the nucleus to trigger additional transcription of genes. In fact, the maintenance of long-term potentiation and the consolidation of long-lasting memories require that the incoming signal eventually reaches the nucleus. The initial burst of protein translation occurring near the spines is necessary for the induction of long-term potentiation (LTP), whereas the maintenance phase of LTP requires further mRNA transcription and protein synthesis. The importance of the induction and maintenance phase of LTP can be demonstrated by the infusion of transcriptional inhibitors into specific brain regions. For example, injection of these inhibitors into the amygdala blocks the consolidation of long-term fear memories, but does not affect short-term fear learning, which does not require gene transcription.

Only a portion of neuronal messages are transported along dendrites and out to the spines. The messages that are transported encode for proteins that are necessary for biochemical tagging and reorganization of synaptic structure [32,33]. FMRP probably is one of the many proteins necessary for this complex process. The transport of messages to the synapses, their inhibition or activation depending on the status of activity at the spines, as well as the scaffolding support for protein synthesis require the interplay of many hundreds of proteins; current estimates are that approximately 400 mRNAs are actively transported to distal dendrites for translation. Based on this model, one could envision that mutations that alter or abolish the function of many proteins along this pathway could disrupt normal synaptic plasticity and produce cognitive deficits in affected individuals.

Having tackled the local translation mechanism, researchers next asked how these transported messages are kept dormant until a synaptic stimulus reaches the spine. Recent studies from various laboratories suggested that one function of FMRP is to inhibit the translation of mRNAs with which it associates [5]. FMRP binds to newly synthesized mRNA molecules in the nucleus and is transported along with these messages along dendrites, all the while preventing their translation into proteins. Two theories have been put forward for how FMRP associates with mRNAs, and each has experimental data to support it. The first showed that a subpopulation of the transported messages contains specific nucleotide sequences (G quartets) to which FMRP binds [33]. The second model showed that FMRP binds to a small RNA molecule (BC1), and, that BC1, in turn, binds to target messages. Together, this triad of proteins and RNAs forms a circular structure that prevents the initiation of translation [34]. How the FMRP-mediated inhibition of translation is removed is an area of active research, but it seems to involve the activation of extracellular signal-regulated protein kinase [35,36].

The model of synaptic translation allows us to make certain predictions about the molecular changes occurring in patients who have FXS. If FMRP plays a role in regulating protein translation at spines, then disruption of FMRP function should interfere with the normal structural remodeling of spines that accompanies synaptic plasticity. This is what Greenough and his colleagues found in anatomic studies in patients who had FXS as well as in animal models in which a mutated *FMR1* gene replaces the normal *FMR1* gene [37,38]. Compared with controls, humans with FXS and the transgenic mice had greater numbers of long, spindly, and immature-looking spines and reduced numbers of mature, short, and mushroom-shaped spines.

Although the expansion of trinucleotide repeats at the *FMR1* gene loci originally was considered to be a genetic aberration unique to FXS, more than a dozen other triplet repeat disorders have been identified. These include Huntington's chorea, Friedreich's ataxia, and myotonic dystrophy [39–41]. In most of these disorders, the phenomenon of anticipation is apparent, but it was explained away in earlier studies as being due to ascertainment bias; however, the discovery of triplet repeat expansions has provided the molecular explanation for its occurrence. The degree of anticipation observed between generations may be dramatic. For example, in muscular dystrophy, the expansion of repeats just above the threshold results in the development of cataracts late in adult life; however, further expansion of these long repeats over several generations results in fatal congenital disorder [42].

Prader-Willi and Angelman syndrome

We derive our genetic complement of 46 chromosomes from our parents, with the mother and father contributing 23 chromosomes each. It was assumed previously that the homologous genes on the maternal and paternal chromosomes were identical and produced comparable amounts of functional protein. It would follow that mutations in one copy of the gene might be overcome by the availability of functional protein obtained from the homologous gene.

Although this mechanism holds true for most genes, recent studies showed that some gene pairs are not functionally equivalent. In these cases, only one copy of the gene is active, whereas the other copy is repressed. Under normal conditions, whether a particular gene product is produced depends on whether the active gene locus was contributed by the mother or father. In certain instances, the maternal genes in a particular chromosomal region are expressed, whereas in others it is the father's genes that are active. This phenomenon by which a subset of genes is expressed based on the parent of origin is called "genomic imprinting."

Most genetic disorders are caused by mutations within the gene sequence that results in loss of protein function; however, in some disorders, chromosomal mutations are not involved. The production of functional protein in these cases is dictated by factors that regulate the pattern of gene expression, not the actual nucleotide sequence. This type of phenomenon is termed "epigenetic." Earlier, we reviewed an example of epigenetic factors when we discussed the methylation of CpG islands in FXS; we continue this discussion below with regards to Rett syndrome. Imprinting is another example of an epigenetic phenomenon.

Genomic imprinting has been identified in about 30 genes. Many of the protein products of these genes are necessary for growth and differentiation of various tissues. Disruption in the genetic imprinting of these genes has been implicated in a variety of cancers and developmental disorders. The latest advances in this field are discussed here related to Prader-Willi syndrome (PWS) and Angelman syndrome, two developmental disorders caused by imprinting defects [43].

PWS is a rare genetic disorder with a prevalence of 1 in 10,000 live births. Individuals with this defect manifest a plethora of symptoms at birth [44]. Newborns show pronounced hypotonia and failure to thrive. In addition, the dietary habits change dramatically within the first couple of years of life and are characterized by hyperphagia and food preoccupations, and the affected individual often become obese [45]. Mild to moderate mental retardation is present, as well as several other behavioral problems, including temper tantrums, aggressive behaviors, and obsessive-compulsive symptoms outside of the compulsive food-related behaviors [46–48].

Angelman syndrome is another rare neurologic disorder with a similar prevalence to PWS. Affected infants also are hypotonic after birth, develop motor delays, and show mild to moderate mental retardation. They have a characteristic facial appearance with a large mandible and an open-mouth expression, stiffened gait, and puppet-like limb movements. They rarely develop speech and exhibit severe learning disabilities and deficits in attention and hyperactivity. Most of the affected children develop abnormal electroencephalograms and epilepsy [49].

By the mid-1980s, the genetic locus associated with both syndromes was identified, and investigators mapped a deletion on chromosome 15 (15q11-13). Cytogenetic and molecular analysis showed that the same region of chromosome 15 was deleted in individuals with either disorder. It was difficult to comprehend how identical deletions could cause two completely different syndromes: Prader-Willi and Angelman [50,51]. Further studies showed that the clinical symptoms depend on whether the chromosome 15q deletion is derived from the mother or father [52]. It was then discovered that most cases of PWS resulted from deletions of the paternal chromosome, whereas Angelman was due to a deletion in the mother's chromosome 15.

The underlying mechanism was clarified further when a smaller segment within the chromosome 15 deletions was identified for each disorder. The segment of the DNA responsible for PWS is discrete, but maps close to the region that is implicated in Angelman syndrome. This explained how the identical chromosomal deletion could lead to the two syndromes. A large deletion of chromosome 15 spans genetic loci for both disorders; the child develops PWS when the paternal chromosome is deleted and Angelman syndrome when the maternal chromosome is deleted.

The genetic imprinting of these two closely inherited regions of chromosome 15 is different. Normally, the paternal chromosome expresses genes within the PWS region, whereas the nearby set of Angelman genes is imprinted or silenced. In contrast, the maternal chromosome expresses the genes within the Angelman region, whereas the adjacent PWS region is repressed [53,54]. Thus, a deletion of the paternal chromosome results in the deletion of the active PWS genes, and the corresponding region on the maternal chromosome does not compensate for the missing gene products: the result is PWS. When the deletion occurs on the maternal chromosome, the active Angelman genes are deleted, and the paternal chromosome remains imprinted and again cannot compensate for the missing genes.

Approximately 70% of cases of PWS and Angelman syndrome are attributed to chromosome 15 deletions; however, a second mechanism exists for these disorders. Occasionally, segregation defects during meiosis result in two copies of chromosome 15 being inherited from one of the parents [55]. This unusual mechanism is called uniparental disomy (UPD). UPD occurs when two copies of a chromosome or a part of the chromosome is inherited from one of the parents, with no contributions from the other. It usually arises because of a trisomy event, where two chromosomes from one parent are inappropriately passed on with one copy from the other parent, resulting in three copies of the chromosome. One of three chromosomes is lost during the formation of gametes. If the initial trisomy happened as a result of two copies of the maternal chromosome and one copy of the paternal chromosome, loss of the paternal chromosome results in maternal UPD with two maternal copies of the chromosome. Conversely, if the initial trisomy event involved two copies of the paternal chromosomes, the loss of the maternal chromosome during gamete formation leads to paternal UPD.

Inheritance of two maternal copies of chromosome 15 results in PWS [56]. In this case, the genes in the PWS region are present on both of the maternal chromosomes, but are repressed because of genomic imprinting; the converse applies for paternal UPD. The PWS genes present on both paternal copies of chromosome 15 are expressed. In contrast, the adjacent region critical for Angelman syndrome is imprinted, resulting in transcriptional silencing and lack of protein expression.

A third mechanism is observed in 2% to 3% of individuals with PWS or Angelman syndrome and involves mutations within the imprinting center [57,58]. The imprinting center regulates gene expression by controlling the level of methylation resulting in heterochromatin spreading for hundreds of kilobases on either side. One of the effects of methylation is to facilitate the compacting chromatin to be tightly packaged; however, a consequence is that this stretch of DNA is inaccessible for transcription. Imprinting of PWS and Angelman critical chromosomal region 15q11-13 is modulated by the same bipartite imprinting center. Mutation within this imprinting center results in a disruption of the normal patterns of paternal or maternal imprinting.

Finally, a fourth molecular mechanism for Angelman syndrome is responsible for about 10% of cases; mutations occur in a specific gene (*UBE3A*) that lies within the Angelman region [59–61]. *UBE3A* encodes a protein called ubiquitin protein ligase that normally is required for regulating the turnover of cellular proteins by ubiquitin-mediated proteolysis. The removal of proteins from the intracellular environment by protein degradation is essential for maintaining proper cellular function. These include signaling proteins that need to be sequestered and degraded quickly. It also is vital to remove damaged proteins before they disrupt the normal cellular processes. Several copies of a small protein molecule (ubiquitin) are added to the protein targeted for proteasomal degradation. The attachment of several ubiquitin molecules requires the function of *UBE3A*, because it one of the enzymes that mediates the addition of ubiquitin tags. Intracellular organelles called proteasomes recognize the ubiquitinated proteins, bind to them, and activate proteases necessary to degrade these proteins into constitutive amino acids. Mutation in *UBE3A* leads to improper accumulation of damaging molecules within the central nervous system (CNS) that interferes with normal synaptic functioning.

In addition to *UBE3A*, several other enzymes are required to catalyze the intermediary steps in the attachment of ubiquitin molecules to protein targeted for proteolysis. It is possible that mutations in these other proteins could result in Angelman syndrome. This would be an excellent example of locus heterogeneity, where mutations in distinctly different genes of the same pathway result in the expression of identical phenotype. Several laboratories are pursuing this line of study. In the case of PWS, mutations in a single gene have not been identified.

Two final points should be made about Angelman syndrome. Recent studies suggested that the maternal chromosomes are differentially imprinted in a brain region–specific pattern [62]. For example, the maternal copy of *UBE3A* is expressed exclusively in the hippocampus and cerebellum. This adds an interesting twist to the imprinting story, because it suggests that some genes are expressed depending on whether they lie on the paternal or maternal copy and that specific brain areas may contribute to expression levels through activation of imprinting mechanisms. Finally, one of the genes encoded by the Angelman critical region is a subunit of the γ-aminobutyric acid (GABA)$_A$ receptor [63]. The aberrant GABA transmission as a result of this mutation is believed to be responsible for the epilepsy that develops in many affected individuals. Patients who have cases of Angelman syndrome in which only a point mutation exists in the *UBE3A* gene do not develop epilepsy.

Rett syndrome

Rett syndrome is characterized by progressive neurologic decline [64]. Children affected by this syndrome develop normally and achieve age-appropriate milestones during the first year of life; parents of these children do not report developmental abnormalities. One of the first observable clinical signs is the loss of voluntary hand movements and the development of stereotypical repetitive behaviors, such as hand wringing. Other symptoms of the disorder soon emerge, including progressive loss of speech, growth retardation that leads eventually to microcephaly, ataxia, and a severe disruption of higher brain functions. The clinical symptoms reach a plateau and stabilize over the next few decades of life [65].

An unusual aspect of this syndrome is that most of the affected individuals are female. The female prevalence was explained by the fact that the mutated gene was on the X-chromosome, and, hence, would cause embryonic lethality in males. There are numerous examples of X-linked disorders in which the males die in utero because they have only one copy of the X-chromosome. In females, the second normal X-chromosome seems to generate enough gene products to provide protection during embryonic development and into the initial phase of postnatal life. Nevertheless, symptoms eventually emerge as a result of haploinsufficiency, because a single copy of the gene is unable to impart lasting protection.

Analysis of affected female siblings led to the mapping of the gene to Xq28, and candidate genes in this region were studied carefully [66]. A systematic comparison of nucleotide sequences from affected and normal individuals excluded a number of genes as possible candidates; however, more recent studies identified a gene that is mutated in several patients who have Rett syndrome [67]. The gene encodes a methyl CpG-binding protein 2 (MeCP2), and mutations in two of its functional domains have been reported.

What is the relevance of MeCP2 mutations to the clinical symptoms? Of an estimated 25,000 to 35,000 genes in the human genome, a third of them are expressed solely in the CNS. A portion of these genes and their gene products are essential for the normal development of the brain, whereas others are required during postnatal development, and the rest are expressed constitutively to perform housekeeping functions. Therefore, it is important to regulate gene expression carefully, such that only those genes are expressed that are required in a particular tissue and during a specific time period.

The protein that is implicated in Rett syndrome plays an important role in regulating gene expression. The accessibility of DNA to transcription factors is determined by the degree of methylation of the regulatory sequences [68]. Methylation is a chemical modification of the DNA, where a methyl group is attached to the cytosines, especially when it occurs within CpG sequences. These CpG islands are found predominantly within the regulatory region of genes termed the "promoter." One of the approaches to identify transcriptional start sites is to look for CpG islands, because they are found often adjacent to transcriptional initiation sites.

It was believed previously that methylation of DNA sequences was sufficient for repressing gene transcription. RNA polymerase II, which is the enzyme that transcribes most DNA to RNA, was believed to be incapable of binding to promoter regions with methylated CpG islands, and, hence, could not initiate transcription of these genes. The mechanism of gene activation and repression turns out to be more complicated.

MeCP2, the protein mutated in Rett syndrome, consists of different functional domains [69]. The amino-terminal methyl CpG binding domain recognizes methylated cytosines and binds to them. The transcriptional repressor domain (TRD) is then activated, leading to the recruitment of other proteins to form a regulatory complex that works together to repress transcription. One of the proteins in this complex is a histone deacetylase. Histones are a family of nuclear proteins that play a role in packaging DNA into higher-order chromatin structures. Modification of histones by methylation and acetylation determines whether the secondary structure of DNA is accessible to transcription factors. The histone deacetylases remove the acetyl groups from histones, resulting in the compaction of DNA around the promoter such that the transcriptional machinery is no longer able to access it. This heterochromatic region effectively represses gene expression. In summary, MeCP2 functions to silence genes to which it binds, and mutations that inactivate it presumably lead to inappropriate transcriptional activation [70].

The first report on MeCP2 mutations identified six types [67]. Several of these were missense mutations that replaced critical amino acids and led to aberrant protein function. Most of the mutations of this kind were mapped to the methyl CpG binding domain, and, thereby, disrupt the ability of MeCP2 to recognize and bind methylated DNA. Other mutations were found in the second critical domain of the protein: the transcriptional repressor domain that is necessary for recruiting histone deacetylases. These mutations included a single nucleotide insertion that leads to a frame shift of the downstream codons. A shift in the codon reading frame results in an altered amino acid sequence downstream of the point of mutation. The second mutation found within the TRD domain was an inappropriate change to a stop codon. This type of mutation leads to the production of shortened or truncated proteins. The proteins produced as a result of these mutations have reduced function or are completely nonfunctional [67].

In the initial study, only certain regions of the MeCP2 locus was sequenced. Only the DNA sequence that encodes for amino acids was sequenced. Generally, these regions of the DNA are analyzed first because they require far fewer nucleotides to be sequenced as compared with the large noncoding sequences that include introns and regulatory elements. For this reason, mutations within the coding regions of the gene are identified earlier, although mutations may occur within the regulatory sequences disrupting the gene function. As additional noncoding sequences were analyzed, more than 80% of the individuals who had Rett syndrome were found to carry mutations in the MeCP2 gene.

Different mutations within the same gene that result in similar phenotypic expression are examples of allelic heterogeneity. In many disorders, identical or closely related clinical phenotypes are observed when different functional domains of the same protein are mutated. This phenomenon of allelic heterogeneity was found in the initial Rett syndrome study in which six mutations in the MeCP2 gene produced individuals with the same clinical disorder [67]. It is likely that additional mutations identified in the MeCP2 gene will produce similar phenotype. In certain cases, mutations to a single gene can produce different clinical manifestations. One example would be mutations that occur in one of the fibroblast growth factor receptors, where several independent mutations result in distinctly different skeletal and growth abnormalities [71].

Conversely, locus heterogeneity refers to the phenomenon by which mutations in different genes produce similar clinical symptoms among affected individuals. This can happen when several proteins are necessary for a series of signaling events. MeCP2, for example, is one member of a large family of proteins that play a role in gene silencing. Two other members of this protein family have been reported to bind DNA and recruit histone deacetylase complex. Various laboratories are examining the function of these proteins in gene repression and whether mutations in them can lead to Rett syndrome or related disorders. Several proteins besides MeCP2 are necessary for maintaining specific genes in a repressed state. The clinical phenotype produced by mutations in these other genes may result in symptoms that are similar to those seen in Rett syndrome. Recently, mutations in two other genes, cyclin-dependent kinase like 5 and netrin G, were reported to result in similar clinical phenotype [72–74].

Recent developments in the field of Rett syndrome have raised several interesting questions. One of the questions relates to the preponderance of neurologic problems in the clinical assessment. MeCP2 expression is not restricted to the brain, but is found in many other tissues; however, symptoms other than the neurologic deficits are not observed commonly. This suggests that the CNS may be especially sensitive to the disruption of MeCP2 protein function. Another disorder with a similar situation is Huntington's chorea, in which the neurologic disruptions are a central component of the disease but the mutated gene is expressed in multiple tissue types.

The second question relates to the normal development that occurs early in life. In many neurodegenerative disorders, the development of clinical signs is delayed and not detected until the fourth or fifth decade of life. One possible explanation for this delay is that toxic molecules need to accumulate over a long period of time before they cause neuronal damage. The neuronal loss due to free radical damage, for example, has been implicated in neurodegenerative disorders, including Huntington's chorea, Parkinson's disease, and Alzheimer's disease. In normal cells, enzymes are present to neutralize the free radicals. Loss of enzymatic activity or reduced amounts of the protein because of mutations can cause toxic compounds to accumulate over time and eventually disrupt the normal neuronal function.

This mechanism may explain what is happening in the brain of patients who have Rett syndrome. The normal function of MeCP2 is to repress the expression of certain genes. The downstream target genes, as well as their function, have not been discovered; however, it is reasonable to propose that mutations in MeCP2 result in inappropriate expression of these genes. These gene products may be toxic and disrupt the functioning of normal cellular proteins over time; however, several laboratories have searched for upregulation of genes using microarray techniques and none have been found.

Summary

The focus of this special issue is on neuropsychiatric disorders, and this article has reviewed several childhood neuropsychiatry disorders with established mutations or deletions. The molecular basis for most common child and adolescent mental disorders has not been determined. Although the reasons for this failure are beyond the scope of this article, one of the major stumbling blocks has been genetic complexity. Many of the genetic disorders discussed, such as Rett syndrome or FXS, exhibit Mendelian patterns of inheritance; however, pedigree analysis of most child and adolescent psychiatric disorders fails to reveal a clear vertical pattern of transmission across generations.

The presence of non-Mendelian patterns of inheritance does not exclude the involvement of genetic factors; rather, it suggests that their role in the transmission or expression of the clinical symptoms is complex. Polygenic disorders are illness in which multiple genes and environmental factors contribute to the expression of an illness. Autism, childhood-onset anxiety disorders, and attention deficit hyperactivity disorder are examples of disorders that likely fall into this category. Estimates for autism, for example, suggest that up to 10 genes may contribute to the etiology of the disorder, with any one of them making only a small contribution. Significant progress has been made in understanding the genetics of complex disorders in several other fields, including breast cancer and hypertension [75,76]. Child psychiatry should take advantage of the knowledge that has become available from these successes.

Technical advances in genomics, molecular genetics, and developmental neurobiology has given us a remarkable list of accomplishments over the past decade, and these advances lay the foundation for further studies into the molecular basis of these disorders. Success in the field ultimately will lead to the genes that cause more complex diseases, such as autism and pervasive developmental disorders. Identification of cellular and molecular components that are responsible for these disorders will prompt advances in drug development, and the promise of gene therapy may be realized for monogenic disorders.

Acknowledgments

This work was funded, in part, by The National Association of Research on Schizophrenia and Depression and the National Institute of Mental Health grants (MH01527) (PJL), and a Brown-Coxe Fellowship (DVV).

References

[1] Kandel ER. A new intellectual framework for psychiatry. Am J Psychiatry 1998;155:457–69.
[2] Neslter EJ, Barrot M, DiLeone RJ, et al. Neurobiology of depression. Neuron 2002;34: 13–25.

[3] Abelson JF, Kwan KY, O'Roak BJ, et al. Sequence variants in SLITRK1 are associated with Tourette's syndrome. Science 2005;310:317–20.

[4] Gupta AR, State MW. Recent advances in the genetics of autism. Biol Psychiatry. 2007;61:429–37.

[5] Bagni C, Greenough WT. From mRNP trafficking to spine dysmorphogenesis: the roots of fragile X syndrome. Nat Rev Neurosci 2005;6:376–87.

[6] Lubs H. A marker X chromosome. Am J Hum Gen 1969;21:231–44.

[7] Fu YH, Kuhl DP, Pizzuti A, et al. Variation of the CGG repeat at the fragile site results in genetic instability: resolution of the Sherman paradox. Cell 1991;67:1047–58.

[8] Hagerman RJ, Staley LW, O'Conner R, et al. Learning-disabled males with a fragile X CGG expansion in the upper premutation size range. Pediatrics 1996;97:122–6.

[9] de von Flindt R, Bybel B, Chudley AE, et al. Short-term memory and cognitive variability in adult fragile X females. Am J Med Genet 1991;38:488–92.

[10] Kemper M, Hagerman R, Ahmad R, et al. Cognitive profiles and the spectrum of clinical manifestations in heterozygous fra(X) females. Am J Med Genet 1986;23:139–56.

[11] Murphy DG, Mentis MJ, Pietrini P, et al. Premutation female carriers of fragile X syndrome: a pilot study on brain anatomy and metabolism. J Am Acad Child Adolesc Psychiatry 1999; 38:1294–301.

[12] Allingham-Hawkins DJ, Babul-Hirji R, Chitayat D, et al. Fragile X premutation is a significant risk factor for premature ovarian failure: The Iinternational Collaborative POF in Fragile X Study- preliminary data. Am J Med Genet 1999;83:322–5.

[13] Jacquemont S, Hagerman RJ, Leehey MA, et al. Penetrance of the fragile X-associated tremor/ataxia syndrome in a premutation carrier population. J Am Med Assoc 2004;291: 460–9.

[14] Jacquemont S, Leehey MA, Hagerman RJ, et al. Size bias of fragile X premutation alleles in late-onset movement disorders. J Med Genet 2006;43:804–9.

[15] Hagerman PJ, Hagerman RJ. Fragile X-associated tremor/ataxia syndrome (FXTAS). Ment Retard Dev Disabil Res Rev 2004;10:25–30.

[16] Nelson D. The fragile X syndromes. Semin Cell Biol 1995;6:5–11.

[17] Oberle I, Rousseau F, Heitz D, et al. Instability of a 550-base pair DNA segment and abnormal methylation in fragile X syndrome. Science 1991;252:1097–110.

[18] Pieretti M, Zhang F, Fu Y-H, et al. Absence of expression of the FMR-1 gene in fragile X syndrome. Cell 1991;66:817–22.

[19] Eichler EE, Richards S, Gibbs RA, et al. Fine structure of the human FMR1 gene. Hum Mol Genet 1993;2:1147–53.

[20] Siomi H, Siomi M, Nussbaum R, et al. The protein product of the fragile X gene, FMR1, has characteristics of an RNA-binding protein. Cell 1993;74:291–8.

[21] Siomi H, Choi M, Siomi MC, et al. Essential role for KH domains in RNA binding: impaired RNA binding mutation in the KH domain of FMR1 that causes fragile X syndrome. Cell 1994;77:33–9.

[22] De Boulle K, Verkerk AJ, Reyniers E, et al. A point mutation in the FMR-1 gene associated with fragile X mental retardation. Nat Genet 1992;3:31–5.

[23] Musco G, Stier G, Joseph C, et al. Three dimensional structure and stability of the KH domain: molecular insights into the fragile X syndrome. Cell 1996;85:237–45.

[24] Khandjian EW, Corbin F, Woerly S, et al. The fragile X mental retardation protein is associated with ribosomes. Nat Genet 1996;12:91–3.

[25] Abitbol M, Menini C, Delezoide AL, et al. Nucleus basalis magno cellularis and hippocampus are the major sites of FMR-1 expression in human fetal brain. Nat Genet 1993;4:147–52.

[26] Mostofsky SH, Mazzocco MM, Aakalu G, et al. Decreased cerebellar posterior vermis size in fragile X syndrome: correlation with neurocognitive performance. Neurology 1998;50: 121–30.

[27] Mostofsky SH, Reiss AL, Lockhart P, et al. Evaluation of cerebellar size in attention-deficit hyperactivity disorder. J Child Neurol 1998;13:434–9.

[28] Reiss AL, Lee J, Freund L. Neuroanatomy of fragile X syndrome: the temporal lobe. Neurology 1994;44:1317–24.

[29] Dutch-Belgian Fragile X Consortium. FMR-1 knock out mice: a model to study fragile X mental retardation. Cell 1994;78:23–33.

[30] Steward O, Schuman EM. Protein synthesis at synaptic sites on dendrites. Annu Rev Neurosci 2001;24:299–325.

[31] Ostroff LE, Fiala JC, Allwardt B, et al. Polyribosomes redistribute from dendritic shafts into spines with enlarged synapses during LTP in developing rat hippocampal slices. Neuron 2002;35:535–45.

[32] Brown V, Jin P, Ceman S, et al. Microarray identification of FMRP-associated brain mRNAs and altered mRNA translational profiles in fragile X syndrome. Cell 2001;107:477–87.

[33] Darnell JC, Jensen KB, Jin P, et al. Fragile X mental retardation protein targets G quartet mRNAs important for neuronal function. Cell 2001;107:489–99.

[34] Zalfa F, Giorgi M, Primerano B, et al. The fragile X syndrome protein FMRP associates with BC1 RNA and regulates the translation of specific mRNAs at synapses. Cell 2003;112:317–27.

[35] Kelleher RJ, Govindarajan A, Tonegawa S. Translational regulatory mechanisms in persistent forms of synaptic plasticity. Neuron 2004;44:59–73.

[36] Kelleher RJ, Govindarajan A, Jung HY, et al. Translational control by MAPK signaling in long-term synaptic plasticity and memory. Cell 2004;116:467–79.

[37] Irwin SA, Patel B, Idupulapati M, et al. Abnormal dendritic spine characteristics in the temporal and visual cortices of patients with fragile-X syndrome: a quantitative examination. Am J Med Genet 2001;98:161–7.

[38] Comery TA, Harris JB, Willems PJ, et al. Abnormal dendritic spines in fragile X knockout mice: maturation and pruning deficits. Proc Natl Acad Sci USA 1997;94:5401–4.

[39] Caskey CT, Pizzuti A, Fu YH, et al. Triplet repeat mutations in human disease. Science 1992;256:784–9.

[40] Nelson D, Warren S. Trinucleotide repeat instability: when and where? Nat Genet 1993;4:107–8.

[41] Warren S. The expanding world of trinucleotide repeats. Science 1996;271:1374–5.

[42] Fu YH, Pizzuti A, Fenwick RG Jr, et al. An unstable triplet repeat in a gene related to myotonic dystrophy. Science 1992;255:1256–8.

[43] Isles AR, Humby T. Modes of imprinted gene action in learning disability. J Intellect Disabil Res 2006;50:318–25.

[44] Prader A, Labhart A, Willi H. A syndrome of adiposity, small stature, cryptorchism, mental retardation and hypotonia in new-born infants [German]. Schweiz Med Wschenschr 1956;86:1260–1.

[45] Holm VA, Cassidy SB, Butler MG, et al. Prader-Willi syndrome: consensus diagnostic criteria. Pediatrics 1993;91:398–402.

[46] Dykens EM, Cassidy SB. Correlates of maladaptive behavior in children and adults with Prader-Willi syndrome. Am J Med Genet 1995;60:546–9.

[47] Dykens EM, Leckman JF, Cassidy SB. Obsessions and compulsions in Prader-Willi syndrome. J Child Psychol Psychiatry 1996;37:995–1002.

[48] State MW, Dykens EM, Rosner B, et al. Obsessive-compulsive symptoms in Prader-Willi and "Prader-Willi-like" patients. J Am Acad Child Adolesc Psychiatry 1999;38:329–34.

[49] Angelman H. 'Puppet children' a report of three cases. Dev Med Child Neurol 1965;7:681–8.

[50] Ledbetter DH, Riccardi VM, Airhart SD, et al. Deletions of chromosome 15 as a cause of the Prader-Willi syndrome. N Engl J Med 1981;304:325–9.

[51] Magenis RE, Brown MG, Lacy DA, et al. Is Angelman syndrome an alternate result of del(15)(q11q13)? Am J Med Genet 1987;28:829–38.

[52] Cassidy SB, Schwartz S. Prader-Willi and Angelman syndromes: disorders of genomic imprinting. Medicine 1998;77:140–51.
[53] Cassidy SB. Prader-Willi syndrome. J Med Genet 1997;34:917–23.
[54] Nicholls RD, Saitoh S, Horsthemke B. Imprinting in Prader-Willi and Angelman syndromes. Trends Genet 1998;14:194–200.
[55] Ledbetter D, Engel E. Uniparental disomy in humans: development of an imprinting map and its implications for prenatal diagnosis. Hum Mol Genet 1995;4:1757–64.
[56] Nicholls RD, Knoll JH, Butler MG, et al. Genetic imprinting suggested by maternal heterodisomy in non-deletion Prader-Willi syndrome. Nature 1989;342:281–5.
[57] Ohta T, Gray TA, Rogan PK, et al. Imprinting-mutation mechanisms in Prader-Willi syndrome. Am J Hum Genet 1999;64:397–413.
[58] Buiting K, Barnicoat A, Lich C, et al. Disruption of the bipartite imprinting center in a family with Angelman syndrome. Am J Hum Genet 2001;68:1290–4.
[59] Kishino T, Lalande M, Wagstaff J. UBE3A/E6-AP mutations cause Angelman syndrome. Nat Genet 1997;15:70–3.
[60] Matsuura T, Sutcliffe JS, Fang P, et al. Novo truncating mutations in E6-AP ubiquitin-protein ligase gene (UBE3A) in Angelman syndrome. Nat Genet 1997;15:74–7.
[61] Nicholls RD. Strange bedfellows? Protein degradation and neurological dysfunction. Neuron 1998;21:647–9.
[62] Albrecht U, Sutcliffe JS, Cattanach BM, et al. Imprinted expression of the murine Angelman syndrome gene, Ube3a, in hippocampal and Purkinje neurons. Nat Genet 1997;17:75–8.
[63] DeLorey TM, Handforth A, Anagnostaras SG, et al. Mice lacking the beta3 subunit of the $GABA_A$ receptor have the epilepsy phenotype and many of the behavioral characteristics of Angelman syndrome. J Neurosci 1998;18:8505–14.
[64] Rett A. On a unusual brain atrophy syndrome in hperammonemia in childhood [German]. Wien Med Wochenschr 1966;116:723–6.
[65] Naidu S. Rett syndrome: natural history and underlying disease mechanisms. Eur Child Adolesc Psychiatry 1997;6:14–7.
[66] Webb T, Clarke A, Hanefeld F, et al. Linkage analysis in Rett syndrome families suggests that there may be a critical region at Xq28. J Med Genet 1998;35:997–1003.
[67] Amir RE, Van den Veyver IB, Wan M, et al. Rett syndrome is caused by mutations in X-linked MECP2, encoding methyl-CpG-binding protein 2. Nat Genet 1999;23:185–8.
[68] Kass SU, Pruss D, Wolffe AP. How does DNA methylation repress transcription? Trends Genet 1997;13:444–9.
[69] Neul JL, Zoghbi HY. Rett syndrome: a prototypical neurodevelopmental disorder. Neuroscientist 2004;10:118–28.
[70] Nan X, Campoy FJ, Bird A. MeCP2 is a transcriptional repressor with abundant binding sites in genomic chromatin. Cell 1997;88:471–81.
[71] Park WJ, Meyers GA, Li X, et al. Novel FGFR2 mutations in Crouzon and Jackson-Weiss syndromes show allelic heterogeneity and phenotypic variability. Hum Mol Genet 1995;4:1229–33.
[72] Weaving LS, Christodoulou J, Williamson SL, et al. Mutations of CDKL5 cause a severe neurodevelopmental disorder with infantile spasms and mental retardation. Am J Hum Genet 2004;75:1079–93.
[73] Evans JC, Archer HL, Colley JP, et al. Early onset seizures and Rett-like features associated with mutations in CDKL5. Eur J Hum Genet 2005;13:1113–20.
[74] Borg I, Freude K, Kubart S, et al. Disruption of Netrin G1 by a balanced chromosome translocation in girl with Rett syndrome. Eur J Hum Genet 2005;13:921–7.
[75] Lifton RP. Molecular genetics of human blood pressure variation. Science 1996;272:676–80.
[76] Miki Y, Swensen J, Shattuck-Eidens D, et al. A strong candidate for the breast and ovarian cancer susceptibility gene BRCA1. Science 1994;266:66–71.

ELSEVIER
SAUNDERS

Child Adolesc Psychiatric Clin N Am
16 (2007) 557–579

CHILD AND
ADOLESCENT
PSYCHIATRIC CLINICS
OF NORTH AMERICA

From Genes to Brain: Understanding Brain Development in Neurogenetic Disorders Using Neuroimaging Techniques

Marie Schaer, MD[a,b,*], Stephan Eliez, MD[a,c]

[a]*Service-Médico-Pédagogique, Department of Psychiatry, University of Geneva, Geneva, Switzerland*
[b]*Signal Processing Institute, Swiss Federal Institute of Technology, Lausanne, Switzerland*
[c]*Department of Genetic Medicine and Development, University of Geneva School of Medicine, Geneva, Switzerland*

The extraordinary burst of acquisition and cognition processes developed during childhood are underlined by major microscopic and macroscopic changes in the brain. First delineated by postmortem studies, MRI has become a powerful tool for studying in vivo the structural correlates of brain maturation. Fascinating studies have revealed the main morphologic tendencies that accompany the development of the superior cognitive functions during childhood [1–4]. These studies revealed the dynamics of the tissular compartment associated with the selection and optimization of brain circuitry, culminating with recent observations that the profile of cortical thickness maturation is closely related to the level of intelligence [5]. As a corollary, neuroimaging studies also have devoted attention to individuals with atypical cognitive and brain development resulting from genetic etiology or environmental injury. In the specific context of relating genes to brain structure and behavior, neurogenetic syndromes were elected as ideal candidates to "reveal insights into neurodevelopmental pathways that might otherwise be obscured or diluted when investigating more heterogeneous pathologies" [6].

This research was supported by grants from Swiss National Research Funds to Dr. Marie Schaer (323500-111165) and Dr. Stephan Eliez (3200-063135, 3232-063134, and PP00B-102864). This work was also supported by a grant from NARSAD to Dr. Eliez.

* Corresponding author. Service Médico-Pédagogique, 16-18 Bd Saint Georges, Case Postale 50, 1211 Geneva 8, Switzerland.

E-mail address: marie.schaer@medecine.unige.ch (M. Schaer).

Behavioral neurogenetics is a research field that has emerged from the observation that neurodevelopmental and neuropsychiatric disturbances are various in their presentation and origins [6,7]. Our opportunity to understand the pathogenesis of abnormal behavioral or cognitive manifestations relies on a narrow definition of homogenous subgroups. Neurogenetic syndromes are considered by researchers as "a window into the understanding of a broader spectrum of learning and developmental disabilities" [7]. Some of these neurogenetic conditions have even been designated as models for broader neurodevelopmental or neurodegenerative pathologies of unclear origin, such as Down syndrome and Alzheimer's disease [8], velocardiofacial syndrome (VCFS) and schizophrenia [9], or fragile X syndrome and autism [10].

Thanks to its incredible ability to quantify structural developmental trajectory, neuroimaging—among other molecular, genetic or endocrine approaches—plays a crucial role in behavioral neurogenetic research. In this article we review some examples of the use of neuroimaging methods to understand neurodevelopmental alterations in genetic conditions. The techniques devoted to image analyses, as used by most clinical studies, are briefly described. We then discuss three syndromes, which were chosen because they illustrate interesting (and different) aspects of the contribution of neuroimaging to the understanding of neurogenetic phenotype. Down syndrome has a long history and exemplifies how neuropathologic and neuroimaging data can be integrated to delineate structural brain alterations. Down syndrome is also of interest because it is often taken as a control group in fragile X or Williams syndrome studies [11–14]. Fragile X provides an example to demonstrate variability in the phenotypic expression related to the range of alterations to the same gene (from premutation to full mutation) [15]. Finally, VCFS (22q11.2 deletion syndrome) represents a developmental model for schizophrenia [9,16] and offers a unique opportunity to identify precursors to the development of psychosis.

Image processing techniques

MRI takes advantage of the magnetic properties of atoms' nuclei (ie, their ability to align along a magnetic field). Contrary to CT, MRI scanners do not use ionizing radiation and are safe for patients. Because of its excellent spatial resolution and contrast, MRI is perfectly adapted for visualizing soft tissue, such as the brain. Different contrasts in the images (T1-weighted, T2-weighted, and diffusion tensor imaging [DTI]) result from modification in the acquisition parameters.

Cerebral MRI datasets typically consist of three-dimensional volume, in which each voxel is attributed an intensity that closely reflects the biologic properties of the tissue. Various methods have been used to exploit the information contained in T1- or T2-weighted MRI. During early brain development, changes in the water content associated with myelination produce quantifiable variations in T1 and T2 intensity values [3]. Pathologic changes in intensities also may reflect white matter lesions, for example, in the fragile X–associated ataxia/tremor syndrome (FXTAS) [17,18]. Except these specific examples, intensity values in the image are preferentially taken as a whole, considering their distribution on the entire volume (histogram). Segmentation algorithms based on the histogram (eventually with prior atlas-based information) are implemented to distinguish between gray and white matter and cerebrospinal fluid (Fig. 1, right). Overall volumes of the different tissue compartment (gray and white matter) are then measured. Semi-automated, atlas-based subdivision or manual landmarks are used to obtain a finer localization in cerebral lobes and cerebellar volumes [19,20]. Smaller regions, such as amygdala and hippocampus, are typically outlined by hand (Fig. 1, left) based on validated protocols [21]. The anatomic boundaries that circumscribe a structure are not always evident, however, which restrains the number of structures that could be delineated reliably. For that purpose, voxel-wise statistical approaches based on whole brain images have proved useful for identifying regional differences in gray matter concentration [22]. Preprocessing in voxel-based morphometry is intended to allow for statistical comparison of gray or white matter density at each voxel between groups. Spatial normalization warps cerebral images to

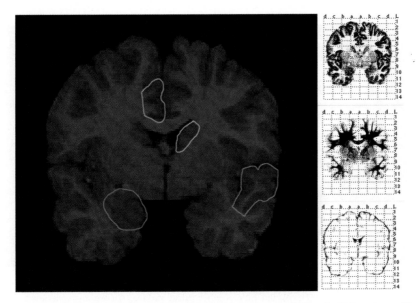

Fig. 1. Volumetric measurements of specific structures. A coronal slice of which regions of interest are manually outlined (*left*). Amygdala is drawn in red, cingulate gyrus in orange, caudate nucleus in green, and superior temporal gyrus in blue. Before delineation, cerebral images are classically reoriented, and strictly validated protocols ensure a maximized reliability between different raters and across the sample of individuals. Measurements are conducted on segmented images (*right*), with Talairach grid overlaid.

match a common template, and smoothing is implemented to cope with interindividual differences in sulcal patterns. As a result of the transformation processes, voxel-based morphometry is highly sensitive to focal differences in gray or white matter concentration but may smooth gross volumetric differences. More recently, measurements of cortical thickness at thousands of points over the cortical surface were developed [23,24] using precise three-dimensional reconstruction of the cortical mantle (Fig. 2). Comparison of the thickness values at each point between individuals uses optimal alignment of the sulcal pattern [25,26], which provides incredible precision in the localization of the alterations. Finally, characterization and quantification of sulcal patterns also received attention, with gyrification index [27], sulcal morphometry [28,29], and local measures of cortical gyrification [30].

A growing interest was also devoted to the development of techniques for analyzing images from DTI, which is particularly adapted for analyzing white matter structure [31] and changes in water content associated with maturation [32]. Fractional anisotropy is a measure of white matter organization (Fig. 3) that was commonly implemented to assess connectivity in neurogenetic syndromes [33,34]. One step farther, fiber tracking offers a promising tool to reconstruct axonal trajectories in the brain from DTI images [35]. Beyond the aesthetics of "virtual axonal dissections" [36],

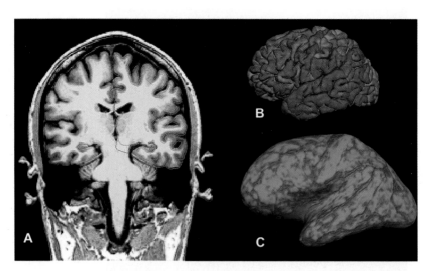

Fig. 2. Example of cortical thickness measurements (using *FreeSurfer* software). (*A*) Coronal section showing inner (*green*) and outer (*red*) cortical surface. Algorithms generating these three-dimensional surfaces are fully automated. Cortical thickness is measured as the distance between both cortical surfaces. (*B*) Three-dimensional reconstruction of the pial surface, with thickness measurements overlaid with a color-coded scale. (*C*) Inflated surface, with the same color overlay, permits visualization of the surface buried into the sulci. Inflated surface is then registered with spherical coordinates for accurate point-to-point comparison of cortical thickness between groups.

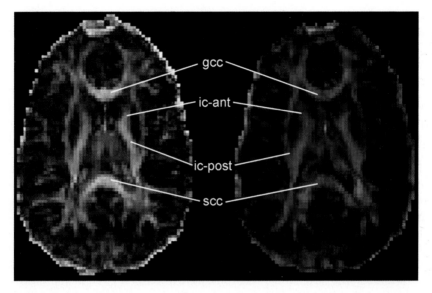

Fig. 3. Axial sections of maps resulting from DTI: On the left, axial section of a fractional anisotropy map, which measures the orientation of white matter tracts. The highly compact corpus callosum (gcc and scc) appears brightly white. On the right, a color-coded map shows the different directions of the axonal tracts. In blue, the genu (gcc) and splenium (scc) of the corpus callosum, which cross from left to right. In green, the rostral limb of the internal capsule (ic-ant) goes to the frontal regions. In red, the posterior limb of the internal capsule (ic-post) goes upward to the parietal regions.

quantitative studies have been developed and potentially will reveal the pattern of axonal connections in the brain of typically developing individuals and patients affected by neurodevelopmental conditions [37].

Down syndrome

Overview

With an average incidence of 1 per 800 live births, Down syndrome is the most common genetic cause of mental retardation. Down syndrome is related to the presence of an extra copy of chromosome 21. Physical characteristics associated with the syndrome include short stature, flat occiput, single transverse palmar crease, bilateral epicanthal folds, and enlarged tongue. Congenital heart defects and gastrointestinal malformations are frequently observed in affected individuals. Mental retardation is typical but is variable and encompasses specific language troubles, short-term memory impairments, and difficulties in changing tasks. Premature aging of the skin and hair is characteristic, along with decreased life expectancy [38] and a high incidence of dementia clinically similar to Alzheimer's disease. Together, neuroimaging and neuropathologic findings in Down syndrome point to intricated mechanisms, in which neurodegenerative processes super-impose neurodevelopmental alterations.

Neonatal period and infancy

As in many syndromes, few neuroimaging studies are conducted during the neonatal period because of the absence of clinical incentive and the technical difficulties associated with the image processing of unmyelinated brains. Our knowledge of early brain development in Down syndrome is mostly derived from postmortem studies. It is of special interest that microcephaly and cerebellar reduction, which are the most consistent findings in the later stage of the syndrome [11,39–42], are not observed at birth, neither under neuro-pathologic examination [39] nor with CT [43]. Despite normal macroscopic appearance, however, cortical alterations are already found upon micro-scopic examination, with a decrease of 25% to 50% in neuronal number [44]. From as early as 3 months after birth, differences in brain size become distinctive between infants affected with Down syndrome and normal con-trols. Infants who have Down syndrome have lower brain weight and shorter anteroposterior diameter driven by a marked reduction of frontal lobe [39]. It has been suggested that this early dissociation between the micro- and macro-scopic observations is driven by a prenatal delay in neurogenesis, which is sub-sequently followed by abnormalities in synaptogenesis that impairs postnatal brain growth [39]. Similar to postnatal deviant brain growth, delayed myeli-nation of the white matter is not observed at birth but only after 2 months of age [45]. As suggested by Nadel and colleagues [46], the delay in the appear-ance of myelination changes seems to parallel the chronology of learning impairment in Down syndrome, with early psychomotor development pre-served in 3-month-old infants [47] but subsequent altered motor learning [48]. Because delayed myelination also has been observed in young children not affected by Down syndrome who died from a congenital heart disease or neoplastic condition [49], further MRI studies assessing myelination devel-opment in infants who have Down syndrome could provide a more compre-hensive understanding of abnormal maturation associated with the syndrome.

Childhood and young adulthood

From the age of 5 to 6 years, patients can achieve sufficient immobility during the MRI acquisition, which allows for scanning them without any need for sedation. This is probably the main reason why there are more neu-roimaging data for all neurogenetic syndromes available for this age range than for infants. The major neuroanatomic changes reported in children who have Down syndrome are decreased cerebellar volume [11,40], reduced frontal lobe [12], preservation of the parietal gray [11,40] and subcortical gray matter [40], and structural changes in the temporal lobe [12,40,50].

As in infants, decreased frontal lobe volume was reported in children when compared with age-matched controls [12,40]. Volume decreases remained significant after controlling for the reduced brain size only in one study, however [12]. The observed frontal volumetric divergence in children may rely on divergences in the measured tissue (gray and white matter [40] versus gray matter only [12]), but it also may illustrate a specific morphology of the brain in Down syndrome. In the brachycephalic brains of individuals who have Down syndrome (ie, with decreased total rostrocaudal length), small differences in placement of landmarks for the posterior subdivision of frontal lobe could particularly affect volumetric measurements. Measurements in adults are more consistent, all reporting a disproportionate reduction in frontal lobe volume or gray matter concentration [41,42]. Decreased sulcal length also has been reported in the frontal lobe [41], which suggests an early abnormal cortical development. The reduction and morphologic alterations of frontal lobe are likely to be partly responsible for impairment in executive functions and language in Down syndrome.

Not observed during gestation and neonatal period [39], a drastic decrease in cerebellar volume is shown in children [11,12,40] and adults who have Down syndrome [42,43,51]. Cerebellar reduction mostly affects posterior vermis [42] and does not undergo massive atrophy with age, even in older affected adults [51]. Because cerebellar growth is typically achieved during the first year of life [52], it has been proposed that a smaller cerebellum in children and adults but not in fetuses who have Down syndrome results from impaired cerebellar growth [42]. As suggested by Shapiro [53], an exaggerated vulnerability of cerebellum may be key in explaining its recurrent alterations in many pathologic processes. Shapiro and colleagues arguably proposed that cerebellar hypoplasia associated with Down syndrome could be related to functional, biochemical, or environmental disturbances rather than a direct genetic effect. In turn, cerebellar reduction in Down syndrome could be responsible for hypotonia, difficulties in motor coordination, and language deficits of multiple origins (eg, articulatory disturbances, verbal fluency, difficulties in syntax) [40].

Temporal lobe structures also have frequently received attention in Down syndrome related to the specific impairment in language skills and short-term memory. The relative preservation of temporal lobe volume [40] contrasts with the underlying divergent volumetric alterations (Table 1). Among those specific alterations, strong hippocampal reduction has been reported consistently in children [50] and adults [41,42,54], with significant atrophy with age [41]. Although hippocampal reduction in children suggests an early abnormal development, it also plays a crucial role in the development of Alzheimer symptomatology in older individuals who have Down syndrome, providing a clear biologic substrate for the impaired mnesic performances. Concomitant with decreased hippocampal size, a surprising enlargement of the adjacent parahippocampal gyrus has been reported repeatedly in young adults who have Down syndrome [41,42]. Parahippocampal enlargement is even more intriguing given the frequent implication of this gyrus in Alzheimer's disease. To the best of our knowledge, an increase in

Table 1
Summary of the major volumetric changes in the brain of patients affected by Down, Williams, fragile X, and velocardiofacial syndromes, as observed by neuroimaging studies

	Down syndrome	Fragile X syndrome	Velocardiofacial syndrome (22q11DS)
Total brain volume	↓ [11,39–42]	Enlarged or preserved [15,66]	↓ [100–102]
Cerebellum	Children: ↓ [11,12,40] Adults: ↓ [42,43,51,127], mostly posterior vermis	↓ vermis [63,66,75]	↓ with prominent reduction of vermis [116,117]
Frontal lobe	Children: ↓ [12,40] Adults: ↓ [41,42]	→ [13]	Children/young adults: ↑ [100,102–104] Adults: ↓ [95,122]
Parietal lobe	↑ gray [11,40]	→ [13]	Children: ↓ [100,102,104]
Temporal lobe	→ [40]	↓ in young children [13], mostly gray; → in children/ young adults [67]	Children: → [110] Adults: ↓ [95,122]
Superior temporal gyrus	↓ gray matter [40,41]	→ [67]	→ [110]
Planum temporale	↓ [128]		
Hippocampus	↓ [41,42,50,54] But enlarged parahippocampal gyrus [41,42]	Children: ↑ [21,67], Adults: → [68]	↓ children [110–112], mainly body adults → compared with IQ matched individuals [114]
Amygdala		→ [67]	→ [110,112]; ↑ [111]
Occipital lobe	→ [40]	→ [13]	Children: → [100] or ↓ [102] Schizophrenic adults: ↓ [122]
Subcortical gray matter	Children: ↑ [12,40] Adults: ↑ [42,129], mostly putamen [129]	↑ Caudate and thalamus children [15,70]	↑ Caudate, mostly head [103,121,130] ↓ Thalamus, prominently posterior [131]
Corpus callosum (area on midsagittal section)	↓ [14,54], mostly affecting rostral part		↑ [96,132]

(continued on next page)

Table 1 (*continued*)

	Down syndrome	Fragile X syndrome	Velocardiofacial syndrome (22q11DS)
White matter organization (fractional anisotropy using DTI)		↓ Fractional anisotropy fronto-striatal pathways and sensory motor tracts [33]	↓ Fractional anisotropy in frontal, parietal and temporal regions [33,104]
Sulcal patterns and cortical complexity	↓ sulcal length in frontal lobe [41]		Decreased gyrification in frontal and parietal lobes [113]
Neuropathologic findings	Calcified basal ganglia [60,61], amyloid senile plaques, and neurofibrillary tangles [56]	Overabundant synapses and numerous dendritic abnormalities [72,73]	

To provide a more exhaustive overview of the structural alterations, findings on white matter organization (fractional anisotropy), cortical complexity, and neuropathologic observations are also presented.

parahippocampal gyrus has not been reported in any other neurodevelopmental conditions. Given its specificity, enlarged parahippocampal gyrus has been proposed as a quantitative marker for Down syndrome [42]. An inverse correlation between parahippocampal volume and general cognitive performance (PIQ score) also has been observed, but underlying mechanisms still remain unclear.

Other preserved structures (ie, enlarged relatively to the overall cerebral reduction) in the brain of children who have Down syndrome include the parietal lobe [12,50] and the basal ganglia [40]. The relative increase in the parietal lobe is related to an increase in the gray matter volume. As suggested by Pinter [40], preservation of the parietal lobe in children may explain the relative strength in visuospatial processing as compared with language skills. Parietal lobe preservation is no more reported into adulthood, but rather a trend for parietal white matter reduction [42]. The splenium of the corpus callosum, which connects parietal association cortices, has been found to be reduced in nondemented adults who have Down syndrome [54]. Decreased connectivity between bilateral association cortices was correlated with cognitive performance and may represent a substrate for the non-mnesic symptomatology associated with dementia.

Dementia and Alzheimer's disease in older individuals who have Down syndrome

Half of older individuals who have Down syndrome develop clinical symptoms of Alzheimer's disease [55], whereas virtually all of them present with diagnostic neuropathologic lesions (amyloid senile plaques and neurofibrillary tangles) [56]. The beta-amyloid precursor protein is coded on chromosome 21 [57], which provides potential explanation for the high incidence of amyloid plaques in Down syndrome. Mann [8] proposed that cerebral aging processes in Down syndrome could give insights into the pathogenesis of Alzheimer's disease. For the first time, a neurogenetic disorder was elected as an excellent example to understand the interaction among the genetic, neural, and environmental influences. Plenty of articles have been published about the relationship between Down syndrome and Alzheimer's disease. Many structures in the brains of individuals who have Down syndrome show similar alterations than in typical Alzheimer's disease (ie, without Down syndrome). For example, hippocampal atrophy with age is observed years before clinical dementia [41,58]. As mentionned by Teipel [59], however, it is important to remember that this "Alzheimer model" develops on top of an abnormally developed brain with its own specificities (eg, the enlarged parahippocampal gyrus). The preceding developmental abnormalities and the neuroanatomic divergences may explain why, when virtually all patients present with the characteristic histologic lesions, only 50% of older adults who have Down syndrome develop clinical dementia [55]. The identification of pathogenic mechanisms responsible for the subsequent development of dementia in Down syndrome will contribute to proposed targeted therapies for individuals who have Down syndrome and for individuals who present with Alzheimer's disease not associated with Down syndrome.

Summary

Together, neuroimaging and neuropathologic studies have contributed to further our understanding of brain development in Down syndrome. The opportunity given by these different techniques to study different age ranges has led to a comprehensive overview of the alterations in the syndrome—from normal volumes at birth, to characteristic pattern of development alterations during childhood, to massive neurodegeneration associated with specific histologic findings associated with dementia in older adults. Even if neuroimaging and neuropathology observations undoubtedly reveal the peculiar dynamic of brain structure in Down syndrome, however, their findings may sometimes be confusing. For example, basal ganglia calcifications were frequently observed by neuropathologists [60,61] or on CT [43]. The timetable of calcium deposit observations diverges between both techniques: postmortem examinations showed massive calcifications in infants and average quantities of calcifications after the fourth decade of life [60]. On the contrary, a linear increase in calcifications after age 5 was observed using CT [43]. This discrepancy nicely illustrated a selection bias in postmortem studies, because the minority of exceptionally affected children who expired during the first years of life provided material for neuropathologic studies and was not included in neuroimaging studies. This emphasizes the value of (longitudinal) neuroimaging studies to characterize the developmental profile presented by most affected individuals rather than exceptional findings found in a few of them.

Fragile X syndrome

Fragile X syndrome is the most common hereditary cause of mental retardation and the second most important genetic cause of mental retardation. The genetic defect responsible for fragile X is an excess of trinucleotide (cytosine-guanine-guanine [CGG]) repeats on the terminal end of chromosome X (Fragile Mental Retardation gene [FMR1]) associated with methylation and silencing of the gene, which results in decreased expression of the FMR protein [62]. An extensive molecular and clinical description of the syndrome is provided in the article by Hall and colleagues elsewhere in this issue. Briefly, mental retardation and delay in language acquisition are often seen in infancy, whereas attention disorders and social deficits with peers are reported during childhood. Although affected boys are often more severely cognitively affected, affected girls demonstrate high frequencies of social disabilities, anxiety, and depression [63]. Longitudinal studies have shown that both genders can experience prepubertal fall in IQ [64,65].

Preserved brain structures in children who have fragile X syndrome

In children affected by fragile X syndrome, increased or preserved volume of several structures has been reported. Overall enlarged brain volumes have been observed in boys and girls with fragile X syndrome [15,66]. The latter finding is consistent with the observation by Kates and colleagues [13] that relatively few cortical volume alterations are found in young children with fragile X syndrome compared with normal controls, which contrasts with the significant reductions observed in children who have delayed developmental language or Down syndrome. A moderate increase in hippocampal volume has been observed in children [21,67] but not adults with fragile X [68]. Although this divergence may be caused by methodologic differences, the normal volumetric increase accompanying hippocampal maturation suggests that abnormal maturation may be responsible for the discrepancies between children and adults [69]. Among subcortical structures, increased caudate and thalamus volumes have been observed in young affected subjects [15,70], with caudate volume being negatively correlated with the production of FMR protein [15]. As normal maturation typically proceeds with volumetric reduction in caudate and thalamus [71], abnormal maturation also may explain their aberrant enlargement in fragile X.

If structural observations of enlarged structures in fragile X syndrome point to abnormal maturation, neuropathologic and molecular studies provide additional clues for understanding the syndrome's pathogenesis. Microscopic examinations of cortex reveal overabundant quantities of synapses, associated with numerous dendritic abnormalities [72,73]. Specifically, long, thin, and tortuous spines with irregular dilatation on the apical dendrites, typical of abnormal synapse elimination, have been observed. Mice studies suggest that the amount of FMR protein is crucial for the protein synthesis at the synapse and synaptic plasticity [74]. Together, molecular and neuropathologic studies suggest that the relationship between decreased FMR protein level and impaired synapse selection may be key to understanding the pathogenesis of fragile X syndrome. Because pruning is the principal microscopic process contributing to macroscopic decreases in gray matter [1], increased volumes in the brain of affected individuals corroborate abnormal synapse elimination. This putative failure to optimize brain circuitry during childhood may be responsible for the prepubertal fall in IQ observed by longitudinal studies [64,65].

Altered brain structures in children who have fragile X syndrome

Abnormal maturation, however, does not fully explain neuroanatomic alterations associated with fragile X syndrome. In particular, hypoplasia of the cerebellar vermis with concurrent enlargement of the fourth ventricle is consistently reported in affected individuals [63,66,75]. This alteration seems to be related to psychopathology in the syndrome, because the size of the cerebellar vermis is negatively correlated with the amount of atypical social behaviors [63]. Similarly, vermis hypoplasia is reported in autism [76], along with increases in total volume [77] and caudate enlargement [78]. A similar explanation of abnormal synapse elimination has been proposed in fragile X and autism, with "early overgrowth followed by premature arrest of growth" [77]. These shared neurodevelopmental characteristics support an evidence for common pathogenic mechanisms leading to impaired social behaviors in these overlapping syndromes [10].

FMR1 premutation carriers and fragile X associated ataxia/tremor syndrome

The full fragile X phenotype is associated with more than 200 CGG repeats on the terminal end of X chromosome, whereas 6 to 54 repeats are found in the typical population [79]. The less-defined interval that falls between the normal population and the full phenotype is known as the premutation. Fragile X premutation carriers are more common than fragile X syndrome, with an average of 1 in 259 women and 1 in 379 men [80]. Premutation carriers were initially believed to be relatively unaffected, aside from a higher incidence of premature ovarian failure in women [81]. A subgroup of older men with intention tremor and gait ataxia has since been identified and associated with the FMR1 premutation, however, leading to the identification of FXTAS [17,82]. FXTAS typically develops in men during the fifth decade of life, with motor impairment and particularly devastating neurodegeneration. FXTAS rarely has been reported in women.

The first published MRI of a 62-year-old patient with FXTAS show pronounced atrophy that affected the frontal and parietal lobes, corpus callosum, cerebellum, and brain stem [82]. Subsequent neuroimaging studies have delineated a pattern of brain alterations associated with FXTAS, among which T2 hyperintensities in the middle cerebellar peduncles were proposed to serve as a major diagnostic criterion for FXTAS [17]. Corroborating qualitative observations of atrophy, volumetric measurements indicate a severe overall brain reduction in FXTAS [18,83]. Upon neuropathologic examination, nuclear inclusions in neurons and astrocytes are apparent [84]; the cause of such inclusions remains unclear. More recent studies emphasize identifying potential risk factors for the development of FXTAS in premutation carriers. Two recent neuroimaging studies showed a strong negative correlation between total brain volume and the number of repeats in older premutation carriers, which suggested that after a certain age, the number of repeats may determine the development of this devastating syndrome [83,85]. Consistent with these observations, the amount of intranuclear inclusions upon neuropathologic examination is also strongly correlated with the number of CGG repeats after the sixth decade of life [84].

Summary

Providing a comprehensive interpretation of the neuroanatomic alterations associated with FMR1 mutation is an ongoing challenge that is directly related to the broad genetic and gender spectrum associated with the mutation. There is increasing evidence that absence of FMR protein during the critical period of synaptic selection may explain an important part of the neuroanatomic and cognitive phenotype associated with fragile X syndrome. In individuals with the premutation, however, alterations are shown to depend on the number of CGG repeats, but the precise pathogenic mechanisms leading to massive atrophy after the fifth decade of life remain to be elucidated.

Velocardiofacial syndrome

VCFS (also known as 22q11 deletion syndrome) is a neurogenetic disorder that affects 1 in 5000 live births [86] and presents with cognitive and learning impairments [87]. A comprehensive clinical description of the syndrome can be found in the article by Burg and colleagues elsewhere in this issue. VCFS has received much attention during the last decade, mostly because of the increased prevalence of numerous psychopathologies in the syndrome. Neuropsychiatric manifestations during childhood include attention problems [88], difficulties in social interactions with avoidant behaviors [89,90], and a high prevalence of anxiety and depression [91]. The main incentive for studying VCFS is probably the high prevalence of affected patients developing psychotic symptoms and schizophrenia, 50% and 30%, respectively, during adolescence or early adulthood [16,92]. VCFS represents the highest genetically homogenous risk known currently for developing schizophrenia and has been proposed as a model for studying the neuroanatomic changes associated with the onset of psychosis [9]. The first neuroimaging studies in VCFS that emphasized qualitative brain anomalies associated with the syndrome have been supplanted by quantitative volumetric studies on larger sample of individuals. More recently, specific structural alterations accompanying or preceding the development of psychotic symptoms received much attention.

Qualitative findings in children and adults who have velocardiofacial syndrome

The first neuroimaging reports in children and adults who have VCFS showed cerebral atrophy [93,94] and cerebellar reduction [93,94]. Nonspecific white matter alterations also were observed, such as a high incidence of bright foci on T2-weighted MRI [93] and cysts around the frontal horn of the ventricle [94]. Midline anomalies, such as enlarged cavum septum pellucidum or cavum vergae, were shown in numerous affected patients [93–96]. Other frequent noncerebral midline malformations in VCFS encompass cleft palate, cardiac malformations, and thymic hypoplasia [87]. Such a high prevalence of midline anomalies in VCFS potentially point to a common cause. The midline tissues that are frequently involved in the syndrome are derived from the rostral neural crest; genetically induced perturbation of early neural crest development may explain the higher incidence of malformations associated with VCFS [97].

Another qualitative finding that may give insight on the origin of brain anomalies in VCFS is severe polymicrogyria, which was frequently reported in the syndrome [98]. Polymicrogyria is a cortical malformation primarily caused by ischemic injury during a critical period of cortical development [99]. Because cardiovascular malformation is one of the cardinal symptoms of the syndrome, genetically induced circulatory disturbances during embryologic development may result in abnormal neuronal migration and subsequent gyral alterations [87].

Quantitative findings in children who have velocardiofacial syndrome

After the first qualitative delineations of cerebral anomalies associated with VCFS, numerous quantitative studies were conducted on larger sample of patients. Cerebral atrophy was confirmed, presenting as overall gray and white matter reduction in children and young adults who have VCFS [100–102]. Further analyses revealed a specific pattern of lobar alterations in children who have VCFS. After adjusting for global reduction, relative frontal enlargement/preservation was observed [100,102–104], along with disproportionate parietal lobe reduction [100,102,104]. Frontal and parietal volumetric alterations may provide explanations for part of the cognitive phenotype associated with the syndrome. Relative frontal lobe preservation has been suggested [100] to allow the maintenance of a borderline IQ in children who have VCFS [89], whereas other disorders with substantial frontal lobe reduction show more severe mental retardation (eg, Rett [105] and Williams [106] syndromes). On the contrary, the significant volumetric decrease of the parietal lobe observed in children who have VCFS is likely to account for part of the cognitive deficits. Specifically, parietal lobe dysfunction may be responsible for visuo-spatial deficits and lower performance in abstract reasoning tasks, such as arithmetic [107,108]. Abnormal functioning of the parietal lobe also may cause learning difficulties in children who have VCFS, and fMRI and positron emission tomographic studies have attributed a crucial role for the parietal cortex in normal mnesic processes [109]. Along with parietal involvement, hippocampal reduction found in children and young adults who have VCFS may explain impaired short-term memory and part of the learning difficulties associated with VCFS [110–112]. Frontal and parietal lobes, which are most frequently associated with volumetric changes, show significant decreased cortical complexity, whereas no significant differences are found in gyral complexity of temporal and occipital lobes [113]. According to Van Essen's tension-based morphogenesis model of cortical development [114], altered gyrification in the frontal and parietal lobes of children who have VCFS is likely to reflect aberrant underlying neural connectivity. DTI observations further corroborate the hypothesis of disturbed white matter organization, with decreased fractional anisotropy found predominantly in the middle and superior frontal gyri [34] and diffusely in the parietal lobe [33,104,115].

Similar to cerebral atrophy, early qualitative observations of cerebellar reduction [93,94] were confirmed by volumetric measurements [116,117]. Qualitative and quantitative studies emphasized a prominent reduction of the vermis [94,116,117]. Reduction of the vermis also was reported in other neurogenetic and neurodevelopmental disorders, such as fragile X syndrome [63,66,75] and autism [76]. Because of typical social difficulties presented in these neurodevelopmental disorders [118] and in VCFS [89,90,119], reduction of the cerebellar vermis may represent an important biologic substrate for avoidant behaviors and communication problems. The enlarged posterior vermis found in overempathic subjects who have Williams syndrome strengthens a hypothetical positive correlation between vermis size and social skills [106,120].

The development of psychosis in adults who have velocardiofacial syndrome

An important challenge that motivates researchers on VCFS is the aim of identifying markers and risk factors for the highly prevalent psychotic symptoms and schizophrenia associated with the syndrome. To date, inferences about specific anomalies associated with schizophrenia in the syndrome are mainly based on comparison of neuroimaging findings obtained by different research groups on children [100,102,104,121] and adults [95,122]. For example, observations of prominent gray matter deficits in the frontal and temporal lobes reported in adults who have VCFS [95,122] contrast with the relative increase of the frontal lobe [100,102–104] and preservation of temporal lobe [100,102] found in children. The latter volumetric divergence may rely on accelerated neurodegenerative processes in the frontal and temporal lobes of affected patients. Findings of disproportionate reduction of frontal and temporal lobes volumes are in agreement with structural abnormalities observed in schizophrenia [123]. Such hypothesis based on the comparison of different studies may be hazardous, however, because of differences in methodology or sample selection (eg, control subjects matched for IQ [95] or typically developing individuals [100,104,122]). Such "children versus adults" comparison designs may not be able to identify specific changes associated with schizophrenia.

Van Amelsvoort and colleagues [124] compared adults who have VCFS with schizophrenia (S-VCFS) and without schizophrenia (NS-VCFS). They reported generalized gray and white matter volume decrease in patients with schizophrenia compared with patients without psychotic symptoms. Significant frontal and temporal lobe reduction was shown in S-VCFS compared with normal controls but not when compared with NS-VCFS. Because frontal and temporal reduction was not found in NS-VCFS compared with controls, frontal and temporal volume decrease may be specifically associated with schizophrenia. A large sample size may be required to evidence localized brain anomalies when comparing schizophrenic to nonpsychotic VCFS patients, however. Alternatively, longitudinal studies offer the possibility to assess intraindividual changes in brain anatomy over time, providing a powerful approach to isolate structural alterations distinctively associated with psychotic evolution. The first longitudinal study on patients who have VCFS was recently published, illustrating the potential of such design to identify risk factors and markers for the development of psychotic symptoms. Gothelf and colleagues [125] prospectively followed 24 children who have VCFS and 23 subjects with idiopathic developmental disorder from childhood to early adulthood, and they identified that decline in prefrontal volume accompanies the emergence of psychosis. They were able to designate the low activity allele of the catechol-O-methyltransferase gene as a major risk factor for the development of psychotic symptoms. The prediction of prefrontal reduction and subsequent psychiatric symptomatology according to catechol-O-methyltransferase polymorphism is likely to rely on modified dopaminergic transmission [126].

Summary

VCFS illustrates how knowledge can evolve rapidly to build promising correlations among genotype, behaviors, and brain structure. Neuroimaging studies have allowed the definition of the pattern of brain alterations that may be responsible for cognitive deficits in the syndrome. Interesting hypotheses about the cause of brain alterations have been proposed, such as abnormal control of the neural crest development and circulatory disturbances in the developing brain. Future postmortem descriptions of the cerebral microarchitecture in VCFS may help to corroborate or affirm assumptions on the pathogenesis of structural brain alterations, however. Finally, the promising identification of a gene dosage effect on psychotic evolution shows potential for outlining risk factors and markers for the development of psychosis and announcing future fascinating longitudinal studies toward a better understanding of schizophrenia.

Summary

Among other neurogenetic syndromes, Down, fragile X, and velocardiofacial syndromes exemplify how neuroimaging studies further our understanding of the gene-brain-behavior relationship (Table 1) as referenced to in [127–132]. Early isolated case reports and qualitative studies of brain structure using MRI have been succeeded by a substantial amount of quantitative studies delineating the volumetric pattern of cerebral alterations in neurogenetic syndromes. Specific developmental profiles were identified in each neurogenetic condition, potentially explaining the cognitive phenotypical differences between the syndromes. Currently, spectacular developments of image processing techniques offer increasingly subtle information about the underlying morphometric processes that contribute to volumetric changes. After almost two decades of research exploiting cerebral MRI, the contribution of neuroimaging studies is far from being fulfilled. Next generation methods offer promising tools to delineate normal and abnormal brain development more precisely, such as the assessment of three-dimensional cortical morphology or the identification and quantification of white matter tracts.

More elaborate image processing techniques applied on a large sample of individuals also will permit explorations of factors such as genetic polymorphism. The identification of genetically distinct subgroups within a neurogenetic condition will put forward insights on the neurodevelopmental pathways that give rise to cognitive and behavioral impairments. Neuroimaging studies in genetic disorders will provide successful attempts at integrating clinical phenotypes in an approach from genes to brain to behavior.

Acknowledgment

The authors would like to thank Bronwyn Glaser for helpful comments on the manuscript.

References

[1] Pfefferbaum A, Mathalon DH, Sullivan EV, et al. A quantitative magnetic resonance imaging study of changes in brain morphology from infancy to late adulthood. Arch Neurol 1994;51(9):874–87.

[2] Giedd JN, Blumenthal J, Jeffries NO, et al. Brain development during childhood and adolescence: a longitudinal MRI study. Nat Neurosci 1999;2(10):861–3.

[3] Holland BA, Haas DK, Norman D, et al. MRI of normal brain maturation. AJNR Am J Neuroradiol 1986;7(2):201–8.

[4] Toga AW, Thompson PM, Sowell ER. Mapping brain maturation. Trends Neurosci 2006; 29(3):148–59.

[5] Shaw P, Greenstein D, Lerch J, et al. Intellectual ability and cortical development in children and adolescents. Nature 2006;440(7084):676–9.

[6] Reiss AL, Eliez S, Schmitt JE, et al. Brain imaging in neurogenetic conditions: realizing the potential of behavioral neurogenetics research. Ment Retard Dev Disabil Res Rev 2000; 6(3):186–97.

[7] Baumgardner TL, Green KE, Reiss AL. A behavioral neurogenetics approach to developmental disabilities: gene-brain-behavior associations. Curr Opin Neurol 1994;7(2):172–8.

[8] Mann DM. The pathological association between Down syndrome and Alzheimer disease. Mech Ageing Dev 1988;43(2):99–136.

[9] Murphy KC, Owen MJ. Velo-cardio-facial syndrome: a model for understanding the genetics and pathogenesis of schizophrenia. Br J Psychiatry 2001;179:397–402.

[10] Hagerman RJ, Ono MY, Hagerman PJ. Recent advances in fragile X: a model for autism and neurodegeneration. Curr Opin Psychiatry 2005;18(5):490–6.

[11] Jernigan TL, Bellugi U. Anomalous brain morphology on magnetic resonance images in Williams syndrome and Down syndrome. Arch Neurol 1990;47(5):529–33.

[12] Jernigan TL, Bellugi U, Sowell E, et al. Cerebral morphologic distinctions between Williams and Down syndromes. Arch Neurol 1993;50(2):186–91.

[13] Kates WR, Folley BS, Lanham DC, et al. Cerebral growth in fragile X syndrome: review and comparison with Down syndrome. Microsc Res Tech 2002;57(3):159–67.

[14] Wang PP, Doherty S, Hesselink JR, et al. Callosal morphology concurs with neurobehavioral and neuropathological findings in two neurodevelopmental disorders. Arch Neurol 1992;49(4):407–11.

[15] Reiss AL, Abrams MT, Greenlaw R, et al. Neurodevelopmental effects of the FMR-1 full mutation in humans. Nat Med 1995;1(2):159–67.

[16] Murphy KC, Jones LA, Owen MJ. High rates of schizophrenia in adults with velo-cardio-facial syndrome. Arch Gen Psychiatry 1999;56(10):940–5.

[17] Brunberg JA, Jacquemont S, Hagerman RJ, et al. Fragile X premutation carriers: characteristic MR imaging findings of adult male patients with progressive cerebellar and cognitive dysfunction. AJNR Am J Neuroradiol 2002;23(10):1757–66.

[18] Jacquemont S, Hagerman RJ, Leehey M, et al. Fragile X premutation tremor/ataxia syndrome: molecular, clinical, and neuroimaging correlates. Am J Hum Genet 2003;72(4): 869–78.

[19] Andreasen NC, Rajarethinam R, Cizadlo T, et al. Automatic atlas-based volume estimation of human brain regions from MR images. J Comput Assist Tomogr 1996;20(1): 98–106.

[20] Bokde AL, Teipel SJ, Zebuhr Y, et al. A new rapid landmark-based regional MRI segmentation method of the brain. J Neurol Sci 2002;194(1):35–40.

[21] Kates WR, Abrams MT, Kaufmann WE, et al. Reliability and validity of MRI measurement of the amygdala and hippocampus in children with fragile X syndrome. Psychiatry Res 1997;75(1):31–48.

[22] Ashburner J, Friston KJ. Voxel-based morphometry: the methods. Neuroimage 2000;11 (6 Pt 1):805–21.

[23] Thompson PM, Hayashi KM, Sowell ER, et al. Mapping cortical change in Alzheimer's disease, brain development, and schizophrenia. Neuroimage 2004;23(Suppl 1):S2–18.

[24] Fischl B, Dale AM. Measuring the thickness of the human cerebral cortex from magnetic resonance images. Proc Natl Acad Sci USA 2000;97(20):11050–5.

[25] Fischl B, Sereno MI, Tootell RB, et al. High-resolution intersubject averaging and a coordinate system for the cortical surface. Hum Brain Mapp 1999;8(4):272–84.

[26] Thompson PM, Hayashi KM, de Zubicaray G, et al. Dynamics of gray matter loss in Alzheimer's disease. J Neurosci 2003;23(3):994–1005.

[27] Zilles K, Armstrong E, Schleicher A, et al. The human pattern of gyrification in the cerebral cortex. Anat Embryol (Berl) 1988;179(2):173–9.

[28] Mangin JF, Riviere D, Cachia A, et al. A framework to study the cortical folding patterns. Neuroimage 2004;23(Suppl 1):S129–38.

[29] White T, Andreasen NC, Nopoulos P. Brain volumes and surface morphology in monozygotic twins. Cereb Cortex 2002;12(5):486–93.

[30] Luders E, Thompson PM, Narr KL, et al. A curvature-based approach to estimate local gyrification on the cortical surface. Neuroimage 2006;29(4):1224–30.

[31] Pierpaoli C, Jezzard P, Basser PJ, et al. Diffusion tensor MR imaging of the human brain. Radiology 1996;201(3):637–48.

[32] Mukherjee P, Miller JH, Shimony JS, et al. Diffusion-tensor MR imaging of gray and white matter development during normal human brain maturation. AJNR Am J Neuroradiol 2002;23(9):1445–56.

[33] Barnea-Goraly N, Eliez S, Hedeus M, et al. White matter tract alterations in fragile X syndrome: preliminary evidence from diffusion tensor imaging. Am J Med Genet B Neuropsychiatr Genet 2003;118(1):81–8.

[34] Barnea-Goraly N, Menon V, Krasnow B, et al. Investigation of white matter structure in velocardiofacial syndrome: a diffusion tensor imaging study. Am J Psychiatry 2003;160(10):1863–9.

[35] Mori S, Kaufmann WE, Davatzikos C, et al. Imaging cortical association tracts in the human brain using diffusion-tensor-based axonal tracking. Magn Reson Med 2002;47(2):215–23.

[36] Hagmann P, Thiran JP, Jonasson L, et al. DTI mapping of human brain connectivity: statistical fibre tracking and virtual dissection. Neuroimage 2003;19(3):545–54.

[37] Molko N, Cohen L, Mangin JF, et al. Visualizing the neural bases of a disconnection syndrome with diffusion tensor imaging. J Cogn Neurosci 2002;14(4):629–36.

[38] Thase ME. Longevity and mortality in Down's syndrome. J Ment Defic Res 1982;26(Pt 3):177–92.

[39] Schmidt-Sidor B, Wisniewski KE, Shepard TH, et al. Brain growth in Down syndrome subjects 15 to 22 weeks of gestational age and birth to 60 months. Clin Neuropathol 1990;9(4):181–90.

[40] Pinter JD, Eliez S, Schmitt JE, et al. Neuroanatomy of Down's syndrome: a high-resolution MRI study. Am J Psychiatry 2001;158(10):1659–65.

[41] Kesslak JP, Nagata SF, Lott I, et al. Magnetic resonance imaging analysis of age-related changes in the brains of individuals with Down's syndrome. Neurology 1994;44(6):1039–45.

[42] Raz N, Torres IJ, Briggs SD, et al. Selective neuroanatomic abnormalities in Down's syndrome and their cognitive correlates: evidence from MRI morphometry. Neurology 1995;45(2):356–66.

[43] Ieshima A, Kisa T, Yoshino K, et al. A morphometric CT study of Down's syndrome showing small posterior fossa and calcification of basal ganglia. Neuroradiology 1984;26(6):493–8.

[44] Wisniewski KE, Laure-Kamionowska M, Wisniewski HM. Evidence of arrest of neurogenesis and synaptogenesis in brains of patients with Down's syndrome. N Engl J Med 1984;311(18):1187–8.

[45] Wisniewski KE, Schmidt-Sidor B. Postnatal delay of myelin formation in brains from Down syndrome infants and children. Clin Neuropathol 1989;8(2):55–62.

[46] Nadel L. Down's syndrome: a genetic disorder in biobehavioral perspective. Genes Brain Behav 2003;2(3):156–66.

[47] Ohr PS, Fagen JW. Conditioning and long-term memory in three-month-old infants with Down syndrome. Am J Ment Retard 1991;96(2):151–62.

[48] Ohr PS, Fagen JW. Contingency learning in 9-month-old infants with Down syndrome. Am J Ment Retard 1994;99(1):74–84.

[49] Dambska M, Laure-Kamionowska M. Myelination as a parameter of normal and retarded brain maturation. Brain Dev 1990;12(2):214–20.

[50] Pinter JD, Brown WE, Eliez S, et al. Amygdala and hippocampal volumes in children with Down syndrome: a high-resolution MRI study. Neurology 2001;56(7):972–4.

[51] Aylward EH, Habbak R, Warren AC, et al. Cerebellar volume in adults with Down syndrome. Arch Neurol 1997;54(2):209–12.

[52] Koop M, Rilling G, Herrmann A, et al. Volumetric development of the fetal telencephalon, cerebral cortex, diencephalon, and rhombencephalon, including the cerebellum in man. Bibl Anat 1986;(28):53–78.

[53] Shapiro BL. Developmental instability of the cerebellum and its relevance to Down syndrome. J Neural Transm Suppl 2001;(61):11–34.

[54] Teipel SJ, Schapiro MB, Alexander GE, et al. Relation of corpus callosum and hippocampal size to age in nondemented adults with Down's syndrome. Am J Psychiatry 2003; 160(10):1870–8.

[55] Lai F, Williams RS. A prospective study of Alzheimer disease in Down syndrome. Arch Neurol 1989;46(8):849–53.

[56] Mann DM, Esiri MM. The pattern of acquisition of plaques and tangles in the brains of patients under 50 years of age with Down's syndrome. J Neurol Sci 1989;89(2–3): 169–79.

[57] Patterson D, Gardiner K, Kao FT, et al. Mapping of the gene encoding the beta-amyloid precursor protein and its relationship to the Down syndrome region of chromosome 21. Proc Natl Acad Sci USA 1988;85(21):8266–70.

[58] Krasuski JS, Alexander GE, Horwitz B, et al. Relation of medial temporal lobe volumes to age and memory function in nondemented adults with Down's syndrome: implications for the prodromal phase of Alzheimer's disease. Am J Psychiatry 2002;159(1):74–81.

[59] Teipel SJ, Hampel H. Neuroanatomy of Down syndrome in vivo: a model of preclinical Alzheimer's disease. Behav Genet 2006;36(3):405–15.

[60] Wisniewski KE, French JH, Rosen JF, et al. Basal ganglia calcification (BGC) in Down's syndrome (DS): another manifestation of premature aging. Ann N Y Acad Sci 1982;396: 179–89.

[61] Takashima S, Becker LE. Basal ganglia calcification in Down's syndrome. J Neurol Neurosurg Psychiatr 1985;48(1):61–4.

[62] Verkerk AJ, Pieretti M, Sutcliffe JS, et al. Identification of a gene (FMR-1) containing a CGG repeat coincident with a breakpoint cluster region exhibiting length variation in fragile X syndrome. Cell 1991;65(5):905–14.

[63] Mazzocco MM, Kates WR, Baumgardner TL, et al. Autistic behaviors among girls with fragile X syndrome. J Autism Dev Disord 1997;27(4):415–35.

[64] Lachiewicz AM, Gullion CM, Spiridigliozzi GA, et al. Declining IQs of young males with the fragile X syndrome. Am J Ment Retard 1987;92(3):272–8.

[65] Wright-Talamante C, Cheema A, Riddle JE, et al. A controlled study of longitudinal IQ changes in females and males with fragile X syndrome. Am J Med Genet 1996;64(2): 350–5.

[66] Mostofsky SH, Mazzocco MM, Aakalu G, et al. Decreased cerebellar posterior vermis size in fragile X syndrome: correlation with neurocognitive performance. Neurology 1998; 50(1):121–30.

[67] Reiss AL, Lee J, Freund L. Neuroanatomy of fragile X syndrome: the temporal lobe. Neurology 1994;44(7):1317–24.

[68] Jakala P, Hanninen T, Ryynanen M, et al. Fragile-X: neuropsychological test performance, CGG triplet repeat lengths, and hippocampal volumes. J Clin Invest 1997;100(2):331–8.

[69] Giedd JN, Vaituzis AC, Hamburger SD, et al. Quantitative MRI of the temporal lobe, amygdala, and hippocampus in normal human development: ages 4–18 years. J Comp Neurol 1996;366(2):223–30.

[70] Eliez S, Blasey CM, Freund LS, et al. Brain anatomy, gender and IQ in children and adolescents with fragile X syndrome. Brain 2001;124(Pt 8):1610–8.

[71] Giedd JN, Snell JW, Lange N, et al. Quantitative magnetic resonance imaging of human brain development: ages 4–18. Cereb Cortex 1996;6(4):551–60.

[72] Irwin SA, Galvez R, Greenough WT. Dendritic spine structural anomalies in fragile-X mental retardation syndrome. Cereb Cortex 2000;10(10):1038–44.

[73] Wisniewski KE, Segan SM, Miezejeski CM, et al. The Fra(X) syndrome: neurological, electrophysiological, and neuropathological abnormalities. Am J Med Genet 1991;38(2–3): 476–80.

[74] Greenough WT, Klintsova AY, Irwin SA, et al. Synaptic regulation of protein synthesis and the fragile X protein. Proc Natl Acad Sci USA 2001;98(13):7101–6.

[75] Reiss AL, Aylward E, Freund LS, et al. Neuroanatomy of fragile X syndrome: the posterior fossa. Ann Neurol 1991;29(1):26–32.

[76] Courchesne E, Saitoh O, Yeung-Courchesne R, et al. Abnormality of cerebellar vermian lobules VI and VII in patients with infantile autism: identification of hypoplastic and hyperplastic subgroups with MR imaging. AJR Am J Roentgenol 1994;162(1):123–30.

[77] Courchesne E, Karns CM, Davis HR, et al. Unusual brain growth patterns in early life in patients with autistic disorder: an MRI study. Neurology 2001;57(2):245–54.

[78] Sears LL, Vest C, Mohamed S, et al. An MRI study of the basal ganglia in autism. Prog Neuropsychopharmacol Biol Psychiatry 1999;23(4):613–24.

[79] Fu YH, Kuhl DP, Pizzuti A, et al. Variation of the CGG repeat at the fragile X site results in genetic instability: resolution of the Sherman paradox. Cell 1991;67(6):1047–58.

[80] Rousseau F, Rouillard P, Morel ML, et al. Prevalence of carriers of premutation-size alleles of the FMRI gene and implications for the population genetics of the fragile X syndrome. Am J Hum Genet 1995;57(5):1006–18.

[81] Conway GS, Payne NN, Webb J, et al. Fragile X premutation screening in women with premature ovarian failure. Hum Reprod 1998;13(5):1184–7.

[82] Hagerman RJ, Leehey M, Heinrichs W, et al. Intention tremor, parkinsonism, and generalized brain atrophy in male carriers of fragile X. Neurology 2001;57(1):127–30.

[83] Loesch DZ, Litewka L, Brotchie P, et al. Magnetic resonance imaging study in older fragile X premutation male carriers. Ann Neurol 2005;58(2):326–30.

[84] Greco CM, Berman RF, Martin RM, et al. Neuropathology of fragile X-associated tremor/ ataxia syndrome (FXTAS). Brain 2006;129(Pt 1):243–55.

[85] Cohen S, Masyn K, Adams J, et al. Molecular and imaging correlates of the fragile X-associated tremor/ataxia syndrome. Neurology 2006;67(8):1426–31.

[86] Tezenas Du Montcel S, Mendizabai H, Ayme S, et al. Prevalence of 22q11 microdeletion. J Med Genet 1996;33(8):719.

[87] Shprintzen RJ, Goldberg RB, Lewin ML, et al. A new syndrome involving cleft palate, cardiac anomalies, typical facies, and learning disabilities: velo-cardio-facial syndrome. Cleft Palate J 1978;15(1):56–62.

[88] Gothelf D, Presburger G, Levy D, et al. Genetic, developmental, and physical factors associated with attention deficit hyperactivity disorder in patients with velocardiofacial syndrome. Am J Med Genet B Neuropsychiatr Genet 2004;126(1):116–21.

[89] Swillen A, Devriendt K, Legius E, et al. Intelligence and psychosocial adjustment in velocardiofacial syndrome: a study of 37 children and adolescents with VCFS. J Med Genet 1997;34(6):453–8.

[90] Swillen A, Devriendt K, Legius E, et al. The behavioural phenotype in velo-cardio-facial syndrome (VCFS): from infancy to adolescence. Genet Couns 1999;10(1):79–88.

[91] Feinstein C, Eliez S, Blasey C, et al. Psychiatric disorders and behavioral problems in children with velocardiofacial syndrome: usefulness as phenotypic indicators of schizophrenia risk. Biol Psychiatry 2002;51(4):312–8.

[92] Baker KD, Skuse DH. Adolescents and young adults with 22q11 deletion syndrome: psychopathology in an at-risk group. Br J Psychiatry 2005;186:115–20.

[93] Chow EW, Mikulis DJ, Zipursky RB, et al. Qualitative MRI findings in adults with 22q11 deletion syndrome and schizophrenia. Biol Psychiatry 1999;46(10):1436–42.

[94] Mitnick RJ, Bello JA, Shprintzen RJ. Brain anomalies in velo-cardio-facial syndrome. Am J Med Genet 1994;54(2):100–6.

[95] van Amelsvoort T, Daly E, Robertson D, et al. Structural brain abnormalities associated with deletion at chromosome 22q11: quantitative neuroimaging study of adults with velo-cardio-facial syndrome. Br J Psychiatry 2001;178:412–9.

[96] Shashi V, Muddasani S, Santos CC, et al. Abnormalities of the corpus callosum in nonpsychotic children with chromosome 22q11 deletion syndrome. Neuroimage 2004;21(4): 1399–406.

[97] Scambler PJ. The 22q11 deletion syndromes. Hum Mol Genet 2000;9(16):2421–6.

[98] Robin NH, Taylor CJ, McDonald-McGinn DM, et al. Polymicrogyria and deletion 22q11.2 syndrome: window to the etiology of a common cortical malformation. Am J Med Genet A 2006;140(22):2416–25.

[99] Barkovich AJ, Rowley H, Bollen A. Correlation of prenatal events with the development of polymicrogyria. AJNR Am J Neuroradiol 1995;16(4 Suppl):822–7.

[100] Eliez S, Schmitt JE, White CD, et al. Children and adolescents with velocardiofacial syndrome: a volumetric MRI study. Am J Psychiatry 2000;157(3):409–15.

[101] Eliez S, Antonarakis SE, Morris MA, et al. Parental origin of the deletion 22q11.2 and brain development in velocardiofacial syndrome: a preliminary study. Arch Gen Psychiatry 2001; 58(1):64–8.

[102] Kates WR, Burnette CP, Jabs EW, et al. Regional cortical white matter reductions in velocardiofacial syndrome: a volumetric MRI analysis. Biol Psychiatry 2001;49(8):677–84.

[103] Kates WR, Burnette CP, Bessette BA, et al. Frontal and caudate alterations in velocardiofacial syndrome (deletion at chromosome 22q11.2). J Child Neurol 2004;19(5):337–42.

[104] Simon TJ, Ding L, Bish JP, et al. Volumetric, connective, and morphologic changes in the brains of children with chromosome 22q11.2 deletion syndrome: an integrative study. Neuroimage 2005;25(1):169–80.

[105] Reiss AL, Faruque F, Naidu S, et al. Neuroanatomy of Rett syndrome: a volumetric imaging study. Ann Neurol 1993;34(2):227–34.

[106] Reiss AL, Eliez S, Schmitt JE, et al. Neuroanatomy of Williams syndrome: a high-resolution MRI study. J Cogn Neurosci 2000;12(Suppl 1):65–73.

[107] Simon TJ, Bish JP, Bearden CE, et al. A multilevel analysis of cognitive dysfunction and psychopathology associated with chromosome 22q11.2 deletion syndrome in children. Dev Psychopathol 2005;17(3):753–84.

[108] Eliez S, Blasey CM, Menon V, et al. Functional brain imaging study of mathematical reasoning abilities in velocardiofacial syndrome (del22q11.2). Genet Med 2001;3(1): 49–55.

[109] Shallice T, Fletcher P, Frith CD, et al. Brain regions associated with acquisition and retrieval of verbal episodic memory. Nature 1994;368(6472):633–5.

[110] Eliez S, Blasey CM, Schmitt EJ, et al. Velocardiofacial syndrome: are structural changes in the temporal and mesial temporal regions related to schizophrenia? Am J Psychiatry 2001; 158(3):447–53.

[111] Kates WR, Miller AM, Abdulsabur N, et al. Temporal lobe anatomy and psychiatric symptoms in velocardiofacial syndrome (22q11.2 deletion syndrome). J Am Acad Child Adolesc Psychiatry 2006;45(5):587–95.

[112] Debbane M, Schaer M, Farhoumand R, et al. Hippocampal volume reduction in 22q11.2 deletion syndrome. Neuropsychologia 2006;44(12):2360–5.
[113] Schaer M, Schmitt JE, Glaser B, et al. Abnormal patterns of cortical gyrification in velo-cardio-facial syndrome (deletion 22q11.2): an MRI study. Psychiatry Res 2006;146(1):1–11.
[114] Van Essen DC. A tension-based theory of morphogenesis and compact wiring in the central nervous system. Nature 1997;385(6614):313–8.
[115] Barnea-Goraly N, Eliez S, Menon V, et al. Arithmetic ability and parietal alterations: a diffusion tensor imaging study in velocardiofacial syndrome. Brain Res Cogn Brain Res 2005; 25(3):735–40.
[116] Eliez S, Schmitt JE, White CD, et al. A quantitative MRI study of posterior fossa development in velocardiofacial syndrome. Biol Psychiatry 2001;49(6):540–6.
[117] Bish JP, Pendyal A, Ding L, et al. Specific cerebellar reductions in children with chromosome 22q11.2 deletion syndrome. Neurosci Lett 2006;399(3):245–8.
[118] Cohen IL, Fisch GS, Sudhalter V, et al. Social gaze, social avoidance, and repetitive behavior in fragile X males: a controlled study. Am J Ment Retard 1988;92(5):436–46.
[119] Golding-Kushner KJ, Weller G, Shprintzen RJ. Velo-cardio-facial syndrome: language and psychological profiles. J Craniofac Genet Dev Biol 1985;5(3):259–66.
[120] Schmitt JE, Eliez S, Warsofsky IS, et al. Enlarged cerebellar vermis in Williams syndrome. J Psychiatr Res 2001;35(4):225–9.
[121] Campbell LE, Daly E, Toal F, et al. Brain and behaviour in children with 22q11.2 deletion syndrome: a volumetric and voxel-based morphometry MRI study. Brain 2006;129(Pt 5): 1218–28.
[122] Chow EW, Zipursky RB, Mikulis DJ, et al. Structural brain abnormalities in patients with schizophrenia and 22q11 deletion syndrome. Biol Psychiatry 2002;51(3):208–15.
[123] Shenton ME, Dickey CC, Frumin M, et al. A review of MRI findings in schizophrenia. Schizophr Res 2001;49(1–2):1–52.
[124] van Amelsvoort T, Daly E, Henry J, et al. Brain anatomy in adults with velocardiofacial syndrome with and without schizophrenia: preliminary results of a structural magnetic resonance imaging study. Arch Gen Psychiatry 2004;61(11):1085–96.
[125] Gothelf D, Eliez S, Thompson T, et al. COMT genotype predicts longitudinal cognitive decline and psychosis in 22q11.2 deletion syndrome. Nat Neurosci 2005;8(11):1500–2.
[126] Mattay VS, Goldberg TE, Fera F, et al. Catechol O-methyltransferase val158-met genotype and individual variation in the brain response to amphetamine. Proc Natl Acad Sci USA 2003;100(10):6186–91.
[127] Weis S, Weber G, Neuhold A, et al. Down syndrome: MR quantification of brain structures and comparison with normal control subjects. AJNR Am J Neuroradiol 1991;12(6):1207–11.
[128] Frangou S, Aylward E, Warren A, et al. Small planum temporale volume in Down's syndrome: a volumetric MRI study. Am J Psychiatry 1997;154(10):1424–9.
[129] Aylward EH, Li Q, Habbak QR, et al. Basal ganglia volume in adults with Down syndrome. Psychiatry Res 1997;74(2):73–82.
[130] Eliez S, Barnea-Goraly N, Schmitt JE, et al. Increased basal ganglia volumes in velo-cardio-facial syndrome (deletion 22q11.2). Biol Psychiatry 2002;52(1):68–70.
[131] Bish JP, Nguyen V, Ding L, et al. Thalamic reductions in children with chromosome 22q11.2 deletion syndrome. Neuroreport 2004;15(9):1413–5.
[132] Antshel KM, Conchelos J, Lanzetta G, et al. Behavior and corpus callosum morphology relationships in velocardiofacial syndrome (22q11.2 deletion syndrome). Psychiatry Res 2005;138(3):235–45.

ELSEVIER
SAUNDERS

Child Adolesc Psychiatric Clin N Am
16 (2007) 581–597

CHILD AND
ADOLESCENT
PSYCHIATRIC CLINICS
OF NORTH AMERICA

Imaging Genetics for Neuropsychiatric Disorders

Andreas Meyer-Lindenberg, MD, PhD, MSc[a,b,c,*],
Caroline F. Zink, PhD[a,c]

[a]Unit for Systems Neuroscience in Psychiatry, 9000 Rockville Pike,
Building 10/Room 3C101, Bethesda, MD 20892, USA
[b]Neuroimaging Core Facility, 9000 Rockville Pike, Building 10/Room 3C101,
Bethesda, MD 20892, USA
[c]Clinical Brain Disorders Branch; Genes, Cognition and Psychosis Program,
National Institute of Mental Health, NIH, DHHS, 10-3C103,
9000 Rockville Pike, Bethesda, MD 20892-1365, USA

The biological complexity of psychiatric genetics is daunting. It is true that for many important illnesses in this area, such as autism, schizophrenia, and anxiety disorders, the heritability is considerable. Unfortunately, however, that does not imply that the genes associated with these disorders are easy to find or characterize. It is clear that psychiatric illnesses are genetically complex in the sense that they are not caused by single genetic mutations of large effect [1]. Instead, multiple genetic variants come together, likely in interaction with each other and with the environment to increase or decrease an individual's susceptibility for these disorders, which may then lead to illness if the relationship of genetic predisposition and environmental and individual stressors is unfavorable. It is still debated how many genes contribute to each of these disorders [2].

Some researchers in psychiatric genetics believe that a handful of common genetic variants, each by itself increasing risk by only a small amount, is the most likely model (the so-called "common disease–common variant hypothesis") [3], whereas others believe that much larger numbers of diverse mutations of higher risk will be found [4]. Either way, identification of genes in this setting by classical linkage approaches is not easy. Such a difficulty in psychiatric genetics is shared with many other common and complex disorders (eg, hypertension and diabetes). A second level of complexity is unique to neuropsychiatry, however [5]: genetic variants that result in molecular

This work was supported by the NIMH/IRP.
* Corresponding author.
E-mail address: andreasm@mail.nih.gov (A. Meyer-Lindenberg).

1056-4993/07/$ - see front matter. Published by Elsevier Inc.
doi:10.1016/j.chc.2007.02.005

changes whose functional impact can only be understood if considered in terms of the effect on arguably the most complex entity known, the human brain. Understanding this process is made even more difficult by the fact that our knowledge about the underlying neurobiology of most of the clinical symptoms is sparse. For example, there is, as yet, no consensus on what underlies delusions or social dysfunction.

One approach that has proven useful in this difficult-to-negotiate terrain is imaging genetics [5]. The power of neuroimaging to characterize various aspects of brain structure and function in vivo is combined with genetic data to link interindividual variation in imaging parameters to genetic variants that these individuals carry. If the genetic variants under study have been associated with neuropsychiatric, behavioral, or cognitive phenotypes, then the identification of neural systems linked to these variants implicates these systems in mediating genetic risk for the disorders to which the genetic variants have been linked. This imaging genetics approach benefits from the fact that genes are likely to have a bigger effect on the level of biologic processing than on emergent mental or social and behavioral phenomena. In other words, the penetrance is likely to be higher on the neural systems level. In this way, imaging genetics leverages the genetic information usually obtained in large-scale association studies to discover neural systems important in heritable psychiatric disorders [5].

Imaging genetics is, at least in current usage, not primarily an approach to find genes but rather a method to identify brain mechanisms to which genes are linked—a "reverse genetics" approach. Precisely because the genetic risk architecture of neuropsychiatric disorders is complex and each individual genetic variant is likely to only contribute a minor fraction to disease risk, it becomes possible to study the impact of genetic variations on the brain in samples of healthy humans. Such healthy samples are much easier to acquire than samples of patient populations and are free of various disease-related confounds that are difficult to control.

In this article, we focus on two applications of this methodology of relevance for child and adolescent psychiatry. First, we present work dissecting a unique neuropsychiatric disorder already manifest in early childhood, Williams syndrome (WS). Research in this area shows unambiguously that imaging genetics can define dissociable neural systems underlying complex behavioral and cognitive phenotypes of genetic origin in WS [6]. Second, we move from this work in patients to discuss studies of genetic risk variants for depression and violence in large samples of healthy human participants, which begins to delineate neural circuitry for a mechanism of critical importance in psychiatric genetics, namely gene-by-environment interactions [7].

Williams syndrome: a unique neuropsychiatric disorder

A fascinating condition that provides a solid starting point for imaging genetics is WS, a neurodevelopmental disorder that presents a unique combination of neuropsychiatric symptoms in the context of a known genetic mechanism (Fig. 1). Unequal homologous recombination at flanking repeats during meiosis [8] leads to a hemizygous deletion (see Fig. 1B) of approximately 1.6 megabases (see Fig. 1C), containing approximately 25 genes, on chromosome 7q11.23. The occurrence of WS is infrequent but may not be as rare as once thought, with new prevalence estimates as high as 1:7500 [9].

WS encompasses various somatic abnormalities, especially in the cardiovascular system, but also in the endocrine, orthopaedic, and gastrointestinal systems, and abnormal facial features (see Fig. 1A) [10]. Many of these symptoms are caused by haploinsufficiency for the *elastin* gene (*ELN*), which leads to connective tissue abnormalities and many of the facial features [11]. Neural involvement is indicated by symptoms such as

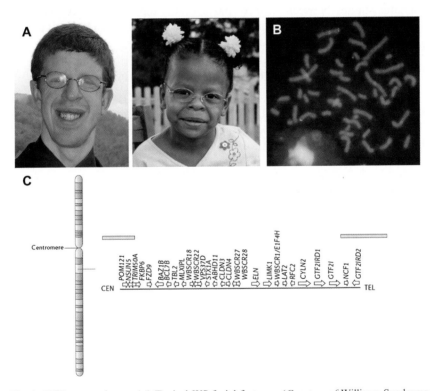

Fig. 1. Williams syndrome. (*A*) Typical WS facial features. (*Courtesy of* Williams Syndrome Association, Clawson, MI; with permission.) (*B*) Chromosomal display during mitosis showing (*in green*) a probe in the WS region present in only one chromosome 7, which indicates its absence on the corresponding chromosome hemideletion. (*Courtesy of* Holly H. Hobart, PhD, Las Vegas, NV.) (*C*) Chromosomal location of the hemideleted region. (*From* Meyer-Lindenberg A, Mervis CB, Berman KF. Neural mechanisms in Williams syndrome: a unique window to genetic influences on cognition and behaviour. Nat Rev Neurosci 2006;7(5):381; with permission.)

hyperreflexia, nystagmus [12], hypersensitivity to sound [10], coordination difficulties, learning difficulties, and mild to moderate mental retardation.

Although many neurodevelopmental disorders impact on multiple somatic and neural systems, a key feature of WS that has attracted considerable attention is its distinctive cognitive profile with a severe visuospatial constructive deficit, combined with relative strengths in verbal short-term memory and language. There is also a pronounced problem with long-term memory. Besides the cognitive symptoms, the second striking neuropsychiatric feature involves high sociability [13,14], social fearlessness, and empathy [14]. Remarkably, this feature goes along with increased anxiety related to nonsocial circumstances, for example phobias. Multimodal neuroimaging allows the delineation of structural and functional alterations in participants with WS compared with normal controls. Although the impact of the condition on IQ usually results in a difference in intelligence and ability to participate in imaging studies between healthy participants and persons with WS, this can be avoided by studying selected subgroups of people with WS and normal intelligence [6].

Structural imaging in Williams syndrome

Structurally, the brain size of people who have WS is reduced [15], particularly in the parietal lobule [16], whereas cerebellar size is preserved [17,18]. These volume changes can be further localized by methods such as voxel-based morphometry, which allows for the mapping of volume changes unconstrained by anatomic landmarks. In our own work, this voxel-based morphometry approach identified circumscribed symmetrical gray matter volume reductions in WS in three regions (Fig. 2A): (1) intraparietal sulcus, (2) around the third ventricle, and (3) orbitofrontal cortex [19]. The intraparietal sulcus finding was recently confirmed in typically functioning children who have WS [20] and was again found together with abnormalities in the superior parietal lobule [16] in typically functioning individuals who have WS [21]. The latter study also had some discrepant findings, especially in the orbitofrontal cortex, but these findings were caused by the specific methodology applied, and the results are convergent if method-related confounds are adequately considered [22]. These regional volume analyses are extended by analyses of cortical shape, which show abnormally increased gyrification in the parietal and occipital lobes [23] and the temporoparietal zone [24], gyral length reductions [25,26], and convergent evidence for reductions in sulcal depth in the intraparietal sulcus in normal IQ participants who have WS [27] and, together with various other symmetric folding abnormalities, in individuals who have mental retardation [28].

Functional neuroimaging in Williams syndrome

Multimodal neuroimaging approaches have been used to identify functional correlates of the aforementioned structural abnormalities in two

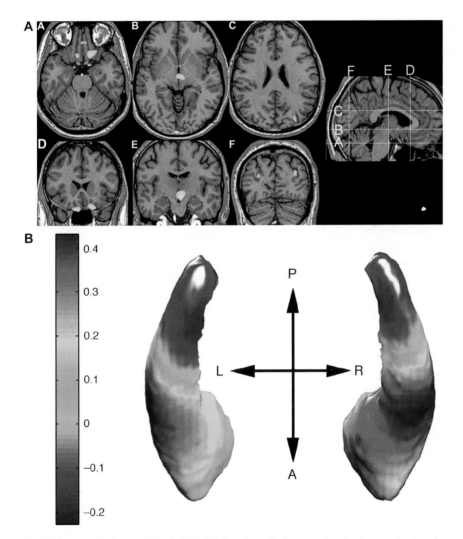

Fig. 2. Structural abnormalities in WS. (*A*) Panel graph shows regional volume reductions in the intraparietal sulcus, hypothalamus, and orbitofrontal cortex of participants with WS compared with normal controls. (*From* Meyer-Lindenberg A, Kohn P, Mervis CB, et al. Neural basis of genetically determined visuospatial construction deficit in Williams syndrome. Neuron 2004;43(5):626; with permission.) (*B*) Map of shape change rendered on an average hippocampal template, posterior view. Negative: relative local volume reduction in WS relative to controls. Positive: relative local volume expansion in WS relative to controls. (*From* Meyer-Lindenberg A, Mervis CB, Sarpal D, et al. Functional, structural, and metabolic abnormalities of the hippocampal formation in Williams syndrome. J Clin Invest 2005;115(7):1889; with permission.)

domains prominently altered in WS: visuoconstruction and social cognition. Disrupted visuospatial construction, "the ability to visualize an object (or picture) as a set of parts and construct a replica of the object from those parts" [29], is a neuropsychological hallmark of WS [30]. Visual processing in human and nonhuman primates is organized into two functionally specialized, hierarchically organized processing pathways—a ventral or "what" stream for object processing and a dorsal or "where" stream for spatial processing [31]. The visuospatial construction disabilities, but relatively good face and object processing skills [32], in WS suggest problems specifically in the dorsal visual processing stream [33–36], with relatively intact ventral stream function (Fig. 3A).

A comprehensive test of the visual processing hierarchy in high-functioning individuals who have WS showed intact ventral stream processing, as measured with functional MRI during passive viewing of pictures, while paying attention to picture identity and during a shape-matching task [19]. In contrast, dorsal stream function was consistently abnormal while participants attended to the spatial locales of the same pictures or performed a two-dimensional puzzle task. Hypofunction was observed immediately adjacent to and anterior to the intraparietal sulcus region in which we had identified decreased gray matter volume and sulcal depth [19,27]. Such results suggested that the structural change may be impeding information flow in the dorsal visual processing stream. We formally tested this hypothesis with path analysis, a method that allows statistical assessment of interactions among regional nodes in a predefined neural system model, which we based on previous path analyses of the visual system. Upon comparison, the only significant difference between the WS group and normal controls was the absence of a path from the structurally abnormal region into lateral (parietal) dorsal stream, which confirmed the hypothesis that this region might be a roadblock that impedes efficient dorsal stream processing in WS.

Functional correlates of the orbitofrontal cortex structural abnormality in WS came into focus in an examination of fear processing related to social cognition. We performed an experiment to study fear-related circuitry [37], with tasks presenting threatening visual stimuli [38] divided into two sets: (1) fearful scenes, which are rarely encountered and socially less relevant, and (2) angry and fearful facial expressions, which are commonly encountered and socially highly relevant. We first focused on amygdala, which is critical for basic emotional—especially fear—processing [39]. The lateral nucleus of the amygdala receives and integrates sensory and prefrontal/limbic inputs and then excites, possibly indirectly, neurons in the central nucleus that evoke fear responses via their projections to brain stem regions, including periaqueductal gray and reticular formation [39]. Amygdala reactivity in WS to threatening socially relevant stimuli was significantly diminished (Fig. 3B) [40], which corresponded to the diminished fear of strangers and consequent social disinhibition [14]. Conversely and again in excellent agreement with the clinical profile of WS, amygdala reactivity abnormally

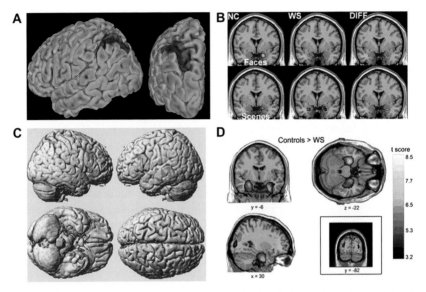

Fig. 3. Functional abnormalities in WS. (*A*) Hypoactivation during various visuospatial tasks (*red, blue, purple*), found directly adjacent to area of structural change in the intraparietal sulcus (*yellow*). (*From* Meyer-Lindenberg A, Kohn P, Mervis CB, et al. Neural basis of genetically determined visuospatial construction deficit in Williams syndrome. Neuron 2004;43(5):627; with permission.) (*B*) Amygdala activation (*P* < .05), corrected for multiple comparisons in amygdala for face (*top row*) and scene (*bottom row*) stimuli, rendered on normal coronal MRI at ± 1 mm to the anterior commissure in neurologic orientation (ie, left+left). First column: normal controls (NC). Second column: participants with WS (WS). Third column: significant differences (DIFF) between groups (blue NC > WS, red WS > NC). (*From* Meyer-Lindenberg A, Hariri AR, Munoz KE, et al. Neural correlates of genetically abnormal social cognition in Williams syndrome. Nat Neurosci 2005;8(8):991; with permission.) (*C*) Regions of significant group difference in cortical reactivity to the faces versus the scenes matching task, rendered in red on standard brain surface. Statistical threshold is *P* < .05, corrected for multiple comparisons. (*From* Meyer-Lindenberg A, Hariri AR, Munoz KE, et al. Neural correlates of genetically abnormal social cognition in Williams syndrome. Nat Neurosci 2005;8(8):992; with permission.) (*D*) Marked reduction of regional cerebral blood flow (measured using positron emission tomography) in the anterior hippocampal formation bilaterally in participants with WS relative to normal controls (*P* < .05), corrected for multiple comparisons. Inset shows reduction in rCBF in the intraparietal/occipitoparietal sulcus in WS (*P* < .001), uncorrected. (*From* Meyer-Lindenberg A, Mervis CB, Sarpal D, et al. Functional, structural, and metabolic abnormalities of the hippocampal formation in Williams syndrome. J Clin Invest 2005;115(7):1890; with permission.)

increased to socially irrelevant stimuli, which offered a potential mechanism for the high rate of nonsocial anxiety in WS [41]. The same study uncovered differences in prefrontal cortical structures regulating the amygdala. Healthy controls differentially activated dorsolateral-prefrontal, medial-prefrontal, and orbitofrontal cortex (OFC), whereas high-functioning participants with WS did not (Fig. 3C). In particular, the OFC did not show any activation versus the control condition in the WS group. Taken together with the structural abnormality in the OFC, this provided convergent evidence for a deficiency of the OFC in the context of social processing. Lesions of OFC are associated with social disinhibition [42]. OFC and OFC-amygdala interactions are critical for stimulus-reinforcement association learning, and in social cognition the role of OFC-amygdala interactions has been hypothesized to link sensory representations of stimuli with the social judgments we make about them on the basis of their motivational value [43]. The disruption of OFC-amygdala circuitry was further substantiated by an analysis of functional interactions between prefrontal cortex and amygdala, which showed that OFC did not interact with amygdala in WS, whereas a significant negative correlation was found in controls. Such a result suggested a primary OFC deficiency that would be predicted to contribute to social disinhibition, reduced reactivity to social cues, and increased tendency to approach strangers, as is typical for individuals who have WS. In contrast, a negative interaction between amygdala and medial prefrontal cortex (perigenual cingulate) was found in healthy controls and subjects who have WS, in whom it was even facilitated by dorsolateral-prefrontal cortex. An important role for this cingulate-amygdala circuit emerged in our further studies that examined genetic variants linked to depression and violence (see later discussion).

We also performed a multimodal study of the hippocampal formation [44], because several cognitive domains that are linked to it are severely affected in WS, including spatial navigation [45,46] and verbal [47] and spatial [48] long-term memory. Structural imaging findings in the hippocampal formation were subtle and restricted to shape changes (Fig. 2B), but functional abnormalities were profound. Baseline blood flow, measured with oxygen-15 water positron emission tomography, was strongly reduced bilaterally in the hippocampal formation, extending into the entorhinal cortex (Fig. 3D). We also used proton magnetic resonance spectroscopy for an in vivo assay of N-acetyl aspartate, a cellular integrity marker and measure of synaptic abundance produced primarily in neurons and related to mitochondrial oxidative phosphorylation [49]. Reduced N-acetyl aspartate (as a ratio to creatine), more pronounced on the left, was found in participants who have WS, which indicated overall depression of hippocampal energy metabolism and synaptic activity in WS. During a functional MRI study of passive viewing of face and house stimuli, no activation was seen in the anterior hippocampal formation in an anatomic locale that corresponds well with the resting positron emission tomography blood-flow reduction, which demonstrated that the hippocampal formation exhibited processing abnormalities under stimulation and changes in resting blood flow and metabolism that might underlie the hippocampal formation–dependent cognitive abnormalities in WS.

Regulatory limbic interactions in depression and gene-by-environment interactions

Multimodal neuroimaging delineated dissociable systems impacted by genetic haploinsufficiency in WS that provided neural mechanisms for the complex neuropsychiatric phenotype in this syndrome. Although in WS the genetic "lesion" is well known and characterized, the phenotype associated with most genetic risk variants in psychiatry is usually only obvious in group comparisons and not on the level of individual subjects. The precise functional impact of variants on gene function is often difficult to quantify, especially for noncoding polymorphisms. Considerable advances have been made in identifying those variants, and imaging genetics has been helpful in defining the associated neural mechanisms. We focus on the aforementioned cingulate-amygdala circuit, which is involved in amygdala regulation, emotional control, and social behavior, because it has emerged as a potential mechanism underlying one of the most important phenomena in psychiatric genetics: gene-by-environment interactions [7].

Clinical experience and patient self-report often suggest a role for environmental adversity in the precipitation of psychiatric episode (eg, depression). Groundbreaking recent epidemiologic evidence has directly demonstrated gene-by-environment interactions for specific susceptibility gene variants linked to serotonergic neurotransmission, SLC6A4 [50], and a variable number of tandem repeats polymorphism in MAO-A (Fig. 4) [51,52]. Because both of these genes impact on the serotonin system, it seems reasonable to expect that studies of neural systems especially responsive to serotonin could be associated with gene-by-environment interactions. In humans, the subgenual cingulate (BA25) displays the highest density of 5-HTT terminals within the human cortex [53] and is impacted by serotonin reuptake inhibitor antidepressants [54]. Even transient alterations in 5-HT homeostasis during early development modify neural connections implicated in mood disorders and cause permanent elevations in anxiety-related behaviors during adulthood [55].

The serotonergic system has been implicated in impulsivity and violent behavior in animals and humans [56]. The subgenual cingulate [57–59] receives strong afferent input from the amygdala and is reciprocally connected to more dorsal parts of the cingulate, which project back to amygdala [60]. Importantly, convergent evidence strongly suggests that amygdala-cingulate interactions represent a functional feedback circuitry regulating amygdala processing of environmental adversity; stimulation of perilimbic prefrontal cortex inhibits amygdala [61], and lesions of this region markedly impair fear extinction [62]. Extinction is the active process by which previously acquired responses to a conditional stimulus are lost if this stimulus is no longer followed by the unconditional stimulus. Because such responses are likely to have arisen through adverse environmental circumstances (eg, a fear response to caregivers after experiencing abuse), neural mechanisms that determine the persistence—or otherwise—of conditioned fear are intriguing candidate mechanisms for gene-by-environment interactions. Specifically, given the hypothesis that the amygdala-cingulate circuit is essential for extinction, serotonergic genetic risk variants acting on this circuit may exhibit gene-by-environment interactions because of abnormal interactions in this regulatory circuitry, impairing the capacity to process

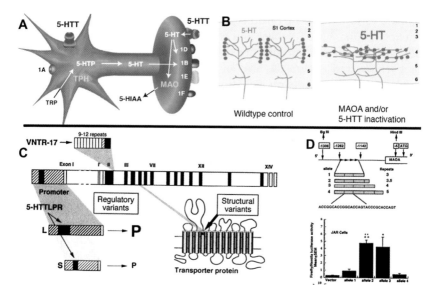

Fig. 4. Serotonergic neurotransmission and associated genetic variants. (*A*) Schematic drawing of serotonergic neuron shows termination of serotonin (5-HT) action by the serotonin transporter (5-HTT) and catabolism by MAO to 5-HIAA and synthesis through tryptophane (TRP) and 5-hyroxytryptophane (5-HTP). Presynaptic serotonin receptors (1A,B,D,E,F) also shown. (*B*) Schematic drawing of neurodevelopmental effects of increased serotonin level caused by inactivation of MAO-A or 5-HTT. (*A, B Adapted from* slide courtesy of K.P. Lesch, MD, Würzburg, Germany.) (*C*) A common variable number of tandem repeat polymorphism in the promoter of the 5-HTT (5-HTTLPR). (*From* Lesch KP, Mossner R. Genetically driven variation in serotonin uptake: is there a link to affective spectrum, neurodevelopmental, and neurodegenerative disorders? Biol Psychiatry 1998;44(3):181; with permission.) Long (L) and short (S) regulatory variants are distinguished, with relatively reduced transcription and activity of the transporter in the S form. (*D*) A common variable number of tandem repeat polymorphism in the promoter of the X-linked MAO-A gene affects transcription, with an optimum range (MAOA-H) of 3.5 or 4 repeats. (*From* Sabol SZ, Hu S, Hamer D. A functional polymorphism in the monoamine oxidase A gene promoter. Hum Genet 1998;103(3):275, 277; with permission.)

contingent negative emotion associations that are bound to arise in the setting of environmental adversity.

The serotonin transporter gene (*SLC6A4*) (see Fig. 4A, C) contains several functional variants, but the one studied most extensively is a variable number of tandem repeats in the 5' promoter region (5-HTTLPR), which influences transcriptional activity and subsequent availability of the 5-HTT [63], with reduced transcription of the 5-HTTLPR short (S) allele in comparison to the long (L) allele. Lower availability of the 5-HTT is predicted to lead to higher levels of synaptic serotonin. Individuals who carry the S allele tend to have increased anxiety-related temperamental traits [63], which are inconsistently related to risk for depression [64]. This is one of the serotonergic variants in which interaction with environmental adversity has been demonstrated [50], whereas main effects of genetic variation were small. In contrast to the results of traditional clinical association, which are largely inconsistent and weak, imaging-based phenotyping has provided strong evidence of a mechanism by which variation in *SLC6A4* could increase biologic risk for anxiety and depression.

The amygdala has been implicated as a centerpiece of this genetic effect because several functional MRI studies have found that S allele carriers evince an exaggerated amygdala response compared with L homozygote individuals [65–67]. These findings suggest that amygdala hyperreactivity might be a neural substrate of trait anxiety predisposing to psychiatric disease. Recent research has made progress toward characterizing the neural circuit contributing to this finding. Using voxel-based morphometry, a reduction in gray matter was found in the sub- and perigenual cingulate regions of healthy carriers of the S allele compared with matched LL homozygotes (Fig. 5C) [57,68]. Analyses of functional and structural connectivity confirmed close interactions of this cingulate region with amygdala and suggested a feedback circuit that inhibits amygdala function and may be involved in fear extinction (Fig. 5D) [57]. The S allele was associated with reduced coupling between amygdala and the subgenual cingulate, and the degree of that coupling predicted close to 30% in the variability of trait anxiety in these normal individuals [57]. Taken together, these results suggested that psychiatric risk associated with 5-HTTLPR is mediated by a weakened circuit for extinction of fear, which offers an attractive potential ("endo") mechanism causally related to amygdala hyperreactivity that, at the same time, provides a neural substrate for the impact of early adversity, which would likely produce the kind of fearful associations that require a functional extinction mechanism to mollify (Fig. 5E). A recent paper by Canli and coworkers [69] directly confirmed for the first time that environmental adversity, stratified by SLC6A4 genotype, impacts on amygdala activation and connectivity. Of interest, another study [67] found increased coupling between more anterior medial prefrontal areas (BA10) and amygdala in S allele carriers, possibly indicating interactions with a brain area implicated in high-order goal maintenance and regulation of the internal milieu [70] that might counteract deficiencies in cingulate-amygdala circuitry. Recent analyses from our laboratory suggested that BA10 may impact on amygdala indirectly though a functional effect on cingulate, a two-layered mechanism that would suggest several levels of hierarchy in amygdala regulation [71].

Convergent evidence for the importance of serotonergic neurotransmission for the amygdala-cingulate circuit comes from studies showing an impact of other functional genetic variants in serotonergic metabolism on amygdala activation and regulation. Two studies have shown that a frequent regulatory variant (G(-844)T) of tyrosine hydroxylase 2 biases the reactivity of the amygdala [72,73]. We recently investigated genetic variation in *MAO-A*, encoding monoamine oxidase A, a key enzyme for the catabolism

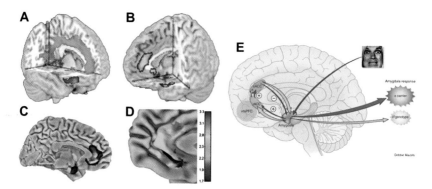

Fig. 5. Neural mechanisms linked to genetic variation in serotonergic risk genes. Structural (using voxel-based morphometry) (*A*) and functional (*Adapted from* Meyer-Lindenberg A, Buckholtz JW, Kolachana B, et al. Neural mechanisms of genetic risk for impulsivity and violence in humans. Proc Natl Acad Sci U S A 2006;103(16):6270; with permission.) (*B*) results (during an emotional faces matching task) show an impact of genetic variation in MAO on amygdala and cingulate volume and function. (*Data from* Meyer-Lindenberg A, Buckholtz JW, Kolachana B, et al. Neural mechanisms of genetic risk for impulsivity and violence in humans. Proc Natl Acad Sci U S A 2006;103(16):6269–74.) Volume is relatively reduced in carriers of the MAOA-L allele implicated in risk for impulsive violence. Amygdala activation is increased, whereas activation of regulatory cingulate regions is decreased. Structural (*C*) and functional (*From* Pezawas L, Meyer-Lindenberg A, Drabant EM, et al. 5-HTTLPR polymorphism impacts human cingulate-amygdala interactions: a genetic susceptibility mechanism for depression. Nat Neurosci 2005;8(6):829; with permission.) (*D*) connectivity (during a faces matching task) are also affected by genetic variation in 5-HTTLPR (*From* Pezawas L, Meyer-Lindenberg A, Drabant EM, et al. 5-HTTLPR polymorphism impacts human cingulate-amygdala interactions: a genetic susceptibility mechanism for depression. Nat Neurosci 2005;8(6):830; with permission.) Carriers of the S allele show relative volume reductions in subgenual cingulate and amygdala and reduced connectivity of amygdala to subgenual cingulate. (*E*) Model drawing of a core circuit for amygdala regulation and fear extinction linking amygdala and cingulate and impacted by serotonergic risk genes. (*Adapted from* Hamann S. Blue genes: wiring the brain for depression. Nat Neurosci 2005;8(6):702; with permission.) Reduced connectivity (5-HTTLPR) or cingulate activation (MAO-A) predict amygdala hyperactivation by reduced feedback inhibition as an endomechanism underlying anxiety and impulsivity associations of these genes. An anterior medial prefrontal area might modulate this effect.

of serotonin and other neurotransmitters during neurodevelopment [74]. The human *MAO-A* gene contains a common variable number of tandem repeats polymorphism that again affects transcriptional efficiency; enzyme expression is relatively high for carriers of 3.5 or 4 repeats (MAOA-H) and lower for carriers of 2, 3, or 5 repeats (*MAOA-L*) (see Fig. 4D) [75]. Although inconsistent evidence exists for the association of genotype with trait impulsivity in human cross-sectional studies [76], a clear and pronounced gene by environment interaction was found in a large longitudinal study of children followed for 25 years in which *MAOA-L* (which is associated with higher levels of synaptic serotonin during neurodevelopment) predicted violent offenses in male subjects with adverse early experience (maltreatment) [51]. Similar to those in 5-HTTLPR, our multimodal imaging results indicated an impact on structure and function of amygdala and perigenual cingulate cortex, which suggested a shared mechanism of emotional regulation under serotonergic control and predicted some overlap in clinical association in risk for depression, as has been observed [74,77]. *MAO-A* showed more extensive effects in structure (Fig. 5A) and activation (Fig. 5B), however, notably affecting more caudal regions of the cingulate associated with cognitive control and orbitofrontal cortex. This may reflect the broader metabolic effect of variation in *MAO-A*, which catabolizes not only serotonin but also other neurotransmitters, notably norepinephrine [56], which is also implicated in limbic system development and emotional experience.

Several additional conclusions emerge from this overview of neural mechanisms related to serotonergic genetic variation. First, it was consistently the variants associated with higher serotonin levels (5-HTTLPR S and MAOA-L) that predicted relatively impaired structure and function. Preclinical data that showed enduring neurodevelopmental abnormalities after transient alterations of serotonin (see Fig. 4B) [55] implicate serotonin signaling in human limbic emotional circuitry development and caution against possible adverse consequences of prenatally increased serotonin levels. That the observed genetic data are likely due to a neurodevelopmental effect and not an acute increase in serotonin during adult life is clear from clinical evidence, which shows that higher levels of serotonin are associated with reduced depression and aggression in adults [78]. Second, multiple serotonergic variants, although they have been predominantly studied for different neuropsychiatric disorders, seem to converge on overlapping neural mechanisms, identifying shared circuitry across conventional diagnostic categories that have implications not only for our understanding of these disorders but also to a more biologically based taxonomy. Finally, one key assumption of the intermediate phenotype concept was clearly confirmed in these studies, namely the hope of increased penetrance on the level of biologic intermediates. Although for all of the genes studied, effect sizes for association with psychiatric disease [51,64,79] and personality traits predisposing to it [80,81] are small and often controversial, the imaging literature is remarkably consistent and provides a degree of biologic validation and mechanistic differentiation unattainable on the level of behavioral association.

Summary

In summary, we have given an overview of contributions of imaging genetics to understanding of the neuropsychiatric phenotypes of relevance to child and adolescent psychiatry, taking WS and genetic risk mechanisms for gene-by-environment interactions as illustrative examples. No attempt has been made to be exhaustive. Important applications of imaging genetics to this area of psychiatry are still only beginning, for example, the examination of genetic variation as it impacts brain maturation across childhood and adolescence [82] or the systems-level study of molecular mediators for attachment, such as the prosocial neuropeptides, in which genetic variation in their receptors has been associated with autism [83,84]. As more genetic variants are being identified and validated in the upcoming whole genome screens of large patient samples, it is to be expected—and hoped—that imaging genetics will be able to contribute an important piece in translational characterization of these disorders that can be used to identify new treatment targets and monitor their efficacy.

References

[1] Menzel S. Genetic and molecular analyses of complex metabolic disorders: genetic linkage. Ann N Y Acad Sci 2002;967:249–57.
[2] Wright AF, Hastie ND. Complex genetic diseases: controversy over the Croesus code. Genome Biol 2001;2(8): COMMENT 2007.1–2007.8
[3] Lander ES, Schork NJ. Genetic dissection of complex traits. Science 1994;265(5181):2037–48.
[4] Terwilliger JD, Haghighi F, Hiekkalinna TS, et al. A biased assessment of the use of SNPs in human complex traits. Curr Opin Genet Dev 2002;12(6):726–34.
[5] Meyer-Lindenberg A, Weinberger DR. Intermediate phenotypes and genetic mechanisms of psychiatric disorders. Nat Rev Neurosci 2006;7(10):818–27.
[6] Meyer-Lindenberg A, Mervis CB, Berman KF. Neural mechanisms in Williams syndrome: a unique window to genetic influences on cognition and behaviour. Nat Rev Neurosci 2006;7(5):380–93.
[7] Caspi A, Moffitt TE. Gene-environment interactions in psychiatry: joining forces with neuroscience. Nat Rev Neurosci 2006;7(7):583–90.
[8] Urban Z, Helms C, Fekete G, et al. 7q11.23 deletions in Williams syndrome arise as a consequence of unequal meiotic crossover. Am J Hum Genet 1996;59(4):958–62.
[9] Strømme P, Bjørnstad PG, Ramstad K. Prevalence estimation of Williams syndrome. J Child Neurol 2002;17(4):269–71.
[10] Committee on Genetics, American Academy of Pediatrics. Health care supervision for children with Williams syndrome. Pediatrics 2001;107(5):1192–204.
[11] Morris CA, Mervis CB, Hobart HH, et al. GTF2I hemizygosity implicated in mental retardation in Williams syndrome: genotype-phenotype analysis of five families with deletions in the Williams syndrome region. Am J Med Genet A 2003;123(1):45–59.
[12] Chapman CA, du Plessis A, Pober BR. Neurologic findings in children and adults with Williams syndrome. J Child Neurol 1996;11(1):63–5.
[13] Klein-Tasman BP, Mervis CB. Distinctive personality characteristics of 8-, 9-, and 10-year-olds with Williams syndrome. Dev Neuropsychol 2003;23(1–2):269–90.
[14] Bellugi U, Adolphs R, Cassady C, et al. Towards the neural basis for hypersociability in a genetic syndrome. Neuroreport 1999;10(8):1653–7.
[15] Jernigan TL, Bellugi U. Anomalous brain morphology on magnetic resonance images in Williams syndrome and Down syndrome. Arch Neurol 1990;47(5):529–33.
[16] Eckert MA, Hu D, Eliez S, et al. Evidence for superior parietal impairment in Williams syndrome. Neurology 2005;64(1):152–3.
[17] Wang PP, Hesselink JR, Jernigan TL, et al. Specific neurobehavioral profile of Williams' syndrome is associated with neocerebellar hemispheric preservation. Neurology 1992;42(10):1999–2002.
[18] Jones W, Hesselink J, Courchesne E, et al. Cerebellar abnormalities in infants and toddlers with Williams syndrome. Dev Med Child Neurol 2002;44(10):688–94.

[19] Meyer-Lindenberg A, Kohn P, Mervis CB, et al. Neural basis of genetically determined visuospatial construction deficit in Williams syndrome. Neuron 2004;43(5):623–31.

[20] Boddaert N, Mochel F, Meresse I, et al. Parieto-occipital grey matter abnormalities in children with Williams syndrome. Neuroimage 2006;30(3):721–5.

[21] Reiss AL, Eckert MA, Rose FE, et al. An experiment of nature: brain anatomy parallels cognition and behavior in Williams syndrome. J Neurosci 2004;24(21):5009–15.

[22] Eckert MA, Tenforde A, Galaburda AM, et al. To modulate or not to modulate: differing results in uniquely shaped Williams syndrome brains. Neuroimage 2006;32(3):1001–7.

[23] Schmitt JE, Watts K, Eliez S, et al. Increased gyrification in Williams syndrome: evidence using 3D MRI methods. Dev Med Child Neurol 2002;44(5):292–5.

[24] Thompson PM, Lee AD, Dutton RA, et al. Abnormal cortical complexity and thickness profiles mapped in Williams syndrome. J Neurosci 2005;25(16):4146–58.

[25] Jackowski AP, Schultz RT. Foreshortened dorsal extension of the central sulcus in Williams syndrome. Cortex 2005;41(3):282–90.

[26] Galaburda AM, Schmitt JE, Atlas SW, et al. Dorsal forebrain anomaly in Williams syndrome. Arch Neurol 2001;58(11):1865–9.

[27] Kippenhan JS, Olsen RK, Mervis CB, et al. Genetic contributions to human gyrification: sulcal morphometry in Williams syndrome. J Neurosci 2005;25(34):7840–6.

[28] Van Essen DC, Dierker D, Snyder AZ, et al. Symmetry of cortical folding abnormalities in Williams syndrome revealed by surface-based analyses. J Neurosci 2006;26(20):5470–83.

[29] Frangiskakis JM, Ewart AK, Morris CA, et al. LIM-kinase1 hemizygosity implicated in impaired visuospatial constructive cognition. Cell 1996;86(1):59–69.

[30] Mervis CB, Robinson BF, Bertrand J, et al. The Williams syndrome cognitive profile. Brain Cogn 2000;44(3):604–28.

[31] Ungerleider LG, Mishkin M. Two cortical visual systems. In: Ingle DJ, Goodale DJ, Mansfield RJW, editors. Analysis of visual behavior. Cambridge (MA): The MIT Press; 1982. p. 549–86.

[32] Landau B, Hoffman JE, Kurz N. Object recognition with severe spatial deficits in Williams syndrome: sparing and breakdown. Cognition 2006;100(3):483–510.

[33] Atkinson J, Braddick O, Anker S, et al. Neurobiological models of visuospatial cognition in children with Williams syndrome: measures of dorsal-stream and frontal function. Dev Neuropsychol 2003;23(1–2):139–72.

[34] Galaburda AM, Holinger DP, Bellugi U, et al. Williams syndrome: neuronal size and neuronal-packing density in primary visual cortex. Arch Neurol 2002;59(9):1461–7.

[35] Nakamura M, Watanabe K, Matsumoto A, et al. Williams syndrome and deficiency in visuospatial recognition. Dev Med Child Neurol 2001;43(9):617–21.

[36] Paul BM, Stiles J, Passarotti A, et al. Face and place processing in Williams syndrome: evidence for a dorsal-ventral dissociation. Neuroreport 2002;13(9):1115–9.

[37] LeDoux J. The emotional brain, fear, and the amygdala. Cell Mol Neurobiol 2003;23(4–5): 727–38.

[38] Hariri AR, Tessitore A, Mattay VS, et al. The amygdala response to emotional stimuli: a comparison of faces and scenes. Neuroimage 2002;17(1):317–23.

[39] LeDoux JE. Emotion circuits in the brain. Annu Rev Neurosci 2000;23:155–84.

[40] Meyer-Lindenberg A, Hariri AR, Munoz KE, et al. Neural correlates of genetically abnormal social cognition in Williams syndrome. Nat Neurosci 2006;8(8):991–3.

[41] Dykens EM. Anxiety, fears, and phobias in persons with Williams syndrome. Dev Neuropsychol 2003;23(1–2):291–316.

[42] Rolls ET, Hornak J, Wade D, et al. Emotion-related learning in patients with social and emotional changes associated with frontal lobe damage. J Neurol Neurosurg Psychiatry 1994; 57(12):1518–24.

[43] Adolphs R. Cognitive neuroscience of human social behaviour. Nat Rev Neurosci 2003;4(3): 165–78.

[44] Meyer-Lindenberg A, Mervis CB, Sarpal D, et al. Functional, structural, and metabolic abnormalities of the hippocampal formation in Williams syndrome. J Clin Invest 2005;115(7): 1888–95.

[45] Nardini M, Breckenridge KE, Eastwood RL, et al. Distinct developmental trajectories in three systems for spatial encoding between the ages of 3 and 6 years. Perception 2004;S33:28.

[46] O'Hearn K, Landau B, Hoffman JE. Multiple object tracking in people with Williams syndrome and in normally developing children. Psychol Sci 2005;16(11):905–12.

[47] Nichols S, Jones W, Roman MJ, et al. Mechanisms of verbal memory impairment in four neurodevelopmental disorders. Brain Lang 2004;88(2):180–9.

[48] Vicari S, Bellucci S, Carlesimo GA. Visual and spatial long-term memory: differential pattern of impairments in Williams and Down syndromes. Dev Med Child Neurol 2005; 47(5):305–11.

[49] Pan JW, Takahashi K. Interdependence of N-acetyl aspartate and high-energy phosphates in healthy human brain. Ann Neurol 2005;57(1):92–7.

[50] Caspi A, Sugden K, Moffitt TE, et al. Influence of life stress on depression: moderation by a polymorphism in the 5-HTT gene. Science 2003;301(5631):386–9.

[51] Caspi A, McClay J, Moffitt TE, et al. Role of genotype in the cycle of violence in maltreated children. Science 2002;297(5582):851–4.

[52] Lesch KP, Mossner R. Genetically driven variation in serotonin uptake: is there a link to affective spectrum, neurodevelopmental, and neurodegenerative disorders? Biol Psychiatry 1998;44(3):179–92.

[53] Varnas K, Halldin C, Hall H. Autoradiographic distribution of serotonin transporters and receptor subtypes in human brain. Hum Brain Mapp 2004;22(3):246–60.

[54] Mayberg HS, Brannan SK, Tekell JL, et al. Regional metabolic effects of fluoxetine in major depression: serial changes and relationship to clinical response. Biol Psychiatry 2000;48(8): 830–43.

[55] Ansorge MS, Zhou M, Lira A, et al. Early-life blockade of the 5-HT transporter alters emotional behavior in adult mice. Science 2004;306(5697):879–81.

[56] Shih JC, Chen K, Ridd MJ. Monoamine oxidase: from genes to behavior. Annu Rev Neurosci 1999;22:197–217.

[57] Pezawas L, Meyer-Lindenberg A, Drabant EM, et al. 5-HTTLPR polymorphism impacts human cingulate-amygdala interactions: a genetic susceptibility mechanism for depression. Nat Neurosci 2005;8(6):828–34.

[58] Drevets WC, Price JL, Simpson JR Jr, et al. Subgenual prefrontal cortex abnormalities in mood disorders. Nature 1997;386(6627):824–7.

[59] Mayberg HS, Liotti M, Brannan SK, et al. Reciprocal limbic-cortical function and negative mood: converging PET findings in depression and normal sadness. Am J Psychiatry 1999; 156(5):675–82.

[60] Paus T. Primate anterior cingulate cortex: where motor control, drive and cognition interface. Nat Rev Neurosci 2001;2(6):417–24.

[61] Stefanacci L, Amaral DG. Some observations on cortical inputs to the macaque monkey amygdala: an anterograde tracing study. J Comp Neurol 2002;451(4):301–23.

[62] Sotres-Bayon F, Bush DE, LeDoux JE. Emotional perseveration: an update on prefrontal-amygdala interactions in fear extinction. Learn Mem 2004;11(5):525–35.

[63] Lesch KP, Bengel D, Heils A, et al. Association of anxiety-related traits with a polymorphism in the serotonin transporter gene regulatory region. Science 1996;274(5292):1527–31.

[64] Lotrich FE, Pollock BG. Meta-analysis of serotonin transporter polymorphisms and affective disorders. Psychiatr Genet 2004;14(3):121–9.

[65] Hariri AR, Mattay VS, Tessitore A, et al. Serotonin transporter genetic variation and the response of the human amygdala. Science 2002;297(5580):400–3.

[66] Hariri AR, Drabant EM, Munoz KE, et al. A susceptibility gene for affective disorders and the response of the human amygdala. Arch Gen Psychiatry 2005;62(2):146–52.

[67] Heinz A, Braus DF, Smolka MN, et al. Amygdala-prefrontal coupling depends on a genetic variation of the serotonin transporter. Nat Neurosci 2005;8(1):20–1.

[68] Hamann S. Blue genes: wiring the brain for depression. Nat Neurosci 2005;8(6):701–3.

[69] Canli T, Qiu M, Omura K, et al. Neural correlates of epigenesis. Proc Natl Acad Sci U S A 2006;103(43):16033–8.

[70] Koechlin E, Basso G, Pietrini P, et al. The role of the anterior prefrontal cortex in human cognition. Nature 1999;399(6732):148–51.

[71] Buckholtz J, Callicott JH, Kolachana B, et al. Genetic variation in MAOA modulates ventromedial prefrontal circuitry mediating individual differences in human personality. Mol Psychiatry, in press.

[72] Brown SM, Peet E, Manuck SB, et al. A regulatory variant of the human tryptophan hydroxylase-2 gene biases amygdala reactivity. Mol Psychiatry 2005;10(9):884–8, 805.

[73] Canli T, Congdon E, Gutknecht L, et al. Amygdala responsiveness is modulated by tryptophan hydroxylase-2 gene variation. J Neural Transm 2005;112(11):1479–85.

[74] Meyer-Lindenberg A, Buckholtz JW, Kolachana B, et al. Neural mechanisms of genetic risk for impulsivity and violence in humans. Proc Natl Acad Sci USA 2006;103(16):6269–74.

[75] Sabol SZ, Hu S, Hamer D. A functional polymorphism in the monoamine oxidase A gene promoter. Hum Genet 1998;103(3):273–9.

[76] Huang YY, Cate SP, Battistuzzi C, et al. An association between a functional polymorphism in the monoamine oxidase A gene promoter, impulsive traits and early abuse experiences. Neuropsychopharmacology 2004;29(8):1498–505.

[77] Yu YW, Tsai SJ, Hong CJ, et al. Association study of a monoamine oxidase A gene promoter polymorphism with major depressive disorder and antidepressant response. Neuropsychopharmacology 2005;30(9):1719–23.

[78] Lesch KP, Merschdorf U. Impulsivity, aggression, and serotonin: a molecular psychobiological perspective. Behav Sci Law 2000;18(5):581–604.

[79] Haberstick BC, Lessem JM, Hopfer CJ, et al. Monoamine oxidase A (MAOA) and antisocial behaviors in the presence of childhood and adolescent maltreatment. Am J Med Genet B Neuropsychiatr Genet 2005;135(1):59–64.

[80] Schinka JA, Busch RM, Robichaux-Keene N. A meta-analysis of the association between the serotonin transporter gene polymorphism (5-HTTLPR) and trait anxiety. Mol Psychiatry 2004;9(2):197–202.

[81] Sen S, Burmeister M, Ghosh D. Meta-analysis of the association between a serotonin transporter promoter polymorphism (5-HTTLPR) and anxiety-related personality traits. Am J Med Genet B Neuropsychiatr Genet 2004;127(1):85–9.

[82] Addington AM, Gornick MC, Shaw P, et al. Neuregulin 1 (8p12) and childhood-onset schizophrenia: susceptibility haplotypes for diagnosis and brain developmental trajectories. Mol Psychiatry 2007;12(2):195–205.

[83] Kim SJ, Young LJ, Gonen D, et al. Transmission disequilibrium testing of arginine vasopressin receptor 1A (AVPR1A) polymorphisms in autism. Mol Psychiatry 2002;7(5):503–7.

[84] Wu S, Jia M, Ruan Y, et al. Positive association of the oxytocin receptor gene (OXTR) with autism in the Chinese Han population. Biol Psychiatry 2005;58(1):74–7.

CHILD AND
ADOLESCENT
PSYCHIATRIC CLINICS
OF NORTH AMERICA

Child Adolesc Psychiatric Clin N Am
16 (2007) 599–616

Cognitive Characteristics of Children with Genetic Syndromes

Tony J. Simon, PhD

University of California, Davis, M.I.N.D. Institute, 2825 50th Street,
Sacramento, CA 95817, USA

The symptoms that are associated with genetic syndromes generally form a large and diverse array of physical and behavioral characteristics. Knowledge about the relationship of these features to each disorder's genotype varies greatly. The cognitive and behavioral phenotypes of most genetic disorders typically are characterized less well than are the physical/medical ones and are linked less clearly to genetic causes. Behavioral scientists have tended to focus on global impairments measured in terms of intelligence quotients (or IQ), whereas clinical geneticists have concentrated on describing physical features, medical complications, salient traits, and the degree of retardation associated with specific genetic etiologies [1]. Recently, much progress has been made in the development of highly characterized behavioral, cognitive, and neurocognitive phenotypes for a range of disorders with known genetic causes and in the establishment of genotype/phenotype relationships. This article concentrates on a particular cognitive phenotype observable in children from several populations that have clearly defined genetic disorders.

Such studies are performed using two complementary sets of tools. Neuropsychologic testing studies use a battery of standardized tests to generate a broad profile of the subject's abilities in the intellectual, academic, and behavioral domains. Normative scores are used to compute the participant's "mental age" for each domain. A percentile score also is generated so that the participant's abilities can be compared between individuals (ie, to the normed population) and within the individual to determine domains of particular strength or weaknesses. Standardized testing has strong

This work was supported by Grants R01HD42974 and R01HD46159 from the National Institutes of Health.

E-mail address: tjsimon@ucdavis.edu

doi:10.1016/j.chc.2007.03.002
childpsych.theclinics.com

descriptive power and enables testing over many domains simultaneously; however, it has weak explanatory power because the behavior measured by such tests is complex and difficult to link directly to the cognitive and neurobiologic substrates that generate it. In other words, it reveals little about the mental representations being used, the manner in which they are processed, the brain circuits upon which those computations depend, and the neurotransmitters involved.

Alternatively, researchers using cognitive experimentation studies develop small sets of experiments, usually in the form of computer-based tasks. They are designed to test hypotheses about how specific cognitive functions work and the nature of the representations that they process. Such experiments are being used increasingly in the context of functional neuroimaging studies to explore relationships between brain structure and cognitive function. Hypotheses are evaluated by determining whether the predicted performance patterns were observed. Typically, new, more detailed hypotheses emerge from such analyses, further experiments are designed, and the process progresses toward an ever more highly specified explanatory account. Such cognitive neuroscience studies can investigate how information is processed, which brain circuits and even neurotransmitters are involved, and how these interact. Of course, there also are limitations to this method. The range of behaviors tested is, by design, limited; the samples tend to be small; and typically, no normed population data are present. Therefore, any individual experiment has weak reliability and needs to bereplicated. Also, the training required for this method means that results are not easily interpretable by other professionals; however, the trade-off is that the explanatory power of this method is high.

Essentially, what experimental cognitive studies of genetic disorders attempt to develop is similar to the idea of an endophenotype, although no hereditary component is necessarily implied. This concept is being used to simplify investigations of the biologic basis of psychiatric disorders by decomposing the entirety of their behavioral manifestations into discrete components more amenable to analysis. Gottesman and Gould [2] defined endophenotypes as "measurable components unseen by the unaided eye along the pathway between disease and distal genotype .... [that] may be neurophysiologic, biochemical, endocrinological, neuroanatomic, cognitive, or neuropsychological .... in nature." This article briefly reviews the phenotypic profiles generated for a small set of genetic disorders with the use of standardized neuropsychologic instruments. It then concentrates on the "cognitive endophenotypes," insofar as they have been described, that attempt to specify the possible causes of impairment in terms of specific cognitive functions and the representations they process. The goal of such studies is to develop explanatory accounts of why particular sets of observed impairments co-occur consistently. From that it is hoped that predictions and inferences about areas of function not directly studied will be possible, along with the generation of hypotheses about the nature and potential efficacy of cognitive and behavioral interventions.

Such cognitive endophenotypes enable the identification of underlying dysfunctions that produce "cascaded effects" in higher-level impairments. This means that the demands of specific mental activities, such as counting, call upon a range of foundational or component processes that vary as a function of the demands of the task. In counting a set of physical objects, these include searching for and identifying a countable item, incrementing a counting list, "marking" the item as counted, disengaging from the counted item, searching for the next countable object, and repeating the necessary steps for that item. Some of these same components are required in other tasks, such as using landmarks to find a specific room in a building. When a component process is dysfunctional, it creates different patterns of impairment in the contexts of the tasks in which it is deployed; however, in all cases, it should be possible to partially explain the difficulty in terms of the dysfunction in the component processes themselves. Because these are likely to develop earlier in life than the actual task in which the difficulty is assessed, it is important to take a developmental approach and to focus on candidate processes that contribute to the cognitive endophenotype. Therefore, accounts developed in terms of basic cognitive processes can generate explanations for impaired functions that are distal in the sense of being much higher level in nature or in what might seem to be a different domain of "behavior." An example of the former is the case of visuospatial attentional dysfunction and impairments in the development of numerical competence. An example of the latter is the relationship between executive attentional impairments and psychiatric disorders from attention deficit disorders to obsessive compulsive disorders to schizophrenia.

One important caveat when considering typical and atypical development is the understanding that structure/function mappings (of brain and mind) change as a function of the interaction between experience, maturation, and the nature of the "start state" of the individual [3,4]. Thus, explanations of impairment are not found in the form of "broken" versions of fully developed cognitive systems or modules, as is the case for adult neuropsychologic single-case studies. For example, inferior parietal damage in typical adults, particularly involving the left angular gyrus, classically induces the Gerstmann syndrome, a component of which is the loss of most or all previously acquired mathematical ability [5,6]; however, it would be wrong to assume that all mathematical disability can be explained by left angular gyrus dysfunction alone. Instead, it is necessary to study the cognitive processing profiles of children with developmental disorders, along with structural and functional assessments of brain development, preferably with the use of longitudinal designs.

This article focuses primarily on several syndromes that tend to get grouped together into the category of "nonverbal learning disorders"

(NLDs) because the consistencies in their cognitive impairments suggest the presence of a shared explanatory intermediate phenotype at some neurobiologic level.

Overview of genetic nonverbal learning disorders

Rourke and colleagues [7] defined NLD as having characteristic primary impairments in tactile and visual perception and complex psychomotor skills, secondary impairments in tactile and visual attention, and tertiary impairments in tactile and visual memory, concept formation, problem solving, and hypothesis testing. Associated psychosocial problems, externalizing in early development and internalizing later, are characteristic.

In fragile X syndrome (FXS), "approximately 50% of females with the full mutation have mental retardation [while the] remaining 50% may manifest borderline to normal intellectual functioning, learning disability, and/or psychosocial difficulties [...]. The majority of males with Fragile X syndrome have mental retardation" [8]. Nevertheless, even "among affected females *without* mental retardation, deficits are seen in measures of visual-spatial skills, attention and 'executive function', and math achievement scores are lower than reading achievement scores [...]. In contrast to math skills performance, verbal skills are relatively spared in females with Fragile X, although girls with Fragile X do have lower verbal skills relative to their unaffected sisters" [8]. Characteristic among the greater impairments seen in males with FXS are "deficits in visual–spatial abilities, visual short-term memory, arithmetic, and processing of sequential information" [9].

Females with Turner syndrome (TS) manifest a specific neurocognitive profile in which verbal ability (including verbal IQ) generally is normal [10–13], whereas nonverbal ability (visual–spatial/perceptual, visual–motor), attention, working memory, motor function, and executive function (planning, organizing) are impaired [14,15]. The risk for learning disabilities, particularly in mathematics, in girls with TS is high [16]. It has been argued that their poor math performance is due to increased operation and alignment errors and decreased fact retrieval, perhaps secondary to slower response time and impaired working memory, executive, and visual–spatial abilities [17,18].

An extensive set of investigations into cognitive functioning has been concerned with Williams syndrome (WS) [19–21]. Most individuals with this disorder rank in the mild to moderately retarded range, with full-scale IQ scores ranging from 40 to 90 with a mean of around 55 and no clinically significant difference between verbal and performance intelligence scores [21]. Individuals with WS demonstrate deficits in cognitive domains, such as basic conceptual knowledge, visual–spatial, and attentional abilities, and they "have difficulty in mathematics and its application to everyday life" [21]. In contrast, the cognitive abilities of individuals with WS are relatively spared in the domains of expressive, but not spatial, language, auditory processing, and face processing.

In the chromosome 22q11.2 deletion or velocardiofacial [22] syndrome (VCFS[1]), a subset of impairments is particularly evident in the areas of visuospatial and arithmetical performance [23–27]. Despite their early language delays, children with VCFS still score higher on standardized tests of verbal abilities than those that test visuospatial abilities. To be more specific, "analysis of the IQ test subtest scores suggest relative strengths in the area of rote verbal knowledge and great weaknesses in the areas of visual-perceptual-spatial abilities and nonverbal reasoning" [28].

The visuospatial, visuomotor, and numerical impairments in WS, TS, FXS, and chromosome 22q11.2 deletion syndromes are striking in their degree of overlap [29] and puzzling in that other commonalities are limited. Because of the intimate connection between space and time, one prediction that flows from the above findings is that impairments also should be found in temporal processing. In fact, the two interdependent domains of function often are described with a single label, that of spatiotemporal cognition. This article examines the small, but growing, set of cognitive experimental studies that attempts to identify the neurocognitive basis for these impairments. Because an important focus is on various functions of the human attention system, a review of several of its key concepts follows.

In their seminal work, Posner and Petersen [30] proposed a subdivision of the concept of attention into three components, each served by a distinct neural network, whose functions and computations can be defined in cognitive terms. The three attentional networks were considered to be those necessary for "(a) orienting to sensory events; (b) detecting signals for focal (conscious) processing, and (c) maintaining a vigilant or alert state." Subsequently, Posner and colleagues [31] developed the attentional networks test (ANT) to evaluate what have become known as the orienting, executive, and alerting networks. The orienting system plays a primary role in responding to cued information in the environment or in the volitional search for and selection of salient information. It is associated with a frontoparietal network that seems to be associated strongly with cholinergic neurotransmitters [31,32]. This network primarily comprises the superior parietal lobule, intraparietal sulcus, pre- and postcentral sulci, and frontal eye fields [33]. The executive system supports the task of detecting and prioritizing signals for conscious processing by engaging in error detection, conflict monitoring, and inhibiting distracting or irrelevant information. It is associated most directly with medial frontal lobe structures, such as anterior cingulate cortex and dorsolateral prefrontal cortex, and depends heavily on the neurotransmitter dopamine. The alerting system supports the complementary functions

---

[1] The abbreviation VCFS is used in this article for consistency with others in this issue. However, because not all children with deletions of chromosome 22q11.2 exhibit velopharyngeal, cardiac, and facial anomalies, the author prefers to refer to the disorder by the more inclusive term of "chromosome 22q11.2 deletion syndrome."

of maintaining vigilance for novel information and the need to concentrate during continuous performance. It is associated with right frontal and parietal regions and depends heavily on the neurotransmitter norepinephrine.

Experimental studies of attentional and spatial processing

The orienting attention system is the most relevant attention system to the "NLD" cognitive phenotype. This is because it plays a role in selecting objects and locations in space for more detailed processing and is likely to support the development of some key early numerical cognitive processes.

Simon and colleagues [34] had children with VCFS and age-matched typical controls complete a visual search task, which was designed to test the orienting attention system. As predicted, children with VCFS had much greater difficulty than typical controls when attention was cued initially to a location other than where a target subsequently appeared. These results indicate that children with VCFS are impaired at navigating the visuospatial environment in the absence of specific indications of where to direct their attention. They are particularly handicapped when previously allocated attentional resources need to be disengaged and reallocated to other locations in a self-directed fashion.

Bish and colleagues [35] compared similar groups of children with VCFS to age-matched typical controls using the ANT, primarily to investigate the executive attention system. For the more reactive orienting test, compared with the more volitional one used in Simon and colleagues' study, there was not a significant difference between groups for what is referred to as the "invalid cue" condition, even though children with VCFS responded more slowly and showed a larger difference between the invalid and valid conditions. Together, the results suggest that children with VCFS suffer from a localized impairment in the ability to volitionally search visual space in a goal-directed fashion.

Scerif and colleagues [36] compared the performance of eight 3- to 4-year-old boys with FXS and eight similarly aged boys and girls with WS to one another and to groups of chronologic and mental age-matched typical controls on a visual search task. Their task required using the orienting system to find target "monsters" hidden behind a subset of disks shown on a touchscreen. Toddlers with either disorder made more errors than did controls. Although the number of errors did not differ between the groups with the two genetic disorders, the error types did. Toddlers with WS searched in inappropriate locations more often did than those with FXS and controls. Toddlers with FXS revisited disks that had not concealed "monsters" more often than toddlers in the other two groups. In each case it is clear that processing goal-directed visual attentional search is less effective in children with FXS or WS; these impairments, although slightly different in nature, can be detected early in development. Munir and colleagues [37] found similar results when they tested 8- to 15-year-old boys with FXS on a similar visuospatial search task. They produced significantly fewer correct target identifications, slower responses, and more incorrect identifications of distractors as targets than did age-matched typical controls, even those selected on the basis of having poor attentional capabilities.

Patterns of impairment in visuospatial processing and their implications for the development of higher-level abilities are not limited to visual search. Several experiments showed that mental manipulation of the spatial characteristics of objects also is impaired in children with genetic disorders. Within the context of a functional MRI (fMRI) experiment, Kesler and colleagues, in Ref. [38] and in an article elsewhere in this issue, tested girls with monosomy TS aged 7 to 18 years on the standardized Judgment of Line Orientation task; they performed more poorly than typical age-matched controls on difficult problems. A similar group of participants also was tested during fMRI scanning by Haberecht and colleagues [39] on a visuospatial memory task. Girls with TS were less accurate and slower than controls when attempting to retain in memory and match spatial information about objects over time. Similar results to both above studies were reported by Hart and colleagues [40] using similar experimental tests before and during fMRI scans. In all of the above cases, reduced activation in parietal lobe areas that typically are associated with spatial processing was observed in the individuals with TS.

Because of the strong contrasts in cognitive strengths and weaknesses and interesting developmental progression, WS has attracted many experimental studies. Landau and colleagues [41] revealed some important strengths and weaknesses regarding visuomotor and visuoconstructive processing in children with WS. Children with WS and typical controls, matched for mental or chronological age, were asked to name everyday objects displayed on a computer screen. The task tested object recognition processes, typically associated with temporal lobe or ventral visual processing functions, and mental rotation processes, which typically depend on parietal or dorsal stream functions. Children with WS performed as accurately as did mental age–matched controls and almost as well as chronological age–matched controls and adults on object recognition; however, they performed significantly more poorly than their chronologically age–matched peers and adults when mental rotation was required. The results indicate that children with WS may require less clarity to recognize objects (ie, they have a relative strength in analyzing an object's features) than other children; however, they are impaired in mentally executing spatial transformations on objects to bring them into a typical "viewpoint" that facilitates recognition. In other words, their impairment seems to be highly selective to the spatial domain.

A related study used the standardized Block Assembly task that requires participants to recreate a geometric pattern using a set of colored blocks. Landau and colleagues [42] compared actions based on "executive mechanisms" (checking for errors, attempting repairs) or "spatial representations" (creating and maintaining a representation of the identity and location of the components of the overall shape). Results indicated that children with WS showed no executive processing impairments compared with mental aged–matched typical controls and adults. Instead, their impairments were attributable to poorer quality mental representations of the characteristics of the component blocks and the spatial relationships among them in the model that they were attempting to reproduce. Consistently, a study with adults who had WS also showed a particular spatial impairment in their ability to determine whether pairs of geometric shapes could be combined to complete a square [43]. By contrast, the ability to detect matches between similar items was not impaired. This study even located the problem within the dorsal stream parietal region by showing lower activation in WS adults in a functional imaging task and reduced gray matter in the adjoining region in a structural imaging study.

Finally, Landau's group [44] showed that visuospatial impairments in children with WS also extend to their use of the orienting attention system to track moving objects. Children with WS performed much more poorly than did mental age–matched typical controls when tracking moving objects, but not on a similar task with static objects. The results suggest that children (and adults) with "NLD"-like disorders suffer from impairments in the mental manipulation of spatial relationships within and between objects.

Simon and colleagues [34,45] contended that such an ability, and, thus, impairments in it, will be related strongly to competence in the higher-level cognitive domain of numerical processing. This is because a range of basic functions in visuospatial attention has been implicated in several numerical subdomains. This is especially true of counting visually presented objects and reasoning about the relationships between different quantities. Quantities acquire ordinal relations that are represented mentally in linear spatial terms (eg, two comes before three, 300 is far beyond 30). Therefore, spatial attention was shown to be a critical component in simple numerical abilities, like counting and magnitude comparison. This small, but growing, literature suggests that the attentional and spatiotemporal impairments described above are specific in nature and limited to particular patterns of processing. Higher-order processes, particularly in the domain of numerical cognition, that depend on these basic functions also show significant impairments; it is likely that this is due to the difficulty of constructing typical higher-level competencies on the foundation of impaired basic ones.

Experimental studies of numerical cognition

Simon and colleagues [34] showed that impaired visuospatial attentional search in children with VCFS likely contributed to poorer performance when counting items randomly arranged in visual displays that did not afford the use of eye movements or other visuomotor actions (like touching) to facilitate the process. This essentially left children only with the tool of visuospatial attention to search for and enumerate items in the display. Because enumeration of approximately one to three items, a process known as subitizing, has been shown to operate independently of, or to depend minimally on, the spatial attention system [46–48], the impairment was not seen until children with VCFS began to use the search-based counting process. They also switched enumeration processes for smaller set sizes (eg, counting from three rather than four items) than was the case for controls. Similar results apparently were found in a similar task with children with WS [44].

In the same study, Simon and colleagues [34] examined a magnitude comparison task where children were asked to determine whether a stimulus representing a specific magnitude (one, two, six, or nine) was larger or smaller than a memorized standard (in this case, five). Magnitudes were depicted as patterns of dots or as Arabic numerals. Typically, such tasks are performed by comparison of one magnitude to another in terms of their position on a mentally represented "number line" with reduced "distance" between the items leading to more uncertainty because of proximity or overlap. There is even evidence that brain regions commonly associated with spatial attention activate when adults and children carry out such a task [49,50]. Results showed that children with VCFS performed more poorly with the spatial dot notation compared with the Arabic notation. Analyses showed that control children demonstrated the typical distance effect for both notations (dots and Arabic numbers) and for small and large numbers. In contrast, children with VCFS demonstrated a significant distance effect for small Arabic numerals only and trended toward a typical distance effect for large numbers of dots. This suggests that the relationships between numerical magnitudes depicted in spatial terms on a putative "mental number line" likely were disturbed in the children with VCFS.

A similar experiment was used by Paterson and colleagues [51] with children and adults with WS whose mental age averaged 6.9 years. Results showed that the individuals with WS did not produce the standard distance effect, even though the trend was in that direction. In contrast, mental age– and chronological age–matched controls did show the effect. This suggests that, like children with VCFS, individuals with WS also suffer from some disturbance of space/number relationships in their mental representations.

Poor visuospatial search and disturbed representations of spatial relationships may not have a detrimental effect only on simple visual counting and approximate numerical reasoning. They also can "cascade" further into negative effects on exact arithmetical computation and several other number-processing tasks. In an extension of their magnitude comparison work, Paterson and colleagues [51] tested the same individuals with WS and controls on nine numerical and arithmetical tasks. Individuals with WS had considerable difficulty with almost all of the tasks, and this impairment generally was much greater than that of another clinical group (individuals with Down's syndrome [DS]). Counting in a nonautomatic fashion (eg, from 25 to 35 or backward) was very difficult for the participants with WS, as was a task asking "What comes before?" and "What comes after?" a given number. Reading multidigit Arabic numbers aloud produced significant impairment as did seriating dot patterns with respect to numerical value and matching dot patterns to Arabic numerals. Few individuals with WS could complete the full set of addition, multiplication, and addition tasks.

In related studies, Ansari and colleagues [52] examined the relative contributions of visuospatial and verbal competence to the development of counting in children with WS and mental age–matched controls. Children with WS understood the cardinality principle of counting (stating the final number word as the magnitude of the counted set) as well as did much younger mental age–matched controls. Also they performed just as well, on the small number, and just as poorly, on the large number components, as controls on a "give a number" task where they were asked to give the experimenter a specific number of marbles from a bowl. The investigators reported that performance on this latter task was accounted for by the visuospatial development (measured as spatial mental age on the British Abilities Scales) of the control children. By contrast, performance of children with WS was accounted for by the language development (measured as verbal mental age on the British Abilities Scales). They stated that "individuals with WS may rely on their relative strength in language to bootstrap or scaffold their understanding of the cardinality principle [whereas] visuospatial ability rather than language predicted success in the control group." This provides further illustrations of impaired visuospatial ability in WS and the relation of that competence to numerical cognition. It also is a clear example of an atypical developmental trajectory to apparently typical performance on a given task.

Little work in this domain seems to have been done using experimental methods with children who have TS, although one study with adults showed some consistency with the above findings. Bruandet and colleagues [53] tested 12 adults with monosomy TS and 13 age-matched typical controls on nine numerical and arithmetical tasks and did not detect many major differences in basic number processing. Adults with TS erred more on estimation questions (eg, "How long is a bus?") particularly on questions regarding length, and always in the direction of underestimating. No differences were found on a magnitude comparison task requiring the choice of the larger of two digits that varied in numerical value differences from one to seven. This finding may have been due to the age of the participants or the particular individuals involved, because a study by Simon and colleagues [54], which included essentially the same task for a similar sized group of children with TS, found very large group differences. In an enumeration task similar to that of Simon and colleagues, described above, Bruandet and colleagues only found differences in the subitizing range. The investigators suggested that adults with TS may have been counting in this range instead of subitizing, but this interpretation may be a result of how the analysis was done. Simon and colleagues' study [54] with children found the major difference between children with TS and controls, but not between children with TS and those with VCFS, was in the counting range, as would be expected. The main results that Bruandet and colleagues reported from their arithmetic tasks were slower response times, but not more errors, in the adults with TS. Despite the difficulty with the interpretation of the results in this paper, it suggested that adults with TS have some problems with basic numerical and arithmetical processing that are consistent with the above findings. Our own studies of younger girls with TS find that the overlap with children who have VCFS and the difference from age-matched controls is significant in tasks where visuospatial abilities strongly underlie numerical performance.

One other study [55] used nonexperimental standardized tests to measure spatial processing in 12- to 22-year-old girls and women with TS and controls who were closely matched by age and other characteristics. Seven of the 13 had monosomy TS, and six had a mosaic form of TS. Females with TS scored significantly lower than controls on many spatial ability tests, which is consistent with the above pattern. Several studies reported impairments in arithmetical processing in individuals with TS [16,18,56], and some related these to brain structure and function differences [57,58].

Studies of temporal cognition

Surprisingly, very few experimental investigations of temporal cognition have been performed with "NLD" populations. In one such study, Debbané and colleagues [59] presented 6- to 39-year-old individuals with VCFS and typical age-matched controls with two temporal judgment tasks. In general, individuals with VCFS were impaired in their representation and processing of temporal information. They were less able to maintain the correct cadence in the finger-tapping task and tended to speed up, which closely paralleled the general tendency to underestimate length in Bruandet and colleagues' [53] study of individuals with TS. In the temporal judgment task, they required larger intervals between two durations than the controls before they could tell them apart as accurately. This finding resembles the "distance effect" results reported for magnitude comparison, where values less close together tend to be confused more easily by affected individuals.

Consistent with these results are the findings from several temporal processing tasks in a study by Silbert and colleagues [55]. Although they did not show significantly poorer performance on similar tapping tasks to the one above, girls with TS were significantly less able to distinguish between pairs of different rhythmic patterns presented at 92 beats per minute each. This indicates that, like individuals with VCFS, these participants with TS also had an impairment in retaining, analyzing, and comparing temporal information.

The results reviewed above provide strong support for the view that impairment in the cognitive endophenotype that comprises a wide range of attentional, spatial, and numerical tasks is not the result of a broken space or number "module" within the neurocognitive system of children from several genetic disorders. Instead, it seems to be the result of a constructive process whereby an impaired outcome emerges as the result of development along an atypical trajectory. Or, as reported by Ansari and colleagues [52], typical performance is produced by the deployment of atypical processes for the task in question. The start state might be constituted such that it can produce typical responses to the simplest tasks. Beyond that, atypical representations and processes soon develop until the resulting competence diverges significantly from that of the typical population. Much evidence presented here suggests that this occurs in the case of early-developing attentional and spatiotemporal cognitive dysfunctions and their interaction with the demands of numerically relevant task processing. The weak foundation cannot support the construction of typical, higher-level representations and the processes required to generate typical outputs from them. As a result, low-level dysfunctions in one or several domains subsequently "cascade" their effects to impairments in a potentially broad range of developmentally distal, higher-level tasks on which their construction depends.

A clear example comes from the work of Paterson and colleagues [60], who showed that 2- to 3-year-olds with WS performed as well as mental and chronological age–matched controls on a simple task requiring numerical change detection between pairs of displays containing one, two, or three objects. Often, variants of this task have been interpreted as evidence for the earliest numerical competence in infants [45,61–64]. At the very least, this shows that, in a domain where the "end state" is recognized as a hallmark of impairment for a particular genetic disorder (ie, numerical competence in WS), one measure of the "start state" indicates no difference at all from the typical population.

Experimental studies of executive function

Because the case was made above that much of the phenotype observed in individuals with "NLD" profiles represents the cascaded effect of attentional and spatiotemporal cognitive impairments, some aspects of what is called "executive function" also should be considered as essential. This is because some executive functions work in tight integration with other components of the attention system. This is especially true of the exercise of cognitive control over the process of goal-directed visuospatial attentional search. The term "executive function" is used broadly to encompass many functions, from planning to problem solving and working memory to inhibitory control, that are associated with functions believed to depend on the frontal lobes of the brain. Discussions here are limited to functions believed to be controlled by the "executive attention system" described earlier (ie, error detection, conflict monitoring, and inhibition).

In an experiment testing a close link between visuospatial search and executive control, Scerif and colleagues [65] found that male toddlers with FXS were impaired, relative to typical age-matched controls, at suppressing eye movements to locations signaled by a cue but not subsequently rewarded with a pleasing visual stimulus. This indicates that the affected toddlers were less able to inhibit irrelevant spatial cue information and effectively manage their eye movements to optimally navigate a visual scene for optimal selection of relevant information. Wilding and colleagues [66] added a response-switching component to an attentional search task so that inhibition of responses to one type of stimulus was required to focus on the other type. The result of this requirement was that boys with FXS (aged 8 to 15 years) performed poorly. They found fewer targets and misidentified more distractors as targets than did mental age–matched controls, even ones selected as having attentional problems. Experiments by Bish and colleagues [35] and Sobin and colleagues [67] showed that children with VCFS were significantly impaired at inhibiting the processing of irrelevant "flankers." Flankers are stimuli on either side of a target stimulus that convey consistent or conflicting information to that carried by the target. Children with VCFS were especially impaired when conflicting flankers were present. This showed that they too have problems processing conflicting information and inhibiting inappropriate responses to it.

By contrast, Landau and colleagues [42] found that individuals with WS demonstrated relatively intact "executive mechanisms" compared with "spatial representations" when attempting to solve block design puzzles. This suggests that they do not suffer from significant impairments in this aspect of cognitive processing. Several results reported by Atkinson and colleagues [68] on "frontal" conflict-based tasks support this conclusion. Finally, although there seems to be a consensus based on standardized testing that some executive dysfunction exists in TS, no experimental studies of specific inhibitory functions seem to have been published.

Comparison with cognitive processing in Down's syndrome

Few other genetic syndromes have been the subject of serious cognitive experimental investigations with the exception of DS, which has been studied extensively. DS probably is the most common neurodevelopmental disorder, with a prevalence estimated to be about 1 in 800 live births. In 95% of cases it results from a full trisomy, or three copies, of chromosome 21. Mental retardation is common and "individuals with Down's syndrome probably comprise the majority of infants and children with mental retardation" [69]. The pattern of strengths and weaknesses in this disorder is less clear, and, thus, less amenable to a generative explanatory framework regarding the neurocognitive basis of impairments than is the case with "NLD" populations. In general, the "caricature" of individuals with DS has been the inverse of "NLD" (ie, extreme deficits in language abilities that exceed impairments in visuospatial and related abilities).

Because of the similarity in global intellectual impairment to individuals with WS and males with FXS in particular, and because of their apparent difference in cognitive profile, individuals with DS often have been studied in cognitive experiments as a comparison group. This is the case in some of the studies described earlier. For example, in Paterson and colleagues' [51] study of individuals with WS, nine individuals with DS were matched to those with WS on the distance effect task. In contrast to the lack of distance effect shown by the individuals with WS, those with DS did "display a robust distance effect," thus reinforcing their relative strength in visuospatial and related numerical domains. In the same study, the difficulty experienced by individuals with DS on the battery of number processing and calculation tasks was less severe than for individuals with WS, although, as expected, their performance was still significantly poorer than that produced by typical controls. Yet, when Paterson and colleagues [60] used a simple numerical change detection task, toddlers with DS showed no evidence of detecting novel numerical set sizes, whereas, surprisingly, those with WS did.

This finding underscores the importance of the developmental approach, because simple tests produced results in two genetic disorder populations that were exactly the opposite of what would be expected based on their "end states." These findings indicate that the characteristic learning and memory impairments in DS, in particular as relates to the language domain, can be found early in childhood, however. Wilding and colleagues' [66] experiment showing executive dysfunction in 8- to 15-year-old boys with FXS also included similarly aged boys with DS. Performance on the single target spatial search task produced similar impairments in boys with DS as in those with FXS, although the latter group's false alarm errors were much more likely to be repetitions of the same object than was the case for boys with DS. In the alternating target search task, which involved an inhibitory component, the results were similar. So in this case, boys with DS showed similar visuospatial and executive impairments to boys with FXS, although they tended to be less perseverative.

Summary

This article presented a cognitive profile associated with the childhood presentation of several common genetic syndromes, all of which have been labeled "NLDs." Characteristic NLD impairments include visual perception and complex psychomotor skills, tactile and visual attention, and tactile and visual memory [7]. To understand and begin to explain the basis for the similar pattern of impairments, the concept of a cognitive endophenotype was introduced as a way to integrate the specific components that contribute to higher-level functions in which the impairments are observed.

The concept also advances the effort to link genes to complex behavioral and cognitive phenotypes more specifically. It has been argued that children with genetic disorders likely begin life with an altered neurocognitive substrate that contributes to an atypical developmental trajectory through the process of acquiring many different domains of cognitive competence. Using the example of several genetic disorders that are associated with "NLDs," the article explored the explanation of diverse impairments in higher-order visual, spatial, temporal, numerical, and executive cognitive competencies deriving from origins in more basic attentional and spatial cognitive dysfunctions. These dysfunctions imply, and a small amount of evidence now demonstrates, that congenital or early developing changes in the neural substrate also exist and contribute to atypical development.

Understanding the cognitive impairments of children with genetic disorders in this way has several implications. Primarily, it provides a more unifying account for understanding the variety of cognitive and behavioral disturbances that are observed in children with genetic disorders. Further, from the perspective of basic science, this approach can help to reduce the complexity in identification of the genetic basis of specific impairments and of structure and function relationships between brain and cognition. From the perspective of translational science, it is hoped that this approach will lead to evidence-based, targeted interventions ranging from pharmacotherapy to early cognitive and behavioral "brain training."

Acknowledgments

The author thanks Joel Johnson, M.D. and Doron Gothelf, M.D. for their thoughtful comments and guidance on drafts of this manuscript.

References

[1] Tager-Flusberg H. An introduction to research on neurodevelopmental disorders from a cognitive neuroscience perspective. In: Tager-Flusberg H, editor. Neurodevelopmental disorders. Cambridge (MA): The MIT Press; 1999. p. 3–24.

[2] Gottesman II, Gould TD. The endophenotype concept in psychiatry: etymology and strategic intentions. Am J Psychiatry 2003;160:636–45.

[3] Johnson MH, Halit H, Grice SJ, et al. Neuroimaging of typical and atypical development: a perspective from multiple levels of analysis. Dev Psychopathol 2002;14(3):521–36.

[4] Karmiloff-Smith A. Development itself is the key to understanding developmental disorders. Trends Cogn Sci 1998;10(2):389–98.

[5] Cipolotti L, Butterworth B, Denes G. A specific deficit for numbers in a case of dense acalculia. Brain 1991;114:2619–37.

[6] Benton AL. Mathematical disability and the Gerstmann syndrome. In: Deloche G, Seron X, editors. Mathematical disabilities: a cognitive neuropsychological perspective. Hillsdale (NJ): Lawrence Erlbaum Associates; 1987. p. 111–20.

[7] Rourke BP, Ahmad SA, Collins DW, et al. Child clinical/pediatric neuropsychology: some recent advances. Annu Rev Psychol 2002;53:309–39.

[8] Mazzocco MM. Advances in research of the fragile X syndrome. Ment Retard Dev Disabil Res Rev 2000;6:95–106.

[9] Mostofsky SH, Mazzocco MM, Aakalu G, et al. Decreased cerebellar posterior vermis size in fragile X syndrome. Neurology 1998;50:121–30.

[10] Rovet JF. The cognitive and neuropsychological characteristics of females with Turner syndrome. In: Bender B, Berch D, editors. Sex chromosome abnormalities and behavior: psychological studies. Bouldor (CO): Westview Press; 1991. p. 39–77.

[11] Robinson A, Bender BG, Linden MG, et al. Sex chromosome aneuploidy: the Denver Prospective Study. Birth Defects Orig Artic Ser 1990;26(4):59–115.

[12] Ratcliffe SG, Butler GE, Jones M. Edinburgh study of growth and development of children with sex chromosome abnormalities. IV. Birth Defects Orig Artic Ser 1991;26(4):1–44.

[13] Stewart DA, Bailey JD, Netley CT, et al. Growth, development, and behavioral outcome from mid-adolescence to adulthood in subjects with chromosome aneuploidy: the Toronto Study. Birth Defects Orig Artic Ser 1990;26(4):131–88.

[14] Waber D. Neuropsychological aspects of Turner syndrome. Dev Med Child Neurol 1979;21: 58–70.

[15] Romans SM, Stefanatos G, Roeltgen DP, et al. Transition to young adulthood in Ullrich-Turner syndrome: neurodevelopmental changes. Am J Med Genet 1998;79(2):140–7.

[16] Rovet J, Szekely C, Hockenberry MN. Specific arithmetic calculation deficits in children with Turner syndrome. J Clin Exp Neuropsychol 1994;16(6):820–39.

[17] Rovet JF. The psychoeducational characteristics of children with Turner syndrome. J Learn Disabil 1993;26(5):333–41.

[18] Temple CM. Arithmetic ability and disability in Turner's syndrome: a cognitive neuropsychological analysis. Dev Neuropsychol 1996;14(1):47–67.

[19] Mervis CB, Morris CA, Bertrand J, et al. Williams syndrome: findings from an integrated program of research. In: Tager-Flusberg H, editor. Neurodevelopmental disorders: contributions to a new framework from the cognitive neurosciences. Cambridge (MA): MIT Press; 1999. p. 65–110.

[20] Bellugi U, Lichtenberger L, Mills D, et al. Bridging cognition, the brain and molecular genetics: evidence from Williams syndrome. Trends Neurosci 1999;22(5):197–207.

[21] Bellugi U, Lichtenberger L, Jones W, et al. The neurocognitive profile of Williams syndrome: a complex pattern of strengths and weaknesses. J Cogn Neurosci 2000;12 (Suppl 1):7–29.

[22] Shprintzen RJ, Goldberg RB, Lewin ML, et al. A new syndrome involving cleft palate, cardiac anomalies, typical faces, and learning disabilities: velo-cardio-facial syndrome. Cleft Palate J 1978;15:56–62.

[23] Bearden CE, Woodin MF, Wang PP, et al. The neurocognitive phenotype of the 22q11.2 deletion syndrome: selective deficit in visual-spatial memory. J Clin Exp Neuropsychol 2001; 23(4):447–64.

[24] Moss EM, Batshaw ML, Solot CB, et al. Psychoeducational profile of the 22q11.2 microdeletion: a complex pattern. J Pediatr 1999;134(2):193–8.

[25] Swillen A, Devriendt K, Legius E, et al. The behavioural phenotype in velo-cardio-facial syndrome (VCFS): from infancy to adolescence. Genet Couns 1999;10(1):79–88.

[26] Wang PP, Woodin MF, Kreps-Falk R, et al. Research on behavioral phenotypes: velocardiofacial syndrome (deletion 22q11.2). Dev Med Child Neurol 2000;42:422–7.

[27] Woodin MF, Wang PP, Aleman D, et al. Neuropsychological profile of children and adolescents with the 22q11.2 microdeletion. Genet Med 2001;3(1):34–9.

[28] Swillen A, Vogels A, Devriendt K, et al. Chromosome 22q11 deletion syndrome: update and review of the clinical features, cognitive-behavioral spectrum, and psychiatric complications. Am J Med Genet 2000;97:128–35.

[29] Bearden CE, Wang PP, Simon TJ. Williams syndrome cognitive profile also characterizes Velocardiofacial/DiGeorge syndrome. Am J Med Genet B Neuropsychiatr Genet 2002; 114:689–92.

[30] Posner MI, Petersen SE. The attention system of the human brain. Annu Rev Neurosci 1990; 13:25–42.

[31] Fossella J, Sommer T, Fan J, et al. Assessing the molecular genetics of attention networks. BMC Neurosci 2002;3(1):14.

[32] Fan J, McCandliss BD, Sommer T, et al. Testing the efficiency and independence of attentional networks. J Cogn Neurosci 2002;14:340–7.

[33] Corbetta M, Shulman GL. Control of goal-directed and stimulus-driven attention in the brain. Nat Rev Neurosci 2002;3(3):201–15.

[34] Simon TJ, Bearden CE, McDonald-McGinn DM, et al. Visuospatial and numerical cognitive deficits in children with chromosome 22q11.2 deletion syndrome. Cortex 2005;41(2): 145–55.

[35] Bish JP, Ferrante S, McDonald-McGinn D, et al. Maladaptive conflict monitoring as evidence for executive dysfunction in children with chromosome 22q11.2 deletion syndrome. Dev Sci 2005;8(1):36–43.

[36] Scerif G, Cornish KM, Wilding J, et al. Visual search in typically developing toddlers and toddlers with fragile X or Williams syndrome. Dev Sci 2004;7:116–30.

[37] Munir F, Cornish KM, Wilding J. A neuropsychological profile of attention deficits in young males with fragile X syndrome. Neuropsychologia 2000;38(9):1261–70.

[38] Kesler SR, Haberecht MF, Menon V, et al. Functional neuroanatomy of spatial orientation processing in Turner syndrome. Cereb Cortex 2004;14(2):174–80.

[39] Haberecht MF, Menon V, Warsofsky IS, et al. Functional neuroanatomy of visuo-spatial working memory in Turner syndrome. Hum Brain Mapp 2001;14(2):96–107.

[40] Hart SJ, Davenport ML, Hooper SR, et al. Visuospatial executive function in Turner syndrome: functional MRI and neurocognitive findings. Brain 2006;129(Pt 5):1125–36.

[41] Landau B, Hoffman JE, Kurz N. Object recognition with severe spatial deficits in Williams syndrome: sparing and breakdown. Cognition 2006;100(3):483–510.

[42] Landau B, Hoffman JE, Reiss JE, et al. Specialization and breakdown in spatial cognition: lessons from Williams syndrome. In: Morris C, Lenhoff H, Wang PP, editors. Williams-Beuren syndrome: research and clinical perspectives. Baltimore (MD): Johns Hopkins Press; 2006. p. 207–36.

[43] Meyer-Lindenberg A, Kohn P, Mervis CB, et al. Neural basis of genetically determined visuospatial construction deficit in Williams syndrome. Neuron 2004;43(5):623–31.

[44] O'Hearn K, Landau B, Hoffman JE. Multiple object tracking in people with Williams syndrome and in normally developing children. Psychol Sci 2005;16(11):905–12.

[45] Simon TJ. Reconceptualizing the origins of number knowledge: a "non-numerical" approach. Cognitive Development 1997;12:349–72.

[46] Piazza M, Giacomini E, Le Bihan D, et al. Single-trial classification of parallel pre-attentive and serial attentive processes using functional magnetic resonance imaging. Proc Biol Sci 2003;270(1521):1237–45.

[47] Piazza M, Mechelli A, Butterworth B, et al. Are subitizing and counting implemented as separate or functionally overlapping processes? Neuroimage 2002;15(2):435–46.

[48] Sathian K, Simon TJ, Peterson S, et al. Neural evidence linking visual object enumeration and attention. J Cogn Neurosci 1999;11(1):36–51.

[49] Dehaene S, Piazza M, Pinel P, et al. Three parietal circuits for number processing. Cogn Neuropsychol 2003;20:487–506.

[50] Temple E, Posner MIP. Brain mechanisms of quantity are similar in 5-year-old children and adults. Proc Natl Acad Sci 1998;95:7836–41.

[51] Paterson SJ, Girelli L, Butterworth B, et al. Are numerical impairments syndrome specific? Evidence from Williams syndrome and Down's syndrome. J Child Psychol Psychiatry 2006; 47(2):190–204.

[52] Ansari D, Donlan C, Thomas MS, et al. What makes counting count? Verbal and visuo-spatial contributions to typical and atypical number development. J Exp Child Psychol 2003; 85(1):50–62.

[53] Bruandet M, Molko N, Cohen L, et al. A cognitive characterization of dyscalculia in Turner syndrome. Neuropsychologia 2004;42(3):288–98.

[54] Simon TJ, Takarae Y, DeBoer TL, et al. Overlapping numerical cognition impairments in chromosome 22q11.2 Deletion and Turner syndromes. 2007, submitted.

[55] Silbert A, Wolff PH, Lilienthal J. Spatial and temporal processing in patients with Turner's syndrome. Behav Genet 1977;7(1):11–21.

[56] Mazzocco MM. A process approach to describing mathematics difficulties in girls with Turner syndrome. Pediatrics 1998;102(2 Pt 3):492–6.

[57] Molko N, Cachia A, Riviere D, et al. Brain anatomy in Turner syndrome: evidence for impaired social and spatial-numerical networks. Cereb Cortex 2004;14(8):840–50.

[58] Kesler SR, Menon V, Reiss AL. Neuro-functional differences associated with arithmetic processing in Turner syndrome. Cereb Cortex 2006;16(6):849–56.

[59] Debbané M, Glaser B, Gex-Fabry M, et al. Temporal perception in velo-cardio-facial syndrome. Neuropsychologia 2005;43:1754–62.

[60] Paterson SJ, Brown JH, Gsodl MK, et al. Cognitive modularity and genetic disorders. Science 1999;286(5448):2355–8.

[61] Xu F, Carey S. Infants' metaphysics; the case of numerical identity. Cognit Psychol 1996;30: 111–53.

[62] Wynn K. Origins of number knowledge. Mathematical Cognition 1995;1:35–60.

[63] Mix KS, Huttenlocher J, Levine SC. Multiple cues for quantification in infancy: is number one of them? Psychol Bull 2002;128(2):278–94.

[64] Simon TJ. The foundations of numerical thinking in a brain without numbers. Trends Cogn Sci 1999;3(10):363–5.

[65] Scerif G, Karmiloff-Smith A, Campos R, et al. To look or not to look? Typical and atypical development of oculomotor control. J Cogn Neurosci 2005;17(4):591–604.

[66] Wilding J, Cornish K, Munir F. Further delineation of the executive deficit in males with fragile-X syndrome. Neuropsychologia 2002;40(8):1343–9.

[67] Sobin C, Kiley-Brabeck K, Daniels S, et al. Networks of attention in children with the 22q11 deletion syndrome. Dev Neuropsychol 2004;26(2):611–26.

[68] Atkinson J, Braddick O, Anker S, et al. Neurobiological models of visuospatial cognition in children with Williams syndrome: measures of dorsal-stream and frontal function. Dev Neuropsychol 2003;23(1–2):139–72.

[69] Nadel L. Down syndrome in cognitive neuroscience perspective. In: Tager-Flusberg H, editor. Neurodevelopmental disorders. Cambridge (MA): MIT Press; 1999. p. 197–221.

Child Adolesc Psychiatric Clin N Am
16 (2007) 617–630

CHILD AND
ADOLESCENT
PSYCHIATRIC CLINICS
OF NORTH AMERICA

ELSEVIER
SAUNDERS

Three Steps Toward Improving the Measurement of Behavior in Behavioral Phenotype Research

Elisabeth M. Dykens, PhD[a,*],
Robert M. Hodapp, PhD[b]

[a]Vanderbilt Kennedy Center, Peabody Box 40, 230 Appleton Place, Nashville,
TN 37203, USA
[b]Vanderbilt Kennedy Center & Department of Education, Peabody Box 328,
230 Appleton Place, Nashville, TN 37203, USA

By all accounts, research on behavioral phenotypes is off and running. Compared with even a decade ago, the number and quality of phenotypic papers have increased dramatically, especially on genetic syndromes associated with intellectual and developmental disabilities. These increases are demonstrated in Table 1, which shows a Web of Science search for articles on ten different syndromes in 1994 to 1995 versus 2004 to 2005. With few exceptions, the numbers of published articles showed exponential increases, usually on the order of 1.5 to 5 times as many articles in 2004 to 2005 as in 1994 to 1995. For example, Williams and velocardiofacial syndromes showed fivefold increases, whereas Rett and Smith-Magenis syndromes showed 2.5-fold increases. Collectively, these publications examined syndromes from many different perspectives: genetic, biochemical, neurologic, cellular, medical, physiologic, developmental, psychiatric, and behavioral.

Behavior is only one way to describe a phenotype, and depictions of behavior vary considerably across the 1000 or more known genetic causes of intellectual disabilities. Many—possibly even most—syndromes feature no or only a few behavioral studies. Others show a flurry of studies that focus intensely on one or two salient behavioral domains (eg, language in Williams syndrome, sleep in Smith-Magenis syndrome). Still other syndromes have experienced steady increases in research across several behavioral

The work summarized in this article was supported by NICHD R01HD35681, R03HD50468, and P30HD15052 to the Vanderbilt Kennedy Center.

* Corresponding author.
E-mail address: elisabeth.dykens@vanderbilt.edu (E.M. Dykens).

Table 1
Number of Web of Science articles on ten genetics syndromes in 1994–1995 and 2004–2005

Syndrome	1994–1995	2004–2005
Angelman syndrome	131	221
Down syndrome	33,658	38,737
Fragile X syndrome	344	412
Prader-Willi syndrome	213	351
Rett syndrome	99	265
Smith-Magenis syndrome	12	42
Velocardiofacial syndrome	21	106
Williams syndrome	83	473
5p- (cri du chat) syndrome	17	23
Cornelia de Lang syndrome	12	33

domains (eg, Prader-Willi syndrome's cognitive profiles, hyperphagia, problem behavior, and compulsivity). The number and complexity of behavioral studies are increasing, but this increase is uneven across syndromes and domains examined.

As the numbers of syndrome-specific behavioral articles continue to grow, now seems a good time to pause and take stock of patterns that are emerging across these many studies. This article takes note of these patterns and summarizes our reading of the behavioral phenotype waters as gleaned from publications, syndrome-based conferences, and informal exchanges with colleagues. Combining these different sources, we propose that there are (at least) three overarching themes that relate to individual differences within syndromes. Together, these themes suggest possible sources of within-syndrome behavioral variability that have yet to be adequately addressed, including the roles of (1) development across the lifespan, (2) gender differences, and (3) other subject and environmental factors. We end with a cautionary note about measures and the need to supplement (alongside weaknesses and psychiatric vulnerabilities) the strengths and positive affect and attributes of individuals who have genetic syndromes.

Within-syndrome behavioral variability: back to basics

At the heart of the entire concept of behavioral phenotype is the notion of probability. In contrast to other, more deterministic definitions [1], Dykens [2] defined a behavioral phenotype as "the heightened probability" that persons with a genetic syndrome will show certain behavioral or developmental sequelae relative to those without the syndrome." Not all children or adults who have a particular genetic disorder show that disorder's "characteristic" behavior(s), but such behaviors are seen more often among individuals who have that disorder. Hence, the notion of increased probabilities. This probabilistic definition invites between-group and within-group studies.

Between-group studies

Between-group comparisons allow researchers to determine the extent to which syndromic behaviors are distinctive or shared. One might ask whether, compared to others with intellectual disabilities, persons who have Prader-Willi syndrome are more likely to show compulsivity or persons who have Williams syndrome show relative strengths in linguistic skills. Between-group studies compare individuals with versus without a particular genetic syndrome, and the task of choosing the "without" group is a science and an art. To date, we have identified many different control or contrast groups used in between-group studies [3]. Some studies compare individuals with a particular syndrome to other genetic etiologies or to groups with no known causes for their intellectual disabilities or to groups with heterogeneous etiologies. Still other studies compare individuals with groups of typical children of the same mental age or, if the behavior of interest is thought to be "spared" (eg, language in Williams syndrome), to typical children of the same chronologic ages. Comparisons sometimes involve group comparisons, sometimes "case-by-case" matching, and, more recently, propensity scores [4].

Several decades of between-group studies have shown the ways that behaviors of different genetic syndromes are sometimes unique and sometimes shared [5]. A few behaviors seem unique to one and only one syndrome. The cat-like cry in 5p- syndrome [6] seems unique to this syndrome, as does hyperphagia and its onset during the early childhood years in persons who have Prader-Willi syndrome [7]. For other behaviors, however, a particular syndrome shows the behavior more than others with intellectual disabilities, but that behavior also may be seen in other genetic syndromes. Hyperactivity is seen among boys who have fragile X and 5p- syndromes [8], and verbal perseveration is common in individuals who have Prader-Willi and Smith-Magenis syndromes [9]. Although these shared features may be qualitatively different, the behavior shows itself in two or more syndromes. Regardless of whether they are unique or shared, etiology-related behaviors typically show individual differences, and this variance is at the heart of most within-syndrome studies.

Within-group studies

Although between-group studies are important and many are ongoing, in some sense they constitute the first generation of behavioral phenotype studies. Arguing against a research culture that did not, until recently, embrace the need to examine different genetic etiologies separately [10], early etiology-oriented researchers needed to prove that genetic conditions did show different behaviors compared to others with intellectual disabilities. By now, however, such between-group differences are well established, and despite residual leeriness or concerns in some disciplines, the importance of phenotypes is increasingly well accepted among behavioral researchers [11]. At this point, researchers are increasingly adopting within-syndrome approaches, and these studies seem to form the heart and soul of phenotypic work. Such studies potentially can describe characteristic behaviors, individual differences in these behaviors, and possible genetic, neurologic, and other sources of within-syndrome variability.

Importantly, families are often the first to note discrepancies in how their child looks or behaves relative to others with the syndrome or to their assumptions about the syndrome. Parents might remark "I know that they say that kids with Down syndrome are friendly, but Johnny really is in his own world"; or "I know in Prader-Willi they are supposed to skin-pick, but we've never had a problem with that." These parental insights are important and, in our own research, have sparked in-depth studies of such topics as jigsaw puzzle skills in Prader-Willi syndrome [12], IQ trajectories in boys who have fragile X syndrome [13], and attraction to music in Williams syndrome [14]. Such parent-generated examples suggest individual differences that have clinical relevance and research implications.

Three underappreciated aspects of within-syndrome variability

Measures of characteristic syndromic behaviors invariably have statistical variance, and unpacking and explaining this variability is the goal of many research programs. Although most people who have Prader-Willi syndrome, for example, show hyperphagia, why is there such wide variability in the severity and course of the drive for food [7]? Young children who have Williams syndrome are keenly attuned to faces, and older individuals show strengths in facial recognition and memory [15], yet why are some individuals better than others with these tasks? Although up to 30% of boys who have fragile X syndrome have co-occurring autism [16], why do others show few autistic behaviors?

To address these questions, researchers increasingly turn to the genetic causes of a given syndrome or to neurologic functioning. Most phenotypic research aims to link genetic, neurologic, and behavioral functioning, ultimately leading to insights about the syndrome itself and possibly to how the involved genes or brain regions might function in the general population. One might explain some of the behavioral variability in Prader-Willi syndrome by comparing hyperphagia, compulsivity, or psychotic illness across persons with paternal deletions of 15q11-q13 versus maternal uniparental disomy [17,18]. One could conduct neuroimaging studies to identify regions involved in face processing in Williams syndrome versus controls [19]. One also might relate autistic symptoms in individuals who have fragile X syndrome to the amount of FMR protein they produce [20].

In the quest to relate syndromic behavior to underlying molecular genetic or neurologic features, however, researchers may have neglected to examine other more basic subject characteristics. These basic characteristics likely interact with genetic or neurologic factors but have yet to be woven into the fabric of most phenotypic studies. These basic features include age and development, gender, and a host of other subject and environmental variables.

Age and lifespan development

Phenotypes are often referred to in a static way, as a characteristic set of behaviors commonly seen in individuals who have a given syndrome. Missing from this formulation is the idea that phenotypes evolve and change over the course of time [21]. Although such an observation seems obvious, the nature of such changes is not, partly because most researchers sample behavior within a given age range and are less apt to measure behaviors longitudinally. Even so, examples abound that show either the earliest glimmerings of characteristic behaviors or changes in these behaviors across time.

Young children

Recent work is delineating the ways that behavioral phenotypes of different genetic disorders develop over a child's earliest years, especially in Williams, fragile X, and Down syndromes. Considering just one of these syndromes, children who have Down syndrome traditionally have been thought to show sociable, outgoing personalities, with such "outer directed" behaviors often overused in attempts to get others to solve problems for them [22,23]. At the same time, children who have Down syndrome, as a group, show specific weaknesses in many cognitive-linguistic areas, most notably expressive language and grammar [24].

Researchers are beginning to join these social personality strengths and cognitive weaknesses. By examining the early development of infant cognitive skills and infant behaviors during mother-child interactions, Fidler and colleagues [25] found that infants who have Down syndrome show particular difficulties in means-ends (ie, instrumental) thinking or in tasks that involve the idea that certain objects (eg, stool) can be used as a means for obtaining other, desired objects (eg, favorite toy). Such deficits likely relate to these children's increased amounts of looking to others for solutions to challenging tasks. Eventually, "the coupling of poor strategic thinking [ie, poor means-ends thinking] and strengths in social relatedness is hypothesized to lead to the less persistent and overly social personality-motivational orientation observed in this population" [26].

Older children

Beyond infancy, many studies describe how phenotypes evolve throughout childhood and adolescence. Boys who have fragile X syndrome, for example, generally show higher-level abilities in simultaneous processing than in sequential processing, yet older boys who have fragile X syndrome show this simultaneous-over-sequential pattern to a much more pronounced degree [13]. In the same way, the percentage of young children who have

Down syndrome showing receptive language abilities in advance of expressive abilities goes up across the childhood years [24,27]. In Williams syndrome, Jarrold and colleagues [28] tested children six times over a 4-year period and showed discrepant slopes between visual-spatial and language tasks. Over time, visuospatial skills developed only slightly, in contrast to the much steeper upward slope in language skills. As a result of these two divergent slopes, an already weak area became progressively weaker and an already strong area became progressively stronger.

Older adults

Although studies remain tipped toward children, the behavioral phenotypes of older adults are occasionally being studied, partly because of demographic changes. Similar to trends in the general population, more persons with intellectual disabilities are living well into their adult years. By 2040, the population of persons with intellectual disabilities aged 65 years and older is expected to double, from approximately 12% to 25% [29]. Such increases are most notable in Down syndrome. Over the past 30 years, the median lifespans of persons who have Down syndrome has increased from approximately 30 years to almost 60 years of age [30]. Such increased life expectancies provide new opportunities for researchers to identify how phenotypes evolve into late adulthood.

Most research on phenotypes in older persons has focused on the well-established ties between Down syndrome and heightened risks of Alzheimer's disease. In addition to ample neurologic and genetic studies on Down syndrome and Alzheimer's disease, a robust behavioral literature also shows age-related changes in adaptive and cognitive skills, personality, psychiatric disorders, and maladaptive behavior in older adults who have Down syndrome [31]. Although adults without symptoms of dementia are sometimes compared to individuals with symptoms, surprisingly little research has examined the behavioral phenotype of older, nondemented adults who have Down syndrome.

Phenotypic data are also sparse on older adults with other syndromes, although findings on three syndromes are promising. First, adults aged 30 years and older who have Williams syndrome have a host of medical complications [32] and increased (often clinically significant) anxiety. Dykens [33] found that adults who have Williams syndrome showed higher levels of anxieties and fears than their younger counterparts, including anticipatory anxiety and specific phobias. Devenny and colleagues [34] identified age-related and chronologically early declines in episodic memory in older adults who have Wllliams syndrome and age-related declines in free recall memory tasks that were similar to adults who have Down syndrome. Medical and cognitive findings suggest mild accelerated aging in Williams syndrome.

In contrast, while examining adults aged 30 to 50 years who have Prader-Willi syndrome, Dykens [35] found significant declines in the severity of their compulsive and problem behaviors and a lessening in the degree to which food seeking interfered with everyday living. The characteristic drive for food, however, seemed relatively stable in older adults [7], which suggested an age-related dampening in certain aspects of the Prader-Willi syndrome phenotype. A final example concerns older adults without intellectual disabilities who carry the fragile X premutation. Recently, these male—and some carrier female—patients have been identified as having fragile X–associated tremor/ataxia syndrome, showing progressive intention tremor and gait ataxia, cognitive decline, and emotional problems [36]. The number of CGG repeats seems to predict neurologic involvement and age of death in these older men.

Even in just these few syndrome examples, it is clear that a syndrome's characteristic behavioral phenotype as measured in children, adolescents, or even young adults may look different when measured in older adults. Older adults may provide new insights on how phenotypic behaviors relate to age-related shifts in hormones, neuropeptides, and health and the effects of chronic stress and long-term intervention efforts.

Gender

Although an overabundance of men with intellectual disabilities has been observed since the last century, we know surprisingly little about the effects of gender on behavior in most genetic syndromes and in others with intellectual disabilities. In a recent review of girls and women with intellectual disabilities, Hodapp and Dykens [37] examined two leading research journals in the field, the *American Journal on Mental Retardation* and the *Journal of Intellectual Disability Research*. In both of these flagship journals, only approximately one fourth of articles published over a 5-year period reported the gender breakdown of their participants and analyzed their behavioral data to determine whether sex differences existed. For most articles in both journals, the gender breakdown of participants was reported, but no mention was made as to whether the researchers looked for possible gender differences. In 10% to 20% of all articles, no mention at all was made of gender. In contrast, such blatant inattention to gender is not found in behavioral studies of typically developing children or adults. From the 1970s [38] until the present, "sex differences" has constituted an area of research specialization in the fields of typical child and adult development. Gender differences are also observed in many psychiatric disorders [39].

Although gender is imbedded in studies of sex-linked disorders, gender is not routinely examined in behavioral studies of non–sex-linked, intellectual disability syndromes. Even so, a few differences have been reported in Down and Williams syndromes. Compared with older men who have Down syndrome, older women may be somewhat more prone to show the clinical symptoms of Alzheimer's disease [40], and this risk may be associated with lowered levels of estrogen.

Most often noted for their relative strengths in aspects of expressive language, children and adults who have Williams syndrome also show heightened anxiety and fears and specific phobias [33,41]. An interaction seems to exist between gender and age, such that girls who have Williams syndrome become increasingly fearful as they get older, whereas boys do not. Comparing 6- to 12-year-old children to adolescents and adults aged 13 to 18 and 18+ years, Dykens [33] found that adolescent girls and adult women became more fearful overall, which suggested an age-related, increased vulnerability in women to anxiety and fears.

A final and more speculative example concerns Prader-Willi syndrome. We find that some persons who have Prader-Willi syndrome have strong desires to take care of others, especially the physical aspects of caregiving. More than others with disabilities, persons may strive to take care of household pets and work with animals or take care of babies and children in schools or daycare centers [42]. We have yet to find gender differences in this "nurturance streak," although anecdotally, women are more apt to express interests in having children. Perhaps interests in caregiving are related to aberrant levels of oxytocin previously reported in Prader-Willi syndrome [43], although it is unknown if gender differences are seen in oxytocin or related neuropeptides.

Because findings are scant or speculative, one might erroneously conclude that gender plays little role in the behavioral phenotypes of non–sex-linked genetic disorders. We contend that because gender has yet to be adequately analyzed or reported in behavioral phenotype studies, gender effects remain an open question and may or may not account for some proportion of within-syndrome behavioral variability.

Other environmental and subject characteristics

In most phenotypic studies, behavioral findings for a particular genetic syndrome are attributed largely to a cascade of effects that stem from that syndrome's underlying genetic anomaly. Many different environmental and subject characteristics also may be associated with the emergence, severity, or course of syndromic behavior. Syndrome-related psychiatric disorders exemplify the importance of these other factors. Although researchers describe a proneness to compulsivity in Prader-Willi syndrome or anxiety in Williams syndrome, we are perhaps too quick to tie these problems to syndrome status and not to other features that we know contribute to these symptoms in people with or without intellectual disabilities.

What are some of these other features and how might they operate in one versus another syndrome? The following factors are among the many "other factors" that have been shown to affect maladaptive behaviors or psychiatric disorders in persons who have intellectual disabilities:

Untreated, undiagnosed, or chronic pain
Low self-esteem
History of failure experiences
Stressors, life events, and transitions

Family psychiatric history
History of institutionalization
History of trauma and abuse

Although these risk factors are discussed elsewhere [44], the last item in this list—trauma and abuse—hints at how one such environmental or personal characteristic may affect persons with a particular genetic disorder. It is well established that children with disabilities suffer from child abuse much more often than nondisabled children. In the best study of this issue, Sullivan and Knutson [45] linked school, department of social service, and court records for all school-aged children in Omaha, Nebraska. They found that in contrast to a 9% rate of child abuse among nondisabled children, 31% of children with disabilities suffered from child abuse. Although rates varied across type of disability, children with disabilities were more likely to be abused and suffer from repeated abuse in multiple forms.

How might child abuse and exploitation in general fit with different genetic disorders? Consider the propensity of many persons who have Williams syndrome to be highly sociable and want to please others. Although such sociability is considered a strength, these individuals are often uninhibited and indiscriminate in their sociability. In one study of 36 children aged 4 to 10 years, Gosch and Pankau [46] found that parents considered 82% to be overly friendly toward strangers. Similarly, Davies and colleagues [47] noted that 94% of adults who have Williams syndrome were considered socially disinhibited, with 59% engaging in inappropriate touching of others.

Currently, the extent to which children and adults who have Williams syndrome are vulnerable to abuse and exploitation remains unknown. In a study of adults by Davies and colleagues [47], 10% of their sample had reported sexual assaults to police, and an additional 10% made allegations of assault that had not been reported. In studies of typical children, rates of sexual abuse are generally twice as high in girls than boys [48]. Although no data currently exist on the prevalence of abuse in individuals who have Williams syndrome, girls may be at higher risk than boys with this syndrome or than girls or boys with other types of intellectual disabilities. A general characteristic of persons with disabilities—increased risks of being abused and exploited—may intersect with features often found in persons who have Williams syndrome. In these ways, abuse histories and life stressors, medical status, pain, and family psychiatric risk factors, all should be taken into account in behavioral phenotype studies.

Cautionary note and new direction

Eclecticism in behavioral measures

In a recent review of measurement [49], we described the type and range of behavioral approaches used to assess behavior in genetic syndromes. These approaches included (1) standardized measures of intelligence, language, maladaptive, and adaptive behavior, (2) videotaped or direct observations of social, linguistic, or other behaviors, (3) parent, informant, or self-report interviews of psychiatric symptoms and social and adaptive behavior, (4) semi-projective techniques, and (5) the use of large-scale administrative medical or other databases. We emphasize a cautionary note: none of these methods is adequate unto itself, and the complexity of most behavioral phenotypes requires a flexible, innovative approach. Novel tasks, questionnaires, or observational methods may need to be developed, and several examples of these approaches exist.

To capture the "self-hugging" behavior often found in persons who have Smith-Magenis syndrome, Finucane and colleagues [50] videotaped such individuals and counted their "upper body spasmodic squeeze" or "self-hugs" across multiple settings. To examine the goal-directed behaviors of toddlers who have Down syndrome, Pitcarin and Wishart [23] analyzed responses of these children to an impossible task, coining the term "party tricks" to describe a set of socially disarming behaviors designed to deflect others' attention away from the task. Examining food ideation in persons who have Prader-Willi syndrome, Dykens [51] developed an interview that tapped persons' ideas about contaminated and oddly combined foods. To elicit referential language in persons who have either fragile X syndrome or Down syndrome, Abbeduto and colleagues [52] developed tasks in which, by putting an opaque "wall" between two speakers, each speaker was unable to see the object being referred to by the other.

These home-grown tasks or measures may be particularly important in describing how behaviors cluster or hang together, forming the behavioral manifestation of so-called "endophenotypes." Endophenotypes represent a putative subset of genetic or pathophysiologic mechanisms involved in a broader phenotype. Endophenotypes are increasingly studied in autism spectrum disorders, and although this concept holds promise for genetic disorders, measuring behaviors associated with endophenotypes requires a flexible blending of standardized and novel measures. For example, a somewhat common behavior in Prader-Willi syndrome—rectal digging—may be a variant of this syndrome's characteristic skin picking, and skin picking seems to be distinct from all other compulsive behaviors in the syndrome [53]. A formal measure of the frequency, severity, and trajectory of rectal digging and skin picking must be developed, because these behaviors may relate to certain genes that are variably deleted in persons who have Prader-Willi syndrome [54]. Behavioral specificity will be increasingly important as researchers strive to link altered genes to behavioral functioning, especially in persons who have unusual or rare genotypes (eg, smaller- or larger-than-usual deletions).

Positive attributes and emotional states

Although we previously noted that behavioral phenotypes need to encompass strengths and weaknesses [2], this recommendation has taken on renewed meaning because of recent advances in the science of positive psychology. Beyond reducing distress associated with psychiatric symptoms or maladaptive behaviors, positive psychology identifies and enhances those emotions, virtues, and states that help people to lead happy, meaningful, and productive lives. As framed by Seligman [55], one might examine positive emotions about the past, present, or future (eg, contentment, forgiveness, savoring, mindfulness, hope), character strengths and virtues (eg, kindness, capacity to love and be loved, curiosity, appreciation of beauty, transcendence), and engagement and meaning (eg, flow, purpose, serving something larger than one's self).

Recently, Dykens [56] applied these concepts to persons who have genetic syndromes and others with intellectual disabilities. We briefly note that behavioral phenotype research holds considerable promise for positive psychologists, because some syndromes have an increased probability of showing certain strengths. Although preliminary, some examples include a proneness toward kindness, forgiveness, and humor in persons who have Down syndrome; nurturance in persons who have Prader-Willi syndrome; and zest and appreciation of beauty, especially music, in individuals who have Williams syndrome. Some syndromes involve behaviors or proficiencies that invite so-called flow or when persons are so engaged with an activity that they lose a sense of self and time [57]. Persons who have Prader-Willi syndrome seem to be in states of flow as they solve jigsaw puzzles, as do musicians who have Williams syndrome as they practice or perform [56]. Increased flow inoculates against depression and enhances well-being.

We end this article with a call to push the envelope even farther in behavioral phenotypic research, including a return to basics and paying greater attention to understudied but important sources of within-syndrome behavioral variability: development across the lifespan, gender, and other participant variables, such as life stressors, pain, and abuse. It also includes a need for more flexible and novel measures of specific behaviors, especially behaviors that might represent endophenotypes or show promising ties to genotypes. Although psychiatric disorders, cognition, and language traditionally have formed the basis of phenotypic studies, so too might positive emotions and states. In addition to existing behavioral domains, perhaps some of these positive attributes will prove just as informative in making connections between genes, brain, and behavior while simultaneously enhancing the well-being of persons who have genetic syndromes.

Acknowledgments

The work summarized in this article was supported by NICHD R01HD35681, R03HD50468, and P30HD15052 to the Vanderbilt Kennedy Center. The authors are grateful for the support of the National Down Syndrome Society, Williams Syndrome Association, and Prader-Willi Syndrome Association in our ongoing work.

References

[1] Flint J, Yule W. Behavioural phenotypes. In: Rutter R, Taylor E, Hersov L, editors. Child and adolescent psychiatry: modern approaches. 3rd edition. London: Blackwell Scientific; 1994. p. 666–87.

[2] Dykens EM. Measuring behavioral phenotypes: provocations from the "new genetics." Am J Ment Retard 1995;99:522–32.

[3] Hodapp RM, Dykens EM. Strengthening behavioral research on genetic mental retardation disorders. Am J Ment Retard 2001;106:4–15.

[4] Blackford JU. Statistical issues in developmental epidemiology and developmental disabilities research: confounding variables, small sample size, and numerous outcome variables. Int Rev Res Ment Retard 2007;33:93–120.

[5] Hodapp RM. Direct and indirect behavioral effects of different genetic disorders of mental retardation. Am J Ment Retard 1997;102:67–79.

[6] Gersh M, Goodart SA, Pasztor LM, et al. Evidence for a distinctive region causing a cat-like cry in patients with 5p deletions. Am J Hum Genet 1995;56:1404–10.

[7] Dykens EM, Maxwell M, Pantino E, et al. Assessment of hyperphagia in Prader-Willi syndrome. 2006; in press.

[8] Sullivan K, Hatton D, Hammer J, et al. ADHD symptoms in children with FXS. Am J Med Genet A 2006;140:2275–88.

[9] Dykens EM, Hodapp RM, Finucane B. Genetics and mental retardation syndromes: a new look at behavior and interventions. Baltimore (MD): Paul H. Brookes Publishing Company; 2000.

[10] Hodapp RM, Dykens EM. Mental retardation's two cultures of behavioral research. Am J Ment Retard 1994;98:675–87.

[11] Dykens EM, Hodapp RM. Research in mental retardation: toward an etiologic approach. J Child Psychol Psychiatry 2001;42:49–71.

[12] Dykens EM. Are jigsaw puzzles "spared" in persons with Prader-Willi syndrome? J Child Psychol Psychiatry 2002;43:343–52.

[13] Hodapp RM, Dykens EM, Ort SI, et al. Changing patterns of intellectual strengths and weaknesses in males with fragile X syndrome. J Autism Dev Disord 1991;21:503–16.

[14] Dykens EM, Rosner BA, Ly T, et al. Music and anxiety in Williams syndrome: a harmonious or discordant relationship? Am J Ment Retard 2005;110:346–58.

[15] Wang P, Doherty S, Rourke SB, et al. Unique profile of visuo-perceptual skills in a genetic syndrome. Brain Cogn 1995;29:54–65.

[16] Philofsky A, Hephburn SL, Hayes A, et al. Linguistic and cognitive functioning and autism symptoms in young children with fragile X syndrome. Am J Ment Retard 2004;109:208–18.

[17] Dykens EM, Cassidy SB, King BH. Maladaptive behavior differences in Prader-Willi syndrome due to paternal deletion versus maternal uniparental disomy. Am J Ment Retard 1999;104:67–77.

[18] Vogels A, Matthijis G, Lugius E, et al. Chromosome 15 maternal uniparental disomy and psychosis in Prader-Willi syndrome. J Med Genet 2003;40:72–3.

[19] Mobbs D, Garrett AS, Menon V, et al. Anomalous brain activation during face and gaze processing in Williams syndrome. Neurology 2004;62:2070–6.

[20] Hatton DD, Sideris J, Skinner M, et al. Autistic behavior in children with fragile X syndrome: prevalence, stability and impact of FMRP. Am J Med Genet A 2006;140:1804–13.

[21] Karmiloff-Smith A. Crucial differences between developmental cognitive neuroscience and adult neuropsychology. Dev Neuropsychol 1997;13:513–24.

[22] Kasari C, Freeman SFN. Task-related social behavior in children with Down syndrome. Am J Ment Retard 2002;106:253–64.

[23] Pitcairn TK, Wishart JG. Reactions of young children with Down syndrome to an impossible task. Brit J Dev Psychol 1994;12:485–9.

[24] Miller J. Lexical development in young children with Down syndrome. In: Chapman R, editor. Processes in language acquisition and disorders. St. Louis (MO): Mosby; 1992. p. 202–16.
[25] Fidler DJ, Philofsky A, Hepburn SL, et al. Nonverbal requesting and problem-solving by toddlers with Down syndrome. Am J Ment Retard 2005;110:312–22.
[26] Fidler DJ. The emergence of a syndrome-specific personality profile in young children with Down syndrome. In: Rondal JA, Perera J, editors. Down syndrome: neurobehavioural specificity. London: John Wiley & Sons; 2006. p. 139–52.
[27] Chapman RS, Hesketh LJ. Behavioral phenotype of individuals with Down syndrome. Ment Retard Dev Disabil Res Rev 2000;6:84–95.
[28] Jarrold C, Baddeley AD, Hewes AK, et al. A longitudinal assessment of diverging verbal and non-verbal abilities in the Williams syndrome phenotype. Cortex 2001;37:423–31.
[29] Davidson P, Prasher V, Janicki MP. Mental health, intellectual disabilities, and the aging process. Oxford (UK): Blackwell Publishing; 2003.
[30] Bittles AH, Glasson EJ. Clinical, social, and ethical implications of changing life expectancy in Down syndrome. Dev Med Child Neurol 2004;46:282–6.
[31] Zigman WB, Schupf N, Wegiel J, et al. Aging and Alzheimer's disease in people with mental retardation. Int Rev Res Ment Retard 2006;34: in press.
[32] Cherniske EM, Carpenter TO, Klaiman C, et al. Multisystem study of 20 older adults with Williams syndrome. Am J Med Genet A 2004;131:255–64.
[33] Dykens EM. Anxiety, fears, and phobias in persons with Williams syndrome. Dev Neuropsychol 2003;23:291–316.
[34] Devenny DA, Krinsky-McHale SJ, Kittler PM, et al. Age-associated memory changes in adults with Williams syndrome. Dev Neuropsychol 2004;26:691–706.
[35] Dykens EM. Maladaptive and compulsive behavior in Prader-Willi syndrome: new insights from older adults. Am J Ment Retard 2004;109:142–53.
[36] Greco CM, Berman RF, Martin RM, et al. Neuropathology of fragile X-associated tremor/ataxia syndrome (FXTAS). Brain 2006;129:243–55.
[37] Hodapp RM, Dykens EM. Problems of girls and young women with mental retardation (intellectual disabilities). In: Bell-Dolan D, Foster S, Mash E, editors. Handbook of behavioral and emotional disorders in girls. New York: Kluwer Academic/Plenum Publishers; 2005. p. 239–62.
[38] Maccoby EE, Jacklin CN. The psychology of sex differences. Stanford (CA): Stanford University Press; 1974.
[39] American Psychiatric Association. Diagnostic and statistical manual of mental disorders. 4th edition-TR. Washington, DC: American Psychiatric Association; 2000.
[40] Ward L. Risk factors for Alzheimer's disease in Down syndrome. Inter Rev Res Ment Retard 2004;29:159–96.
[41] Einfeld SL, Tonge BJ, Florio T. Behavioral and emotional disturbances in individuals with Williams syndrome. Am J Ment Retard 1997;102:45–53.
[42] Dykens EM, Rosner BA. Refining behavioral phenotypes: personality-motivation in Williams and Prader-Willi syndromes. Am J Ment Retard 1999;104:158–69.
[43] Martin A, State M, Anderson GM, et al. Cerebrospinal fluid levels of oxytocin in Prader-Willi syndrome: a preliminary report. Biol Psychiatry 1998;44:1349–52.
[44] Dykens EM. Annotation: psychopathology in children with intellectual disability. J Child Psychol Psychiatry 2000;41:407–17.
[45] Sullivan PM, Knutson JF. Maltreatment and disabilities: a population-based epidemiological study. Child Abuse Negl 2000;24:1257–73.
[46] Gosch A, Pankau R. Personality characteristics and behavior problems in individuals of different ages with Williams syndrome. Dev Med Child Neurol 1997;39:527–33.
[47] Davies M, Udwin O, Howlin P. Adults with Williams syndrome. Br J Psychiatry 1998;172:273–6.

[48] Cutler SE, Nolen-Hoeksema S. Accounting for sex differences in depression through female victimization: childhood sexual abuse. Sex Roles 1991;24:425–38.

[49] Hodapp RM, Dykens EM. Measuring behavior in genetic disorders of mental retardation. Ment Retard Dev Disabil Res Rev 2005;11:340–6.

[50] Finucane BM, Konar D, Haas-Givler B, et al. The spasmodic upper-body squeeze: a characteristic behavior in Smith-Magenis syndrome. Dev Med Child Neurol 1994;36:78–83.

[51] Dykens EM. Contaminated and unusual food combinations: what do people with Prader-Willi syndrome choose? Ment Retard 2000;38:163–71.

[52] Abbeduto L, Murphy MM, Richmond EK, et al. Collaboration in referential communication: comparison of youth with Down syndrome or fragile X syndrome. Am J Ment Retard 2006;111:170–83.

[53] Feurer ID, Dimitropoulos A, Stone W, et al. The latent variable structure of the compulsive behaviour checklist in people with Prader-Willi syndrome. J Intellect Disabil Res 1998;42: 472–80.

[54] Bittell DC, Kibiryeva N, Butler MG. Expression of 4 genes between chromosome 15 breakpoints 1 and 2 and behavioral outcomes in Prader-Willi syndrome. Pediatrics 2006;118.

[55] Peterson C, Seligman M. Character strengths and virtues: a handbook and classification. New York: Oxford University Press; 2004.

[56] Dykens EM. Toward a positive psychology of mental retardation. Am J Orthopsychiatry 2006;76:185–93.

[57] Csikszentmihali M. Flow: the psychology of optimal experience. New York: Harper & Row; 1990.

ELSEVIER
SAUNDERS

Child Adolesc Psychiatric Clin N Am
16 (2007) 631–647

CHILD AND
ADOLESCENT
PSYCHIATRIC CLINICS
OF NORTH AMERICA

Social Phenotypes in Neurogenetic Syndromes

Carl Feinstein, MD*, Sonia Singh

*Department of Child & Adolescent Psychiatry, Lucile Packard Children's Hospital,
401 Quarry Road, MC 5719, Stanford, CA 94305, USA*

A major factor in the quest to define behavioral phenotypes has been the identification of a substantial and growing number of specific gene deletion or mutation syndromes that result in genetic neurodevelopmental disorders (GNDDs). These GNDDs are characterized by distinctive patterns of cognitive and behavioral features and congenital medical sequelae. Specific genotypes, defined by the biologically validated presence of known mutated or deleted genes, seem to result in distinctive behavioral phenotypes. In this article we focus on the distinctive social traits of several GNDDs. We begin by summarizing some of the trends and controversies in research to date. This step is necessary to explain why, for several disorders, social features were not mentioned in the earlier versions of some of the behavioral phenotypes and only recently have been studied in a systematic fashion.

Phenotype and behavioral phenotype: definitions

In this article, we rely on the general definition of a phenotype provided by Gottesman and Gould [1] as: "observable characteristics of an organism, which are the joint product of both genotypic and environmental influences." Although there are a handful of known, highly invariant genotype-to-behavioral phenotypic trait linkages, we rely on the definition of a behavioral phenotype provided by Dykens and Cassidy [2]: "The heightened probability or likelihood that people with a given syndrome will exhibit certain behavioral and developmental sequelae relative to those without the syndrome," in recognition of the behavioral heterogeneity generally present in all GNDDs. The clinical neuroscience research approach that has focused

---

* Corresponding author.
E-mail address: carlf@stanford.edu (C. Feinstein).

1056-4993/07/$ - see front matter © 2007 Elsevier Inc. All rights reserved.
doi:10.1016/j.chc.2007.03.006

on the developmental unfolding of behavioral phenotype in neurogenetic syndromes has been termed "behavioral neurogenetics" [3,4]. This approach is predicated on the concept that in individuals with a defined, biologically validated gene disorder, it is possible to follow the ontogeny of the resulting brain–cognitive-behavioral phenotype over the course of development from earliest childhood to adulthood.

Distinctions between "psychiatric phenotypes" and "behavioral phenotypes"

The major impetus driving research in the behavioral phenotypic expression of GNDDs followed from the distinctive behavioral features described in children with these disorders soon after their genetic etiology was confirmed [5]. In the first generation of reporting discoveries in behavioral phenotypes, clinically oriented researchers created a detailed narrative account of the characteristic behavioral traits for a given GNDD based on direct observation and clinical experience [5]. In many cases, this account was followed by a second generation of research that entailed widely used and standardized "off the shelf" structured and semi-structured research diagnostic interviews that used Diagnostic and Statistical Manual (DSM) and World Health Organization diagnostic criteria and behavioral checklists eliciting standardized behavior symptom data for well-accepted dimensions of psychopathology. The findings from this research approach generated prevalence rates for the various established DSM/World Health Organization psychiatric disorders in the various GNDDs. In some cases in which these data were the main source of behavioral information regarding a given syndrome, the resulting patterns might more accurately have been called "psychiatric phenotypes" to distinguish them from true behavioral phenotypes, because there is more to behavior than psychiatric symptoms.

There are major problems with this second-generation "psychiatric phenotype" approach. Most importantly, psychiatry's diagnostic classification system describes disorders increasingly acknowledged to be heterogeneous, lacking biologic validation, and having multifactorial, polygenic origins [1]. In contrast, the GNDDs, although influenced phenotypically by environmental factors, have a biologically validated, far better understood genotypic origin and phenotypic specificity than the less-validated DSM psychiatric disorders from which they are reported to suffer. There is a conceptual mismatch between the specificity and biologic validity of the GNDD disorders and the heterogeneity and lack of biologic validity of the DSM disorders that have been superimposed as the "psychiatric phenotype" on these GNDDs. An additional mismatch arises from the fact that several of the GNDDs meet criteria for multiple DSM disorders, whereas different GNNDs may have applied to them the same "psychiatric phenotype" (eg, attention deficit hyperactivity disorder, anxiety disorder, autistic disorder).

Another problem with applying DSM-based psychiatric phenotypes to GNDDs is that many of the most significant and distinctive behaviors found for some of the neurodevelopmental disorders have no representation in the DSM. Consequently, behaviors that uniquely distinguish the behavioral phenotypes of the GNDDs are not accounted for in a DSM-based psychiatric phenotyping approach. As seen in the discussion of specific GNDDs, there are situations in which there seems to be a cleavage within specific GNDDs—even in the presence of a behavioral phenotype—between individuals who have a major psychiatric disorder (eg, schizophrenia, autism) and individuals who do not.

Social trait aspects of behavioral phenotypes

Distinctive social phenotypes have only gradually become recognized for most of the GNDDs, with two significant exceptions: fragile X syndrome and Williams syndrome. For these two conditions, the social abnormalities were so prominent that the early clinical observations leading to the initial formulation of their behavioral phenotypes highlighted them. Study of these two syndromes has led the way in the exploration of neurogenetic influences on social cognition and social behavior.

Advances in the understanding of the social phenotype in other GNDDs were likely delayed by several interrelated issues: The failure of most standardized psychiatric phenotyping studies to ascertain symptoms for autistic spectrum disorders (the diagnostic category in which most attention is paid to social impairment), controversies interpreting the presence of autistic (social deficit) symptoms when they are found, the frequent omission of measures of adaptive behavior in defining behavioral phenotypes, and controversies as to whether all significant social deficits must be based on a comorbid diagnosis of an autistic spectrum disorder.

Diagnostic overshadowing: attributing social deficits solely to cognitive deficiency

Diagnostic overshadowing [6,7] also remains an unfortunate tendency to attribute the cause of behavior problems and social deficits in GNDDs solely to cognitive deficiencies rather than to social influences, co-occurring psychiatric disorders, or independent genetic influences on social cognition. Deficits in social functioning found in individuals with lower-than-average IQ are particularly likely to be attributed uncritically to cognitive deficits, even if they are distinctive features of a GNDD. It is not easy, however, to decide whether a pattern of poor social skills for any given GNDD is part of a particular behavioral phenotype—a common downstream effect of psychosocial disadvantage and stigmatization—or is secondary to reduced cognitive capacity.

Distinctions between commonly occurring social impairments and autistic spectrum symptoms

Many cognitively normal children who do not have a GNDD or autism spectrum disorder still have social impairments [8]. Over decades, sociometric studies repeatedly have confirmed that approximately 15% of all children are considered unpopular, have problematic social skills, and are avoided by their peers [8]. Cognitively normal children with psychiatric disorders (eg, attention deficit hyperactivity disorder) repeatedly have been shown to have poor social functioning that may not respond to standard treatment for that disorder [9]. When social deficits are present in the GNDDs, it is not entirely clear whether they are caused by the genotypic abnormality or simply reflect the range of social competence found in all groups of children.

Paucity of adaptive behavior data regarding social functioning

It is not clear why adaptive behavior scales were used so rarely in studies of behavioral phenotypes. Possibly they were viewed by researchers as nonspecific, downstream indicators of cognitive deficiency rather than as sources of information about behavior pertinent to distinctive behavioral phenotypes. As a result, social adaptive information for some of the GNDDs has been lacking, such as could have been provided by the Vineland Adaptive Behavior Scale [10]. The failure to use adaptive behavior measures was also unfortunate because abundant normative social functioning data were available for developmentally disabled children with which the findings of any specific disability group could have been compared.

Distinctions between endophenotypic traits and formal psychiatric diagnoses

A further conceptual issue complicates deciding whether a behavior phenotypic trait found in a GNDD is interpretable as a part of a psychiatric diagnosis. This issue concerns the concept of the endophenotype in psychiatry, which was given little attention until the last few years. Endophenotypes refer to measurable traits associated with underlying susceptibility genes. These traits are associated with illness, are heritable and state independent (present even when the illness is not active), and co-segregate within families of probands. Endophenotypes for heritable disorders occur more frequently in nonaffected family members of probands than in the general population [1]. Specifically, these endophenotypic traits, although they may bear resemblance to symptom criteria for the illness being studied, may not meet criteria for that illness. For the scientific understanding of behavioral phenotypes in GNDDs it may be more heuristic to view these phenotypes as endophenotypes rather than as psychiatric disorders.

The concept of an endophenotype has been particularly relevant to studying the behavioral phenotype in 22q11 deletion syndrome, in which a critical issue has been determining which 30% of children with this condition will develop a schizophrenic disorder by young adulthood [11–14]. In research directed at finding the vulnerable 30%, it could be stated that the cognitive-behavioral phenotype in children with velocardiofacial syndrome (VCFS) is an endophenotype for prodromal schizophrenia.

The concept of endophenotype was used more recently in elucidating possible familial mechanisms to explain the puzzling fact that approximately 7% to 10% of children who have Down syndrome—typically a syndrome associated with high sociability—are autistic [15]. Recent reports of high rates of autistic spectrum disorder symptoms (and attention deficit hyperactivity disorder) in premutation carriers for fragile X [16] suggested that such traits might constitute an autism susceptibility endophenotype associated with fragile X premutation carriers.

Fragile X syndrome

Fragile X syndrome is the most common genetic cause of mental retardation and developmental delay. It occurs in approximately 1 in every 4000 boys and 1 in every 6000 to 8000 girls and is caused by an expansion mutation of the FMR1 gene of the X chromosome [17]. Symptoms are typically more severe in boys than girls, because girls retain one X chromosome, whereas boys who have fragile X syndrome have none. The behavioral phenotype of fragile X syndrome includes several cognitive deficits and behavioral anomalies, such as attention deficits, gaze aversion, hand flapping, and hand biting [18–20].

The social phenotype of fragile X syndrome, especially in boys, is characterized by social withdrawal, anxiety, high emotionality, poor eye contact, and atypical speech [21]. Although girls usually suffer from milder impairments, social anxiety and withdrawal are still relatively common, even in individuals with IQs in the normal range, which implies that their social dysfunction is not merely a consequence of general cognitive disability but also involves specific problems in social cognition [22–24]. Girls with normal IQs and full mutations have impairments in social interaction, organization difficulties, impulsivity, shyness, and moodiness [25,26]. Children who have fragile X syndrome also have theory of mind impairments that are qualitatively different from groups with other learning abilities [27].

Social gaze is strikingly impaired in boys with fragile X syndrome. Greeting behavior is characterized by distinct avoidance of eye contact, even when initiating a handshake or offering a salutation [28]. In tasks such as determining gaze direction of people in photos, boys with fragile X syndrome fare poorly compared with matched controls. Neuroimaging, electrophysiologic, and neuroendocrine studies have demonstrated neuronal dysfunction involving the fusiform gyrus plus clear evidence that direct gaze is processed abnormally. Studies also have shown that face-to-face gaze and eye contact are associated with hyperarousal and a high level of stress [29–32].

A substantial percentage of children, especially boys, who have fragile X syndrome meet DSM criteria for autism. Numerous studies document a rate of autism in fragile X syndrome between 25% and 47%, using various diagnostic methods [33–38]. Some investigators found that the severity of autistic symptoms declines with age [39]; however, other studies indicated high rates of autism at all ages [40]. Recently, behavioral phenotyping studies of carriers of the premutation for fragile X syndrome have been associated with an increased rate of autistic symptoms [16,41].

There has been much debate as to whether "autism" found in fragile X syndrome is truly the same as that seen in idiopathic autism [42]. The key point is that fragile X syndrome is a biologically validated, extensively studied condition with a highly specific behavioral phenotype (in boys), whereas autism is a somewhat more phenotypically heterogeneous disorder that seems to involve many genes [43]. Currently, it is difficult to say more than that the mutation responsible for the autistic-like behaviors in fragile X syndrome is probably one of many genetic configurations that can lead to the DSM categorical diagnosis of autism. In this sense, fragile X syndrome presents one behavioral genetic model of how autism can occur. If it differs in some ways from the autism phenotype seen in "idiopathic" autism, it is likely that as other gene mechanisms are discovered, numerous slightly different biologically validated phenotypic varieties of autism will be identified.

Down syndrome

Down syndrome is caused by trisomy of all or a critical portion of chromosome 21 [44]. It is the most common chromosomal cause of mental retardation and occurs in 1 in 1000 live births, with the incidence increasing with maternal age. Down syndrome is associated with distinctive facial features, congenital heart disease, duodenal stenosis, and mental retardation [44–46].

In most cases, children who have Down syndrome tend to be engaging and affectionate [47]. Compared with adults with learning disabilities matched on age and developmental quotient, a group of adults who have Down syndrome had lower prevalence of aggression, antisocial behavior, property destruction, disturbing others at night, attention seeking, untruthfulness, excessive activity, and excessive noise [48]. Despite language impairments, social communication and relationships seem to be comparable to normally developing controls [49]. Some social processing deficits have been found in recognizing facial expression overall, particularly surprise and fear.

In an investigation of the verbal communication, play, and language skills of children who have Down syndrome, Sigman and colleagues [50] found that the children "engaged in more functional and symbolic play than normal children of equal mental and language age." The children also requested objects and help with objects more frequently than the control group. Similarly, in study of task-related social behavior, Kasari and Freeman [51] found that children who have Down syndrome "looked to an adult and requested help more frequently" than normally developing children and children with idiopathic mental retardation.

In contrast to the more prevalent phenotype of strong sociability observed in Down syndrome is the repeated finding that 7% to 10% of people who have Down syndrome have autistic traits that meet diagnostic criteria for DSM autism [52–58]. This finding indicates that something about Down syndrome confers approximately a tenfold increased risk for autism. Ghaziuddin [15] studied first-degree relatives of individuals who have autistic Down syndrome and compared them with first-degree relatives of individuals who have Down syndrome who had no autistic traits. The author found that the relatives of the individuals who have autistic Down syndrome had a significantly higher rate of traits of the broader autism phenotype. This finding suggested that either Down syndrome is a potent risk factor for autism when other risk genes for autism are present or that something about the chromosomal abnormality predisposes toward autistic traits.

Prader-Willi syndrome

Prader-Willi syndrome is a genetic disorder that usually involves a deletion or uniparental disomy in chromosome 15. Prader-Willi syndrome affects approximately 1 in 10,000 to 15,000 births and is characterized by hyperphagia, hypotonia, hypogonadism, diminished fetal activity, obesity, muscular hypotonia, mental retardation, short stature, hypogonadotropic hypogonadism, small hands and feet, developmental delays, and distinct facial features [59].

Although many studies have considered the behavioral phenotype of Prader-Willi syndrome, few have focused exclusively on the social deficits associated with the syndrome. A study by Dykens and Cassidy [2] found higher frequencies of stubbornness, tantrums, disobedience, and talking too much in children who have Prader-Willi syndrome. Thirty-four percent of tantrums that were reported involved a physical attack of others. Other antisocial behaviors noted in Prader-Willi syndrome include lying, stealing, and hiding, often to obtain or hoard food [60,61]. Research also shows that patients who have Prader-Willi syndrome frequently suffer from compulsive and impulsive-aggressive behaviors [62]. High rates of specific obsessive-compulsive behaviors not related to food—mainly compulsions concerning a need to tell or ask (ie, repeated questioning)—have been identified [63,64].

A survey by Greenswag [65] described solitary behavior, social withdrawal, and poor peer relations in Prader-Willi Syndrome personalities. A later study estimated that most patients preferred being alone, observing that many patients displayed argumentative, verbally abusive, and aggressive behavior toward others [66]. Keonig and colleagues [67] described the performance of patients who have Prader-Willi syndrome on an experimental task, the Social Attribution Task, which measures a specific ability necessary for interpreting social information. The poor performance of the individuals who have Prader-Willi syndrome compared to a cognitively matched group suggested that individuals who have Prader-Willi syndrome have difficulty recognizing social cues and interpreting social situations. In semi-structured interviews of 28 individuals who have Prader-Willi syndrome, many mentioned the importance of friendship; however, most of the participants had few actual friendships and few of them referred to a "best friend." It is important to note that hyperphagia and obesity often restrict the lives of patients who have Prader-Willi syndrome to secluded environments, which leaves them fewer opportunities and more limited social contexts in which to develop and interact [68].

Smith-Magenis syndrome

Smith-Magenis syndrome is a genetic disorder associated with a deletion of band 17p11.2. The typical phenotype of an individual who has Smith-Magenis syndrome includes brachycephaly, midface hypoplasia, prognathism, hoarse voice, speech delay with or without hearing loss, psychomotor and growth retardation, and behavior problems [69]. The prevalence of Smith-Magenis syndrome is estimated to be as high as 1 in every 25,000 births [70].

In a study on maladaptive behaviors of children and adolescents who have Smith-Magenis syndrome, Dykens and Smith [71] reported affective lability, property destruction, impulsivity, nervousness, physical aggression, and argumentative behavior in most participants. The study also revealed a stronger demand for one-on-one attention among patients who have Smith-Magenis syndrome compared to individuals who have Prader-Willi syndrome and mixed intellectual ability. In an article based on interviews with teachers and caregivers of children who have Smith-Magenis syndrome, Barbara Haas-Givler [72] described the following:

> "Children with Smith-Magenis syndrome are very adult-oriented, with a sometimes insatiable need for individualized attention from the teacher (and other adults); when this is denied, aggression toward others, behavioral outbursts, tantrums, and self-injurious behavior frequently result. Individuals with Smith-Magenis syndrome have engaging and endearing personalities (impish smile, selfhugging, good eye contact), are eager to please, and often have a well-developed sense of humor. They enjoy and thrive on adult attention. In the classroom, they are able to learn, remember and recall all the names of fellow teachers and other students."

In our direct clinical experience, the intense attention-seeking behavior directed at adults by individuals who have Smith-Magenis syndrome—with the attendant rage outbursts when the individualized attention is not forthcoming or is withdrawn—is also a manifestation of intense egocentrism and an inability to see the perspective or subjective needs of the other. Although an as-yet untested hypothesis, this pattern suggests deficits in theory of mind.

Turner syndrome

Turner syndrome is a genetic disorder associated with partial or complete absence of one of the two X chromosomes in a phenotypic girl [73]. It occurs in approximately 1 in 2000 live female births. The physical phenotype includes short stature and abnormal pubertal development and a webbed neck, renal dysgenesis, and cardiac malformation [74]. Women who have Turner syndrome are also at high risk of premature ovarian failure [75].

Several studies have pinpointed distinct psychosocial difficulties associated with Turner syndrome, particularly in the areas of social maturity, social cognition, social relationships, and self-esteem [76,77]. According to parental report, girls who have Turner syndrome have lower self-esteem and fewer friends and generally engage in fewer social activities than age-matched controls [76]. The question of whether these social deficits are the result of other aspects of the Turner syndrome phenotype also has been addressed by several studies. Downey and colleagues [78] found that women who have Turner syndrome have more impairment in social functioning than women with constitutional short stature. A study by Schmidt and colleagues [79] compared women with premature ovarian failure, women who have Turner syndrome, and normal controls on scales of shyness, social anxiety and self-esteem. They found that women with premature ovarian failure and women who have Turner syndrome had significantly lower scores on all three scales. They did not, however, find a significant difference between the Turner syndrome group and the premature ovarian failure group. In a study that compared girls who have Turner syndrome to their sisters, the affected girls had more social, thought, and attention problems and poor adaptive socialization skills compared to their own sisters [77]. Reports also have found that girls who have Turner syndrome who undergo hormone treatment typically experience an increase in self-concept though the course of adolescence [80].

An investigation by Lawrence and colleagues [81] into gaze processing in Turner syndrome uncovered other impairments associated with social functioning. Although women who have Turner syndrome performed normally on facial recognition tasks, they showed significant impairment in classification of expression from the upper face, particularly for expressions of "fear" from the eyes. Researchers hypothesized that this impairment is the result of overresponsiveness of the amygdala (because of its enlarged size) to direct gaze or fear in faces [81,82].

Williams syndrome

Williams syndrome is a rare genetic disorder caused by a microdeletion on chromosome 7q11.23 [83–85]. It is characterized by infantile hypercalcemia, hyperacusis, distinctive facial features, and abnormalities of the heart, muscles, and kidneys, usually accompanied by mild to moderate mental retardation [86]. The brain morphology of Williams syndrome has distinctive alterations, some of which can be correlated with distinctive neurocognitive deficits in visual-spatial processing [85].

Hypersociability is a hallmark of the social phenotype of Williams syndrome. Despite initial delays in vocabulary acquisition, grammar use, and gesturing, individuals who have Williams syndrome exhibit a strong interest in social interaction throughout their lives. As infants they are unusually interested in faces, sometimes staring and smiling at the experimenters or administrators of psychological evaluations rather than completing the assigned task [87,88]. As children they are commonly described as "overly friendly." Children who have Williams syndrome often approach strangers and attempt to engage them in conversation, which concerns parents [89,90]. Studies have shown that individuals who have Williams syndrome consistently rate unfamiliar faces more approachable compared with normal and mentally disabled controls, regardless of facial expression [91].

A study by Doyle and colleagues [92] that compared the social behavior of children who have Williams syndrome to typically developing children and children who have Down syndrome concluded that the sociability characteristic of Williams syndrome cannot be attributed to the cognitive impairments associated with the disorder. Individuals who have Williams syndrome consistently scored higher than individuals who have Down syndrome who are also cognitively impaired and normally developing individuals on nearly every aspect of sociability measured, which implied that it is not merely a "lack of understanding of the social conventions governing contact with others."

Despite their highly sociable nature, individuals who have Williams syndrome are generally more socially anxious, and by adulthood, many of them experience failure to develop and maintain friendships and suffer from social isolation and maladaptive and unsatisfying peer interactions [93–96]. It seems that individuals who have Williams syndrome rely primarily on superficial signals but fail to recognize more subtle social cues in their interactions with others [97]. Impairments in theory of mind and limitations in the capacity to interpret more complex facial emotional expressions are the rule [87,95,98,99]. Individuals who have Williams syndrome generally have fewer friends and have difficulty establishing and maintaining friendships with peers. Other studies reported generalized and anticipatory anxiety in most patients who have Williams syndrome, with 96% showing specific phobias [93].

The pattern of strengths and deficits that comprise the social phenotype in Williams syndrome illustrates that social functioning has several dimensions that can be disassociated from each other, including affiliativeness (which is a strength in Williams syndrome), empathy and intersubjective awareness (also a relative strength), and higher order theory of mind involving perspective taking and the incorporation of social contextual cues (a pronounced deficit in Williams syndrome) [95]. In the words of these authors: "...the behavioral and personality profile of people with WBS has produced a complex picture, suggesting a paradoxical combination of high sociability and empathy but poor social relationships and difficulties in social functioning."

Velocardiofacial syndrome

VCFS is associated with a microdeletion at the chromosome region 22q11.2 [100]. The prevalence of VCFS is approximately 1 in 4000, with most cases being de novo mutations [101,102]. Symptoms include cleft palate, velopharyngeal insufficiency, cardiac defects, and distinctive facial features [103–105]. Individuals who have VCFS are likely to have somewhat reduced intelligence, with a mean IQ of approximately 70, and a dramatic delay in early language development. They have receptive and higher order language deficits, abstract reasoning deficits, and visual-spatial deficits [106,107]. The behavioral phenotype for younger children who have VCFS is characterized by mood lability, social withdrawal, awkwardness and shyness, attentional problems, overactive and disinhibited behaviors, and many anxiety symptoms [12,101,108,109].

Approximately 30% of individuals who have VCFS develop psychosis—generally schizophrenia or schizo-affective disorder—by adolescence or young adulthood, which accounts for approximately 2% of all cases of schizophrenia [13,110–113]. VCFS has been referred to as a neurodevelopmental model for schizophrenia, because childhood prodromal cognitive and behavioral features (eg, attentional problems, language problems, social deficits, and learning disabilities) that are characteristic of VCFS have been found consistently in studies of children and adolescents at high risk for schizophrenia [11,114].

The social skills difficulties found in individuals who have VCFS have been widely reported and include communication difficulties, withdrawn and shy behavior, difficulties initiating interactions, and decreased repertoire of facial expressions [115–117]. This finding has led some researchers to consider whether children with this social and communication phenotype have autistic spectrum disorder. Fine and colleagues [115] approached this problem with the premise that applying standard research interviews, such as the Autism Diagnostic Interview-Revised, could clarify the question of autism as a feature of VCFS. This approach raised interesting questions. Social and communication deficits are shared features of autism spectrum disorders and schizophrenia (including premorbid schizotypal states).

Currently, there is no clarity as to how social and communication deficit traits seen in these different neurodevelopmental disorders (autism and schizophrenia) might be the same or different or what the implications might be. It is also not known what the findings would be if assessment instruments for autism were to be applied to a highly vulnerable or prodromal preschizophrenic or schizophrenic population. Some prodromal schizophrenic individuals possibly would exceed the threshold for the diagnosis of autism on the tests. What would that finding mean, however? In our view, parsimony dictates that if an individual meets criteria for schizophrenia or develops schizophrenia within a reasonable time period after autism testing, then a positive finding for autism should be considered a false-positive result. This methodologic quandary is ultimately less interesting than a finding that the social communications deficits seen in these two disorders—autism and schizophrenia—are, in some cases, indistinguishable from each other.

Summary

A review of the social phenotypes seen in GNDDs indicates many subtle variations and complex features that distinguish the conditions from each other. The net effect is to remind us that social functioning is not a monolithic trait but a complex set of interacting operations. A wide variety of social functioning profiles that result from selective central nervous system social substrate "hits" (secondary to the specific gene–brain features of any given GNDD) seems to be emerging from the science of behavioral neurogenetics, which may serve to illuminate the mechanisms of sociability in nonimpaired humans.

References

[1] Gottesman IL, Gould TD. The endophenotype concept in psychiatry: etymology and strategic intentions. Am J Psychiatry 2003;160(4):636–45.
[2] Dykens EM, Cassidy SB. Correlates of maladaptive behavior in children and adults with Prader-Willi syndrome. Am J Med Genet 1995;60(6):546–9.
[3] Reiss AL, Eliez S, Schmitt JE, et al. Brain imaging in neurogenetic conditions: realizing the potential of behavioral neurogenetics research. Ment Retard Dev Disabil Res Rev 2000; 6(3):186–97.
[4] Reiss A, Dant C. The behavioral neurogenetics of fragile X syndrome: analyzing gene-brain-behavior relationships in child developmental psychopathologies. Dev Psychopathol 2003;15(4):927–78.
[5] Hodapp RM, Dykens EM. Measuring behavior in genetic disorders of mental retardation. Ment Retard Dev Disabil Res Rev 2005;11(4):340–6.
[6] Jopp DA, Keys CB. Diagnostic overshadowing reviewed and reconsidered. Am J Ment Retard 2001;106(5):416–33.
[7] Reiss SS, Szykzko J. Diagnostic overshadowing and professional experience with mentally retarded persons. Am J Ment Defic 1983;87(4):396–402.
[8] Hymel S, Vaillancourt T, McDougall P, et al. Peer acceptance and rejection in childhood. In: Smith P, Hart C, editors. Handbook of child social development. Oxford (UK): Blackwell Publishing; 2002. p. 265–79.
[9] Hoza B, Gerdes A, Mrug S, et al. Peer-assessed outcomes in the multimodality treatment study of children with attention deficit hyperactivity disorder. J Clin Child Adolesc Psychol 2005;34(1):74–86.

[10] Sparrow S, Balla D, Cicchetti D. Vineland Adaptive Behavior Scales. Circle Pines (MN): American Guidance Service; 1984.
[11] Eliez S, Feinstein C. Velo-cardio-facial syndrome (deletion 22q11.2): a homogeneous neurodevelopmental model for schizophrenia. In: Keshavan M, Kennedy J, Murray R, editors. Neurodevelopment and schizophrenia. Cambridge (UK): Cambridge University Press; 2004. p. 121–37.
[12] Feinstein C, Eliez S, Blasey C, et al. Psychiatric disorders and behavioral problems in children with velocardiofacial syndrome: usefulness as phenotypic indicators of schizophrenia risk. Biol Psychiatry 2002;51(4):312–8.
[13] Gothelf D, Eliez S, Thompson T, et al. COMT genotype predicts longitudinal cognitive decline and psychosis in 22q11.2 deletion syndrome. Nat Neurosci 2005;8(11): 1500–2.
[14] Baker KD, Skuse DH. Adolescents and young adults with 22q11 deletion syndrome: psychopathology in an at-risk group. Br J Psychiatry 2005;186:115–20.
[15] Ghaziuddin M. Autism in Down's syndrome: a family history study. J Intellect Disabil Res 2000;44(Pt 5):562–6.
[16] Farzin F, Perry H, Hessl D, et al. Autism spectrum disorders and attention-deficit/hyperactivity disorder in boys with the fragile X premutation. J Dev Behav Pediatr 2006;27(2 Suppl):S137–44.
[17] Hagerman R. Clinical and molecular aspects of fragile X syndrome. In: Tager-Flusberg H, editor. Neurodevelopmental disorders. Cambridge (MA): MIT Press; 1999. p. 27–42.
[18] Eliez SFC. The fragile X syndrome: bridging the gap from gene to behavior. Curr Opin Psychiatry 2001;14:443–9.
[19] Hagerman R. Physical and behavioral phenotype. In: Hagerman R, Hagerman P, editors. Fragile X syndrome: diagnosis, treatment, and research. Baltimore (MD): The Johns Hopkins University Press; 2002. p. 3–109.
[20] Mazzocco M. Advances in research on the fragile X syndrome. Ment Retard Dev Disabil Res Rev 2000;6:96–106.
[21] Baumardner T, Reiss A, Freund L, et al. Specification of the neurobehavioral phenotype in males with fragile X syndrome. Pediatrics 1995;95:744–52.
[22] Lachiewicz AM. Abnormal behaviors of young girls with fragile X syndrome. Am J Med Genet 1992;43(1–2):72–7.
[23] Freund LS, Reiss AL, Abrams MT. Psychiatric disorders associated with fragile X in the young female. Pediatrics 1993;91(2):321–9.
[24] Mazzocco MM, Pennington BF, Hagerman RJ. Social cognition skills among females with fragile X. J Autism Dev Disord 1994;24(4):473–85.
[25] Sobesky WE, Taylor AK, Pennington BF, et al. Molecular/clinical correlations in females with fragile X. Am J Med Genet 1996;64(2):340–5.
[26] Mazzocco MM, Pennington BF, Hagerman RJ. The neurocognitive phenotype of female carriers of fragile X: additional evidence for specificity. J Dev Behav Pediatr 1993;14(5): 328–35.
[27] Cornish K, Burack JA, Rahman A, et al. Theory of mind deficits in children with fragile X syndrome. J Intellect Disabil Res 2005;49(Pt 5):372–8.
[28] Wolff PH, Gardner J, Paccla J, et al. The greeting behavior of fragile X males. Am J Ment Retard 1989;93(4):406–11.
[29] Garrett AS, Menon V, MacKenzie K, et al. Here's looking at you, kid: neural systems underlying face and gaze processing in fragile X syndrome. Arch Gen Psychiatry 2004;61(3): 281–8.
[30] Hessl DBB, Dyer-Friedman J, Reiss AL. Social behavior and cortisol reactivity in children with fragile X syndrome. J Child Psychol Psychiatry 2006;47(6):602–10.
[31] Belser R, Sudhalter V. Arousal difficulties in males with fragile X syndrome: a preliminary report. Developmtal Brain Dysfunction 1995;80:270–9.

[32] Miller LJ, McIntosh DN, McGrath J, et al. Electrodermal responses to sensory stimuli in individuals with fragile X syndrome: a preliminary report. Am J Med Genet 1999;83(4): 268–79.

[33] Hatton DD, Sideris J, Skinner M, et al. Autistic behavior in children with fragile X syndrome: prevalence, stability, and the impact of FMRP. Am J Med Genet A 2006; 140(17):1804–13.

[34] Rogers S, Wehner E, Hagerman R. The behavioral phenotype in fragile X: symptoms of autism in very young children with fragile X syndrome, idiopathic autism, and other developmental disorders. J Dev Behav Pediatr 2001;22:409–17.

[35] Turk J, Grahan P. Fragile X syndrome, autism and autistic features. Autism 1997;1:175–97.

[36] Bailey D, Mesibov G, Hatton D, et al. Autistic behavior in young boys with fragile X syndrome. J Autism Dev Disord 1998;28:499–507.

[37] Demark J, Feldman M, Holden J. Behavioral relationship between autism and fragile X syndrome. Am J Ment Retard 2003;108:314–26.

[38] Kaufmann W, Corell R, Kau A, et al. Autisms spectrum disorder in fragile X syndrome: communication, social interaction, and specific behaviors. Am J Med Genet A 2004;129: 225–34.

[39] Reiss A, Freund L. Behavioral phenotype of fragile X syndrome: DSM-III-R autistic behavior in male children. Am J Med Genet 1992;43:35–46.

[40] Bailey D, Hatton D, Skinner M, et al. Autistic behavior, FMR1 protein, and developmental trajectories in young males with fragile X syndrome. J Autism Dev Disord 2001;31:165–74.

[41] Cornish K, Kogan C, Turk J, et al. The emerging fragile X premutation phenotype: evidence from the domain of social cognition. Brain Cogn 2005;57(1):53–60.

[42] Feinstein C, Reiss A. Autism: the point of view from fragile X studies. J Autism Dev Disord 1998;28(5):393–405.

[43] Szatmari P, Paterson AD, Zwaigenbaum L, et al. Mapping autism risk loci using genetic linkage and chromosomal rearrangements. Nature Genetics 2007;39(3):319–28.

[44] Korenberg JR, Chen XN, Schipper R, et al. Down syndrome phenotypes: the consequences of chromosomal imbalance. Proc Natl Acad Sci U S A 1994;91(11):4997–5001.

[45] Epstein CJ, Korenberg JR, Anneren G, et al. Protocols to establish genotype-phenotype correlations in down syndrome. Am J Hum Genet 1991;49(1):207–35.

[46] Roizen NJ, Patterson D. Down's syndrome. Lancet 2003;361(9365):1281–9.

[47] Moore DG, Oates JM, Hobson RP, et al. Cognitive and social factors in the development of infants with Down syndrome. Downs Syndr Res Pract 2002;8(2):43–52.

[48] Collacott RA, Cooper SA, Branford D, et al. Behaviour phenotype for Down's syndrome. Br J Psychiatry 1998;172:85–9.

[49] Laws G, Bishop D. Pragmatic language impairment and social deficits in Williams syndrome: a comparison with Down's syndrome and specific language impairment. Int J Lang Commun Disord 2004;39(1):45–64.

[50] Sigman M, Ruskin E, Arbeile S, et al. Continuity and change in the social competence of children with autism, Down syndrome, and developmental delays. Monogr Soc Res Child Dev 1999;64(1):1–114.

[51] Kasari C, Freeman SF. Task-related social behavior in children with Down syndrome. Am J Ment Retard 2001;106(3):253–64.

[52] Rasmussen P, Borjesson O, Wentz E, et al. Autistic disorders in Down syndrome: background factors and clinical correlates. Dev Med Child Neurol 2001;43(11):750–4.

[53] Capone GT, Grados MA, Kaufmann WE, et al. Down syndrome and comorbid autism-spectrum disorder: characterization using the aberrant behavior checklist. Am J Med Genet A 2005;134(4):373–80.

[54] Starr EM, Berument SK, Tomlins M, et al. Brief report: autism in individuals with Down syndrome. J Autism Dev Disord 2005;35(5):665–73.

[55] Kent L, Evans J, Paul M, et al. Comorbidity of autistic spectrum disorders in children with Down syndrome. Dev Med Child Neurol 1999;41(3):153–8.

[56] Howlin P, Wing L, Gould J. The recognition of autism in children with Down syndrome: implications for intervention and some speculations about pathology. Dev Med Child Neurol 1995;37(5):406–14.

[57] Bregman JD, Volkmar FR. Autistic social dysfunction and Down syndrome. J Am Acad Child Adolesc Psychiatry 1988;27(4):440–1.

[58] Ghaziuddin M. Autism in Down's syndrome: family history correlates. J Intellect Disabil Res 1997;41(Pt 1):87–91.

[59] Wattendorf DJ, Muenke M. Prader-Willi syndrome. Am Fam Physician 2005;72(5): 827–30.

[60] Einfeld SL, Smith A, Durvasula S, et al. Behavior and emotional disturbance in Prader-Willi syndrome. Am J Med Genet 1999;82(2):123–7.

[61] Akefeldt A, Gillberg C. Behavior and personality characteristics of children and young adults with Prader-Willi syndrome: a controlled study. J Am Acad Child Adolesc Psychiatry 1999;38(6):761–9.

[62] Stein DJ, Keating J, Zar HJ, et al. A survey of the phenomenology and pharmacotherapy of compulsive and impulsive-aggressive symptoms in Prader-Willi syndrome. J Neuropsychiatry Clin Neurosci 1994;6(1):23–9.

[63] Clarke DJ, Boer H, Whittington J, et al. Prader-Willi syndrome, compulsive and ritualistic behaviours: the first population-based survey. Br J Psychiatry 2002;180:358–62.

[64] Dykens EM, Leckman JF, Cassidy SB. Obsessions and compulsions in Prader-Willi syndrome. J Child Psychol Psychiatry 1996;37(8):995–1002.

[65] Greenswag LR. Adults with Prader-Willi syndrome: a survey of 232 cases. Dev Med Child Neurol 1987;29(2):145–52.

[66] Dykens EM, Kasari C. Maladaptive behavior in children with Prader-Willi syndrome, Down syndrome, and nonspecific mental retardation. Am J Ment Retard 1997;102(3): 228–37.

[67] Koenig K, Klin A, Schultz R. Deficits in social attribution ability in Prader-Willi syndrome. J Autism Dev Disord 2004;34(5):573–82.

[68] Plesa-Skwerer D, Sullivan K, Joffre K, et al. Self concept in people with Williams syndrome and Prader-Willi syndrome. Res Dev Disabil 2004;25(2):119–38.

[69] Smith AC, McGavran L, Robinson J, et al. Interstitial deletion of (17)(p11.2p11.2) in nine patients. Am J Med Genet 1986;24(3):393–414.

[70] Greenberg F, Guzzetta V, Montes de Oca-Luna R, et al. Molecular analysis of the Smith-Magenis syndrome: a possible contiguous-gene syndrome associated with del(17)(p11.2). Am J Hum Genet 1991;49(6):1207–18.

[71] Dykens EM, Smith AC. Distinctiveness and correlates of maladaptive behaviour in children and adolescents with Smith-Magenis syndrome. J Intellect Disabil Res 1998;42(Pt 6):481–9.

[72] Haas-Givler B. Educational implications and behavioral concerns of SMS: from the teacher's perspective. Spectrum (Newsletter of PRISMS) 1994;1(2):3–4.

[73] Turner H. A syndrome of infantilism, congenital webbed neck and cubitus valgus. Endocrinology 1938;28:566–74.

[74] Ranke MB, Saenger P. Turner's syndrome. Lancet 2001;358(9278):309–14.

[75] Ross JL, Stefanatos GA, Kushner H, et al. The effect of genetic differences and ovarian failure: intact cognitive function in adult women with premature ovarian failure versus Turner syndrome. J Clin Endocrinol Metab 2004;89(4):1817–22.

[76] McCauley E, Ito J, Kay T. Psychosocial functioning in girls with Turner's syndrome and short stature: social skills, behavior problems, and self-concept. J Am Acad Child Psychiatry 1986;25(1):105–12.

[77] Mazzocco MM, Baumgardner T, Freund LS, et al. Social functioning among girls with fragile X or Turner syndrome and their sisters. J Autism Dev Disord 1998;28(6):509–17.

[78] Downey J, Ehrhardt AA, Gruen R, et al. Psychopathology and social functioning in women with Turner syndrome. J Nerv Ment Dis 1989;177(4):191–201.

[79] Schmidt PJ, Cardoso GM, Ross JL, et al. Shyness, social anxiety, and impaired self-esteem in Turner syndrome and premature ovarian failure. JAMA 2006;295(12):1374–6.

[80] Ross JL, McCauley E, Roeltgen D, et al. Self-concept and behavior in adolescent girls with Turner syndrome: potential estrogen effects. J Clin Endocrinol Metab 1996;81(3):926–31.

[81] Lawrence K, Campbell R, Swettenham J, et al. Interpreting gaze in Turner syndrome: impaired sensitivity to intention and emotion, but preservation of social cueing. Neuropsychologia 2003;41(8):894–905.

[82] Elgar K, Campbell R, Skuse D. Are you looking at me? Accuracy in processing line-of-sight in Turner syndrome. Proc Biol Sci 2002;269(1508):2415–22.

[83] Ewart AK, Morris CA, Atkinson D, et al. Hemizygosity at the elastin locus in a developmental disorder, Williams syndrome. Nat Genet 1993;5(1):11–6.

[84] Morris C. The dysmorphology, genetics, and natural history of Williams-Beuren syndrome. In: Morris C, Lenhoff H, Wang P, editors. Williams-Beuren syndrome: research, evaluation, and treatment. Baltimore (MD): The Johns Hopkins University Press; 2006. p. 3–17.

[85] Feinstein C, Reiss A. The neurobiology of Williams-Beuren syndrome. In: Morris C, Lenhoff H, Wang P, editors. Wiilliams-Beuren syndrome: research, evaluation, and treatment. Baltimore (MD): The Johns Hopkins University Press; 2006. p. 309–24.

[86] Greenberg F. Williams syndrome. Pediatrics 1989;84(5):922–3.

[87] Laing E, Butterworth G, Ansari D, et al. Atypical development of language and social communication in toddlers with Williams syndrome. Dev Sci 2002;5:233–46.

[88] Mervis CB, Robinson BF. Expressive vocabulary ability of toddlers with Williams syndrome or Down syndrome: a comparison. Dev Neuropsychol 2000;17(1):111–26.

[89] Gosch A, Pankau R. Personality characteristics and behaviour problems in individuals of different ages with Williams syndrome. Dev Med Child Neurol 1997;39(8):527–33.

[90] Jones W, Bellugi U, Lai Z, et al. Hypersociability in Williams syndrome. J Cogn Neurosci 2000;12(Suppl 1):30–46.

[91] Bellugi U, Adolphs R, Cassady C, et al. Towards the neural basis for hypersociability in a genetic syndrome. Neuroreport 1999;10(8):1653–7.

[92] Doyle TF, Bellugi U, Korenberg JR, et al. "Everybody in the world is my friend" hypersociability in young children with Williams syndrome. Am J Med Genet A 2004;124(3): 263–73.

[93] Dykens EM. Anxiety, fears, and phobias in persons with Williams syndrome. Dev Neuropsychol 2003;23(1–2):291–316.

[94] Gosch A, Pankau R. Social-emotional and behavioral adjustment in children with Williams-Beuren syndrome. Am J Med Genet 1994;53(4):335–9.

[95] Plesa-Skwerer D, Tager-Flausberg D. Social cognition in Williams-Beuren syndrome. In: Morris C, Lenhoff H, Wang P, editors. Williams-Beuren syndrome: research, evaluation, and treatment. Baltimore (MD): The Johns Hopkins University Press; 2006. p. 237–53.

[96] Davies M, Udwin O, Howlin P. Adults with Williams syndrome: preliminary study of social, emotional and behavioural difficulties. Br J Psychiatry 1998;172:273–6.

[97] Frigerio E, Burt DM, Gagliardi C, et al. Is everybody always my friend? Perception of approachability in Williams syndrome. Neuropsychologia 2006;44(2):254–9.

[98] Sullivan K, Tager-Flusberg H. Second-order belief attribution in Williams syndrome: intact or impaired? Am J Ment Retard 1999;104(6):523–32.

[99] Gagliardi C, Frigerio E, Burt DM, et al. Facial expression recognition in Williams syndrome. Neuropsychologia 2003;41(6):733–8.

[100] Shprintzen RJ. Velo-cardio-facial syndrome: a distinctive behavioral phenotype. Ment Retard Dev Disabil Res Rev 2000;6(2):142–7.

[101] Papolos DF, Faedda GL, Veit S, et al. Bipolar spectrum disorders in patients diagnosed with velo-cardio-facial syndrome: does a hemizygous deletion of chromosome 22q11 result in bipolar affective disorder? Am J Psychiatry 1996;153(12):1541–7.

[102] Ryan AK, Goodship JA, Wilson DI, et al. Spectrum of clinical features associated with interstitial chromosome 22q11 deletions: a European collaborative study. J Med Genet 1997; 34(10):798–804.

[103] Shprintzen RJ, Higgins AM, Antshel K, et al. Velo-cardio-facial syndrome. Curr Opin Pediatr 2005;17(6):725–30.

[104] Cohen E, Chow E, Weksberg R, et al. Phenotype of adults with the 22q11.2 deletion syndrome. Am J Med Genet 1999;86:359–65.

[105] McDonald-McGinn D, Kirschner R, Goldmuntz E. The Philadelphia story: the 22q11.2 deletion: report on 250 patients. Genetic Counselling 1999;10:11–24.

[106] Moss E, Batshaw M, Solot C. Psychoeducational profile of the 22q11.2 microdeletion: a complex pattern. J Pediatr 1999;134:193–8.

[107] Gerder M, Solot C, Wang P. Cognitive and behavior profile of preschool children with chromosome 22q11.2 deletion. Am J Med Genet 1999;85:127–33.

[108] Feinstein C, Eliez S. The velocardiofacial syndrome in psychiatry. Curr Opin Psychiatry 2000;13:485–90.

[109] Swillen A, Devriendt K, Legius E. The behavioral phenotype in velo-cardio-facial syndrome (VCFS): from infancy to adolescence. Genetic Counselling 1999;10(1):79–88.

[110] Bassett A, Chow E. 22q11 deletion syndrome: a genetic subtype of schizophrenia. Biol Psychiatry 1999;46:882–91.

[111] Murphy K, Jones L, Owen M. High rates of schizophrenia in adults with velo-cardio-facial syndrome. Arch Gen Psychiatry 1999;56:940–5.

[112] Gothelf D, Feinstein C, Thompson T, et al. Neuropsychiatric risk factors for the emergence of psychotic disorders in adolescents with 22q11.2 deletion syndrome. American Journal of Psychiatry 2007;164(4):663–9.

[113] Usiskin S, Nicolson R, Krasnewich D. Velocardiofacial syndrome in childhood-onset schizophrenia. J Am Acad Child Adolesc Psychiatry 1999;38:1536–43.

[114] Kravanti E, Dazzan P, Fearon P, et al. Can one identify preschizophrenia children? In: Keshavan M, Kennedy J, Murray R, editors. Neurodevelopment and schizophrenia. Cambridge (UK): Cambridge University Press; 2004. p. 415–31.

[115] Fine SE, Weissman A, Gerdes M, et al. Autism spectrum disorders and symptoms in children with molecularly confirmed 22q11.2 deletion syndrome. J Autism Dev Disord 2005; 35(4):461–70.

[116] Niklasson L, Rasmussen P, Oskardottir S, et al. Chromsome 22q11 deletions syndrome (CATCH 22); neuropsychiatric and neuropsychological aspects. Dev Med Child Neurol 2002;44:44–50.

[117] Woodlin M, Wang P, Aleman D, et al. Neuropsychological profile of children and adolescents with the 22q11.2 microdeletion. Genet Med 2001;3:34–9.

ELSEVIER
SAUNDERS

Child Adolesc Psychiatric Clin N Am
16 (2007) 649–661

CHILD AND
ADOLESCENT
PSYCHIATRIC CLINICS
OF NORTH AMERICA

Bioethical Issues in Neuropsychiatric Genetic Disorders

Joaquin Fuentes, MD[a],*,
M. Concepción Martín-Arribas, RN, PhD[a,b]

[a]Service of Child & Adolescence Psychiatry, Policlinica Guipúzcoa,
GAUTENA Autism Society, San Sebastián, Spain
[b]Research Institute of Rare Disorders, (National) Institute of Health Carlos III,
Madrid, Spain

Neurogenetic disorders are conditions that can be labeled as "rare" disorders, because each one of them affects less than 1 per 2000 persons. Despite the rarity of each rare disease, it is always a surprise to discover that in the 25 European Union countries alone, approximately 30 million people have a "rare" disease, which means that between 6% and 8% of the total European Union population are patients who have rare diseases. This figure is equivalent to the combined populations of the Netherlands, Belgium, and Luxembourg [1]. In an era of expanding research and clinical care, the bioethics related to research and care for individuals with these rare disorders goes well beyond the bioethics envisioned in an earlier era.

If we consider the characteristics of rare disorders, we see that approximately 80% of them are genetic in origin (100% in the conditions reviewed in this issue). It may be informative to consider other common characteristics of rare disorders, however, as they apply to neuropsychiatric genetic disorders. Rare diseases are also characterized by the broad diversity of disorders and symptoms that vary not only from disease to disease but also within the same disease [2]. For many diagnoses, there are subtypes of the same disease that affecting in a different way the physical aptitudes, mental abilities, behavior, and sensorial capacities of these patients. Rare diseases also differ widely in terms of seriousness: some are life threatening, whereas others are compatible with a normal life if diagnosed in time and managed properly. In general, rare diseases and neurogenetic syndromes

* Corresponding author. Servicio de Psiquiatría Infanto-juvenil. Policlínica Guipúzcoa. Paseo de Miramón 174, 20009 San Sebastián, Spain.
    E-mail address: jfuentes@ipeuropa.com (J. Fuentes).

1056-4993/07/$ - see front matter © 2007 Elsevier Inc. All rights reserved.
doi:10.1016/j.chc.2007.02.003   *childpsych.theclinics.com*

have the following characteristics: (1) they are frequently associated with disability, (2) they appear during infancy (although often these patients suffer from diagnostic delay), (3) they face limited availability to research, case registries, and epidemiologic surveillance, (4) they cannot be cured and have no known specific treatment, (5) they generate a negative impact in the life of persons affected by them and their families, (6) they require a multidisciplinary contribution to care, and (7) they benefit from the collaboration of a patient's societies.

With neurogenetic disorders, we often must make decisions knowing that evidence-based medicine provides limited guidance. Patients and their families are exposed to conflicting information as to which interventions are the best options to follow, lack of resources to support the affected individual through the life cycle is the norm in most places of the world, and a good quality of life, as defined by the person—or his or her legal representatives and friends—is the ultimate goal. Informed consent for research and care for individuals who have neurogenetic disorders is a challenge for bioethical committees that may be uninformed about the complexities associated with efforts to screen or use novel treatments in these disorders, and the attempts to identify underlying phenotypic and genetic conditions may affect and influence the lives of not formally involved third parties. The purpose of this article is to consider the diverse bioethical concerns related to these rare disorders from the point of view of clinical practice and research. Bioethical considerations must consider the person affected by these conditions and the society in which individuals must cope with neuropsychiatric disability.

Bioethics context

In 1969, the first code of patient's rights was published, and it contained innovative aspects such as "informed consent," which restructured the roles in the therapeutic relationship by establishing that doctors have the information, patients have the choice, and society has the task of ensuring fairness in conducting this transaction. Four classical bioethics principles have been proposed: (1) no malfeasance (avoiding wrongdoing), (2) justice (ensuring equality of all persons), (3) autonomy (deciding with knowledge and without coercion), and (4) beneficence (maximizing good and minimizing harm to individuals and society). In terms of prioritizing them, the first two principles— no malfeasance and justice—are classified as level one and the other two principles—autonomy and beneficence—belong to a second level.

In the new millennium, bioethical principles underscore the importance of human dignity and integrity, solidarity, nondiscrimination, respect for privacy, confidentiality, freedom of research, integrity of research, intellectual honesty, updated scientific knowledge guiding practice, and the impact of medical care on the person, exemplified by the concept of quality of life. New issues propel bioethical discussion, such as cultural and religious differences, human genetic data and other personal health care data, genetic enhancement, gene therapy and genetic modification, genetic modification of organisms (animals, plants) and environments, commercialization of human tissue, including the human genome, moral status accorded to embryos, using embryonic stem cells, donation of human organs, tissue, cells, and gametes, right to consent and refuse treatment and research, anonymity of organ donors, xenotransplantation, reproduction and the beginning of life, euthanasia and end-of-life decisions, the right of infringing drug patents, globalization of biomedical research, intellectual property protection, and many more challenging areas.

An even wider vision has been offered by the United Nations Educational, Scientific, and Cultural Organization Universal Declaration on Bioethics and Human Rights [3], a comprehensive universal instrument on bioethics that states that bioethics also deals with the persistent and critical conditions of human beings all over the world, such as the ethical and legal reflections on birth, child exploitation, gender equality, equality between different human populations, access to cures, disease prevention, death, ecology, the protection of the environment, and the responsibilities toward future generations.

Consent versus assent

In their seminal paper, Chen and colleagues [4] from the National Institutes of Mental Health made an in-depth analysis of strategies in autism research that also fully apply to neurogenetic syndromes. They established seven ethical requirements to be applied for evaluating clinical research in autism spectrum disorders (ASD): social or scientific value, scientific validity, fair subject selection, favorable risk-benefit ratio, independent review, informed consent, and respect for potential and enrolled research participants.

A basic condition for research is the free and informed participation of the involved person, which should be reflected on a written "consent" document. In agreement with the United Nations Educational, Scientific, and Cultural Organization declaration, the consenting person must be mentally competent and reach the legal age for adulthood [5]. Available recommendations and regulations indicate that research in vulnerable subjects (minors or persons who are unable to give consent) is performed only when the results of research may generate a direct benefit on the health of the subjects, there is minimal risk, the research cannot be performed in other subjects competent to produce their consent, and the legally authorized representatives of the vulnerable persons have signed a written consent document. When a vulnerable person is an adult, he or she should participate in the consent procedure in the best possible way. The positive opinion of minors (defined as "assent") should be taken into account, always considering their age and maturity degree. In the same way, the refusal of these persons to take part in research process should be respected [6].

In reference to the consent concept applied to children, different considerations are established. When a minor is not intellectually or emotionally capable to understand the full aspects of the proposed actions, consent should be provided by the legal representative after listening to his or her opinion (assent) if the child is at least 12 years old. When the minor does not have a disability or has not been incapacitated or he or she is emancipated or is at least 16 years old, consent cannot be produced by representation [7–10].

Since 1995, the Joint Commission for Accreditation of Healthcare Organizations [11], the accreditation agency for health institutions in the United States, included as a criterion for accreditation of any hospital the availability of some formal mechanism established to support health care professionals, patients, and their families when dealing with ethical conflicts that may present during clinical practice. This model has been influential in many countries, leading to the establishment of consulting ethical committees for clinical care.

Bioethics committees should accept that there is no single "truth" in itself. Truth must be pluralistically searched, developed, and shared with caution. To do so, different steps are normally considered: (1) identifying the situation that generates conflict, (2) defining the problem and analyzing the factors and possibilities involved, (3) debating the issues in an intersubjective way and being ready to accept the input of other persons, and (4) agreeing on a plan of action.

Common ethical challenges raised by clinical practice in neurogenetic syndromes

There is a relative paucity of research on evolutionary trajectories and treatments for behavioral neurogenetic conditions. In contrast, much more "basic science" research is available on the brain structure and function and molecular mechanisms of these syndromes. This discrepancy constitutes a significant concern, especially for clinicians and disability societies, and should orient the provision of appropriate funding by governmental agencies.

Neuropsychiatric genetic disorders affect brain functioning, with a likely resulting cognitive impairment that makes the person part of the vulnerable populations: individuals whose autonomy, dignity, or integrity can be threatened. In general, because they have limitations for consent and for assent, this situation mandates a careful consideration of risk/benefit of the interventions contemplated. Current bioethical views maintain that these persons should be supported in terms of autonomy, dignity, or integrity as human beings and should receive the appropriate assistance to enable them to realize their full potential.

Often in clinical practice limited evidence is available to orient the practitioner and the patient or his or her legally authorized representative. New information technologies are facilitating the transmission of knowledge in a way that was difficult to imagine not so many years ago. As always, progress brings good and bad consequences. Many persons are subjected to false or misleading information, sometimes oriented to profit making, although sometimes this information is generated by honest persons who simply want to provide information about something that they felt was good for them. In Internet forums, persons give all kind of recommendations—without knowing the other person—based on their personal experience, something that does not have scientific value but is powerful from an emotional point of view.

ASD is a set of heritable complex disorders frequently embedded in conflict. There is compelling evidence for genetic determinants and little or no support for environmental influence [12]. Although there is common scientific agreement on this, its genetic ingredients are yet to be discovered. Clinically, ASD constitutes the paradigm for heated debate and risky decision making. To help patients and practitioners in following a sound and bioethically correct clinical practice, we have proposed several complementary measures in international meetings organized by Autism-Europe, including the use of official framework reports from prestigious national or international scientific institutions and the development of practice parameters, such as the guides of good practice recently developed by the Autism Spectrum Disorder Study Group of the (National) Institute of Health Carlos III of Spain, for early detection, diagnosis, and treatment in autism [13–15].

In their effort to achieve excellence, some programs have predefined their clinical procedures, documenting what and how practitioners are doing when performing a good practice in the framework of an ongoing quality system that, by performing internal and external audits, explores the conformity between what should be done and what is actually done, searching for continuous improvement with full transparency toward patients and their legal representatives, who are active members of a quality system committee or its equivalent. An example of this approach in vulnerable patients who are taking psychotropic medication is the Protocol PHARMAUTISME [16], which forms part of a more complex ISO-9001 quality-oriented system followed in the GAUTENA Program in the Basque Country, Northern Spain [17].

Those initiatives are salutary examples of how to structure the presence and participation of the agents and the receivers of medical care, truly empowering patients while providing a framework of accepted practice for professionals.

Common ethical challenges raised by research in neurogenetic syndromes

Given the characteristics of neurogenetic syndromes and their clinical variability, diverse levels of capacity to provide informed consent are met—from children and adults with marked degree of disability, with whom any participation in research must be with consent from parents or legal representatives, to subjects in whom cognitive skills would permit an assent and a standard consent procedure. As far as possible, informed assent should be sought, providing information about the objective of the research, potential benefit, and possible risks and discomfort, all in a language easily understood by the individual. Visual aids, augmented communication systems, and "easy reading texts" are of paramount importance in the population with associated cognitive or communicative impairments.

In the same way that has been proposed for other vulnerable populations and regarding participation of children in pharmacotherapy clinical trials in general, ethical committees should include permanent or "ad hoc" experts who can review and assess the appropriateness of the adapted forms and documents that are used for consent and assent procedures in this population. Stringent criteria also should be enforced to ensure, for example, that a patient who has responded on a clinical trial to a new drug continues to receive free medication until the product is commercialized.

In all cases, researchers must obtain the approval of an ethical committee for any project that includes persons who, because of their age or behavioral disorder, are not able to provide informed consent.

Access to research and treatment

These individual safeguards may reduce the likelihood of accessing research for these groups of patients, but in behavioral neurogenetics the syndromes may be used as models for understanding psychiatric disorders or brain development. For example, in velocardiofacial and Williams syndromes, many studies use brain imaging and neurocognitive testing. Understanding these populations will lead to better treatment of subjects who have neurogenetic syndromes, but there is a long and uncertain way to go. These persons, whose behavioral disorders or disabilities make them unfit to produce informed consent, should not be deprived of the possible benefits generated by the research, especially if there no therapies or preventive methods exist that may have equivalent or superior results to the one that is being researched [18].

As the Council of Europe has established, it is essential that research conducted with children—and other vulnerable subjects—is guided by the likelihood of direct benefit to the child. In exceptional cases, through significant improvement in the scientific understanding of an individual's condition, disease, or disorder, research has the aim of contributing to the ultimate attainment of results capable of conferring benefit to the person concerned or to other persons in the same age category or afflicted with the same disease or disorder or having the same condition [19]. It should not be interpreted that acting in the best interest of the subject means excluding the person from research but rather that a careful enforcement of all the guarantees protects human rights by using the described mechanisms.

Challenges raised by screening and genetic counseling in neurogenetic syndromes

Diverse neurogenetic syndromes show full autistic symptoms and have bordering cognitive, communicative, or behavioral characteristics similar to those described in ASD. Angelman syndrome, Prader-Willi syndrome, 15q11-q13 duplication, fragile X syndrome, fragile X premutation, deletion of chromosome 2q, XYY syndrome, Smith-Lemli-Opitz syndrome, Apert syndrome, mutations in the ARX gene, De Lange syndrome, Smith-Magenis syndrome, Williams syndrome, Rett syndrome, Noonan syndrome, Down syndrome, velocardiofacial syndrome, myotonic dystrophy, Steinert disease, tuberous sclerosis, Duchenne's disease, Timothy syndrome, 10p terminal deletion, Cowden syndrome, 45,X/46,XY mosaicism, Myhre syndrome, Sotos syndrome, Cohen syndrome, Goldenhar syndrome, Joubert syndrome, Lujan-Fryns syndrome, Moebius syndrome, hypomelanosis of Ito, neurofibromatosis type 1, CHARGE syndrome, and HEADD syndrome have been reviewed in terms of their relationship with ASD [20].

Screening

There is a growing need in the current scientific world to decide whether we are facing an autism epidemic and to determine risk in children who manifest symptoms and signs at an early age. If this were the case, there would be a spectacular social and economic increase in the cost of caring for ASD in our communities [21,22]. Because early intervention shows its biggest effect when started early and the most recent data show that autism can be identified with enough guarantees at approximately 2 years of age, there is a widespread interest in developing reliable screening methods and instruments, such as the modified checklist for autism in toddlers [23].

Challenges involved in research pertain not only to the knowledge of the causation of these disorders but also to the design of good screening tools that support the establishment of early diagnosis and consequent early biomedical and socioeducational treatments. In this area, professionals must assume the responsibility of ensuring that the subject (or his or her legal representatives) understands the difference between screening and clinical care. Research screening programs should clarify this aspect when recruiting people and express clearly when there is no guarantee of potential benefits for the participating subject.

Screening programs must not only consider the screening instruments being studied but also describe the subsequent diagnostic protocol—to discard or confirm diagnosis—offered to subjects classified as positives in the screening phase and later provision of treatment or support services offered to individuals who eventually obtain a positive diagnosis. In the case of neurogenetic syndromes associated with ASD symptoms, we propose that early intervention, as in cases of idiopathic cause, although not curative, will improve the outcome for most cases and generate a better quality of life for all involved persons, patients [24], and relatives [25].

Given the current scientific knowledge, diagnostic protocols for developmental disorders include genetic tests aimed at identifying neurogenetic conditions. This option brings new possibilities and ethical, social, and legal

challenges to clinicians and researchers that should be considered in the informed consent procedure and in genetic counseling. The policy statement
of the American Academy of Pediatrics on ethical issues related to genetic
testing in pediatrics, later reaffirmed in 2005, constituted an excellent guiding document for practitioners and policy makers [26].

All screening programs, especially if they involve genetic tests, require informed consent. Although it is true that the screening process or diagnosis is
often initiated in the framework of a clinic visit, where the signature of an
informed consent document would not be mandatory, it is an indication
of good clinical practice to tackle these themes, following the general recommendations guiding informed consent and genetic counseling [9,27].

In this sense, the information provided to the person must mention the
validity and viability of the screening and diagnostic tests, the possibility
of obtaining false-positive results, the temporal discomfort to which the persons may be subjected until a final diagnosis is established or discarded, the
possibilities of preventing or treating the condition once it is discovered, and
the possible distress and adverse effects of the preventive, diagnostic, or
therapeutic measures. If a person is recruited in a screening protocol in research phase, he or she should be informed about the uncertainties that remain until the research is finished and stress his or her voluntary
participation for the general advancement of the field.

Implications of screening

Ethical challenges are generated when information produced by the results may affect third parties, including family members not directly involved in the process. During the research process there may be
unexpected findings or foreseeable incurable conditions (eg, the identification of carriers of the fragile X gene). Some genetic tests, performed for diagnostic confirmation, may inform about the carrier condition of serious
genetic anomalies in parents or among relatives.

An additional aspect that merits consideration is the frequent absence of
tests that allow estimated risk of transmission and facilitate reproductive
decisions. The concept of risk must be approached in genetic counseling;
currently, however, clinicians can only talk about group—not individual—
considerations in most cases. For example, in ASD, genetic counselors
cannot predict individual risk unless a specific neurogenetic disorder has
been identified and can be searched in the fetus or in vitro fertilization. In
the absence of this possibility, all that can be said is that the group probability
of having a second child with ASD is between 2% and 8% [28], whereas the
risk of having a child with ASD in the general population is much lower
[29,30].

In relation to screening, the lack of training of many clinicians must be
stressed, especially in cases of rare disorders. Health care professionals
must be prepared to interpret the outcome of research and transmit proper

information. The application of evidence-based medicine in the field of genetic testing often remains questionable, because rare diseases imply a difficulty to meet the criteria required in terms of sample size for clinical trials or sound genetic research.

Even if we know the genes involved and the loci associated with the condition, this does not mean that we have an immediate specific line of treatment. This mismatch between risk information and the possibility of effective treatment is one of the sources of ethical, legal, and social conflicts with which researchers and clinicians should be familiar.

A genetic test must be valid from an analytical and clinical viewpoint, which means being able to predict clinical phenotype based on genotype [31]. A given test may identify a group of mutations in a gene, but it may carry a low clinical validity if penetration is low, other loci are involved, or environmental factors are acting in the unfolding of the condition. It is easy to think that a complex (or ignored) condition, such as ASD, can generate high numbers of false-positive or false-negative results. Therefore, clinicians must know the validity of the tests and how to interpret the results.

These considerations must be systematically considered by researchers, clinicians, and bioethical committees when defining protocols, procedures, and materials for informed consent, especially considering the principle of no malfeasance.

Recommendations for improving clinical and research practice from a bioethical point of view

Promoting a personal services portfolio

Much in the same way that most countries fully recognize—theoretically—what kind of health and education persons with disabilities are entitled to, the same does not occur in relation to habilitation and rehabilitation services. A client must be involved in planning for his or her social inclusion and achieving a good quality of life. This principle implies making people aware of the portfolio of services to which they are entitled (ensuring availability in accordance to public laws) and giving the person a real voice in deciding what to receive and how to express satisfaction.

In Spain, FEAPS (the Confederation of Societies in favor of Persons with Intellectual Disability) goes beyond the accessibility of health and education provision and proposes the universal acceptance of 13 kinds of services [32] that, supported by public funding, should be made available for ethical reasons to every subject of the community who requires them because of intellectual disability (Box 1). (We must remember that neuropsychiatric genetic disorders frequently generate an intellectual disability.)

National laws often do not formally recognize the entitlement of citizenship to this provision of essential and interrelated services, in contrast to laws that define mandatory education or access to national health services.

Box 1. Public services that should be made available to persons who have intellectual disability

Early intervention

Intermediation for social and work insertion

Support for social and professional development at the sheltered
   employment schema

Support for social and professional development in regular jobs

Support to families

Occupational therapy

Day programs

Support for full independent living

Support for intermittently supervised living

Support for continuous living supervision

Access to multiprofessional diagnosis, follow-up, assessment,
   planning, and coordination

Guardianship

Leisure time

This lack of recognition underlies the need to enforce an ethical approach in the provision of support services and medical and research activities.

Establishing and supporting bioethical committees

Over the last 40 years, attitudes and behavior among people regarding participation in clinical trials have changed. This change reflects the active position of patients and research participants, in sharp contrast with the passive attitude that was the standard among previous generations. In a parallel way to these changes, formal measures aimed at protecting rights and welfare of patients and persons participating in research have been the outcome of clinical and research ethical committees.

The committees for ethical care and ethical research enjoy specific functions and roles that involve legal repercussions. Clinical ethics committees are basically consulting bodies that produce advisory reports for persons who request them: medical doctors, nurses, or patients. The research ethics committees have a different function, because they authorize and maintain the follow-up of the research projects that involve human beings. Their resolutions reflect the mandates of the institution where the research is conducted.

The ethical committees should protect the rights of the persons recruited for research, including individuals characterized as vulnerable subjects, and ensure that it will not diminish the opportunities for research that can be beneficial for them. This protection requires delineating what areas of research must be incorporated in the general research policies. The ethical committees must judge the benefits/risks ratio before the study, but it must be recognized that decision making in science has changed from being a unilateral business to a more participative model. Ethical committees are instruments for debate, education, and awareness of the general public on bioethical issues, and they are expected to foster empowerment and participation. There are growing experiences in participative models, in which equilibrium between autonomy and paternalism is sought, especially when persons recruited for research purposes can be classified as vulnerable subjects.

There is the need for a permanent dialog among patients, interested professionals, and society at large. A public debate, pluralistic and informed, in which all pertinent opinions are expressed should be promoted. As the Article 19 of the United Nations Educational, Scientific, and Cultural Organization Universal Declaration on Bioethics and Human Rights postulated, ethics committees should foster debate, education, and public awareness of and engagement in bioethics. Many of the difficulties that arise in research ethics review might be ameliorated if a partnership model in which patient groups, financing agencies or industries, and researchers—perhaps in liaison with research ethics committees—could be applied and, in this framework, used in the design and monitoring of research projects [33].

Reviewing and improving ethical aspects in research initiatives in this population

As a model practice, the (National) Institute of Health Carlos III in Spain established an ASD study group that operated during from 2002 to 2005. It produced a guideline for good practice in research in the field of autism that included methodologic and ethical recommendations [34]. This study group stressed the need to justify the relevance, quality, and feasibility of any research project submitted and defined nine indicators that may help bioethical committees and autism societies assess project proposals before granting authorization and participation. Informed consent and related issues were considered, as was the need for confidentiality and compliance with national laws for personal data protection and the recommendation for independent assessment and follow-up of research projects in vulnerable populations.

Fostering and empowering client participation and representation

To support populations with neurogenetic syndromes, there is a need for institutional initiatives such as committees and experts groups, in which patient societies should be represented. To complement these initiatives, there is a need for individual representation ("never about me without me") through legally authorized representatives. Representatives should try to place themselves in the position of the person and ensure that they can control the processes of research or clinical practice and ask themselves what they would do if consent were feasible. Representatives also should evaluate themselves to determine the "goodness of fit" with the involved person and request, when applicable, their substitution for another person who may be in a better position to represent the vulnerable person.

Summary

Bioethics is becoming an area we cannot neglect, and we need to consider bioethics globally, locally, and personally. It is clear that we should profit from transnational good practice and sound initiatives and remain open and ready to discuss difficult issues. We have many biomedical activities that need improvement, but the biggest challenge is how to apply the medical ethical tradition to the personal support services arena, an essential area in the lives of persons who have genetic neuropsychiatric disorders and their families that is yet to be fully clarified and valued as a fundamental service delivered by our society.

Acknowledgments

The authors gratefully acknowledge the critical review and suggestions made by Dr. Myron Belfer, Professor of Psychiatry, Harvard Medical School.

References

[1] EURORDIS -European Organization for Rare Diseases. Rare diseases: understanding this public health priority. Available at: http://www.eurordis.org/IMG/pdf/princeps_document-EN.pdf. Accessed January 8, 2007.
[2] EURORDIS -European Organization for Rare Diseases. European conference on rare diseases 2005: report. Available at: http://www.eurodis.org. Accessed January 8, 2007.
[3] UNESCO. Universal Declaration on Bioethics and Human Rights. Available at: http://unesdoc.unesco.org/images/0014/001461/146180E.pdf. Accessed January 8, 2007.
[4] Chen DT, Miller FG, Rosenstein DL. Ethical aspects of research into the etiology of autism [review]. Ment Retard Dev Disabil Res Rev 2003;9(1):48–53.
[5] Establishing Bioethics Comités. Division of ethics of science and technology: guide 1. Paris: UNESCO; 2005.
[6] International Bioethics Committee (IBC). Project of declaration on universal norms on bioethics. Paris: UNESCO; 2005.
[7] Council of Europe. Additional protocol to the convention on human rights and biomedicine concerning biomedical research. ETS N° 195. Strasbourg: Council of Europe; 2005.
[8] Medical Research Council. Medical research involving children. MRC Ethics Guide 2004.
[9] Act 41/2002, of 14 November. A basic regulation of the autonomy of the patient and of the rights and duties of providing information and clinical documentation. Spain.
[10] Convention for the Protection of Human Rights and Dignity of the Human Being with regard to the Application of Biology and Medicine. Council of Europe; 1997.
[11] Joint Commission for Accreditation of Healthcare Organization. Accreditation manual for hospitals. Oakbrook Terrace (IL): Joint Commission for Accreditation of Healthcare Organization; 1992.

[12] Veenstra-Vanderweele J, Christian SL, Cook EH Jr. Autism as a paradigmatic complex genetic disorder. Annu Rev Genomics Hum Genet 2004;5:379–405.

[13] Hernández J, Artigas J, Martos J, et al. Guía de buena práctica para la detección temprana de los trastornos del espectro autista [Spanish]. Rev Neurol 2005;41(4):237–45.

[14] Díez-Cuervo A, Muñoz-Yunta JA, Fuentes J, et al. Guía de buena práctica para el diagnóstico de los rrastornos del espectro autista [Spanish]. Rev Neurol 2005;41(5):299–310.

[15] Fuentes J, Ferrari MJ, Boada L, et al. Guía de buena práctica para el tratamiento de los trastornos del espectro autista [Spanish]. Rev Neurol 2006;43(7):425–38.

[16] Fuentes J, Gallano I. Tratamiento médico de los trastornos generalizados del desarrollo [Spanish]. Rev Neurol 2001;33(3):208–10.

[17] Fuentes J, Barinaga R, Gallano I. Applying TEACCH in developing autism services in Spain. Int J Ment Health 2000;29:78–88.

[18] International Ethical Guidelines for Biomedical Research Involving Human Subjects. Guideline 15. Switzerland: Council for International Organizations of Medical Sciences (CIOMS); 2002.

[19] Council of Europe. Additional protocol to the convention on human rights and biomedicine concerning biomedical research. Article 15.2. ETS N° 195. Strasbourg: Council of Europe; 2005.

[20] Artigas-Pallares J, Gabau-Vila E, Guitart-Feliubadalo M. Syndromic autism: II. Genetic syndromes associated with autism. Rev Neurol 2005;40(Suppl 1):S151–62.

[21] Fombonne E. Epidemiological surveys of autism and other pervasive developmental disorders: an update. J Autism Dev Disord 2003;33(4):365–82.

[22] Department of Developmental Services, Sacramento, California. Autistic spectrum disorders: changes in the California caseload. An update: 1999 through 2002. April 2003.

[23] Robins D, et al. The Modified Checklist for Autism in Toddlers: An initial study investigating the early detection of autism and pervasive developmental disorders. J Autism Dev Disord 2001;31(2):131–44.

[24] Turner LM, Stone WL, Pozdol SL. Follow-up of children with autism spectrum disorders from age 2 to age 9. Autism 2006;10(3):243–65.

[25] Tonge B, Brereton A, Kiomall M. Effects on parental mental health of an education and skills training program for parents of young children with autism: a randomized controlled trial. J Am Acad Child Adolesc Psychiatry 2006;45(5):561–9.

[26] American Academy of Pediatrics. Ethical issues with genetic testing in pediatrics. Pediatrics 2001;107(6):1451–5.

[27] Council of Europe. Additional protocol to the convention on human rights and biomedicine concerning biomedical research. Article 19. ETS N° 195. Strasbourg: Council of Europe; 2005.

[28] Muhle R, Trentacoste SV, Rapin I. The genetics of autism. Pediatrics 2004;113(5):e472–86.

[29] Simonoff E. Genetic counseling in autism and pervasive developmental disorders [review]. J Autism Dev Disord 1998;28(5):447–56.

[30] McMahon WM, Baty BJ, Botkin J. Genetic counseling and ethical issues for autism [review]. Am J Med Genet C Semin Med Genet 2006;142(1):52–7.

[31] Burke W, Zimmern RL. Ensuring the appropriate use of genetic tests. Nat Rev Genet 2004; 5(12):955–9.

[32] FEAPS presenta su cartera de servicios sociales. Confederación Española de Organizaciones en favor de las personas con discapacidad intelectual (FEAPS) 2006. Available at: http://www.feaps.org/actualidad/cartera_servicios.htm. Accessed December 15, 2006.

[33] The Genetic Interest Group, the Oxford Genetics Knowledge Park and the Oxford Centre for Ethics and Communication in Health Care Practice (Ethox). Research and rare genetic differences: frequently asked questions. The Genetic Interest Group, the Oxford Genetics Knowledge Park and the Oxford Centre for Ethics and Communication in Health Care Practice (Ethox, Oxford, UK); 2005.

[34] Belinchón M, Posada M, Artigas J, et al. Guía de buena práctica en la investigación de los trastornos del espectro autista [Spanish]. Rev Neurol 2005;41(6):371–7.

ELSEVIER
SAUNDERS

Child Adolesc Psychiatric Clin N Am
16 (2007) 663–675

CHILD AND
ADOLESCENT
PSYCHIATRIC CLINICS
OF NORTH AMERICA

Fragile X Syndrome: Assessment and Treatment Implications

Allan L. Reiss, MD, Scott S. Hall, PhD*

Center for Interdisciplinary Brain Sciences Research, Department of Psychiatry and Behavioral Sciences, 401 Quarry Road, Stanford University, Stanford, CA 94305-5975, USA

Fragile X syndrome (FraX) is the most common known cause of inherited mental impairment. *FMR1* gene mutations, the cause of FraX, lead to reduced expression of *FMR1* protein (FMRP) and an increased risk for a particular profile of cognitive, behavioral, and emotional dysfunction. Because of the similarity of these features to important (idiopathic) *Diagnostic and Statistical Manual of Mental Disorders, Fourth Edition* diagnoses, the study of individuals with FraX provides a unique window of understanding into important disorders such as autism, social phobia, cognitive disability, and depression. The study of FraX also is a portal to the realization of innovative interdisciplinary research that spans multiple clinical and basic scientific domains [1]. Such research provides new insights into understanding how genetic and environmental factors contribute to complex variations in typical and atypical human behavior [1,2].

Genetics

FraX occurs in approximately 1 in every 4000 live births. The syndrome arises from the disruption in expression of the fragile X mental retardation gene 1 (*FMR1*), most commonly caused by amplification of a CGG repeat in the 5′ untranslated region. Physical manifestations associated with the syndrome include macroorchidism, long face, large ears, prominent jaw, and mild features of connective tissue dysplasia, such as joint hyperextensibility, soft skin, and mitral valve prolapse. External physical features are not

This work was supported by National Institute of Mental Health grants MH50047 and MH64708 and the Canel Family Fragile X Research Fund.

* Corresponding author.

E-mail address: hallss@stanford.edu (S.S. Hall).

always reliable indicators of the presence of the condition, however, particularly in prepubertal children and women.

In 1991, Verkerk and colleagues [3] reported that a single gene on the X chromosome, *FMR1*, was associated with the symptoms of FraX. Subsequently, it was determined that persons with FraX showed dramatically increased numbers of triplet CGG repeats in the 5′ untranslated region of the first exon of *FMR1* on the long arm of the X chromosome (locus Xq27.3). FraX is one of several disorders caused by a dynamic gene mutation resulting in instability and subsequent expansion of trinucleotide repeats through generations. In normal alleles, the CGG repeats vary from 6 to 50, whereas expansions of approximately 50 to 200 repeats are associated with the "premutation" form of the gene seen in carrier women and men. Larger expansions of more than 200 (up to several thousand) CGG repeats are considered "full mutations" and typically are associated with excessive methylation of cytosines in the *FMR1* promoter region. This modification extinguishes transcription of the *FMR1* gene into mRNA, stopping translation of the fragile X mental retardation protein (FMRP) (Fig. 1).

Cognition and behavior

Studies from our laboratory and others indicate that the most common problem behaviors observed in FraX consist of attentional dysfunction and hyperactivity, hyperarousal, disturbance in language/communication, and social anxiety (see Ref. [1] for a recent review). In boys, problematic behaviors often take the form of social deficits with peers, qualitative abnormalities in communication, unusual responses to sensory stimuli, stereotypic behavior, self-injurious behavior (SIB), aggression, social avoidance, gaze aversion, inattention, impulsivity and hyperactivity. Girls with FraX also seem to exhibit high rates of emotional disturbance and maladaptive behaviors, including problems with depression, social anxiety, and withdrawal and attention deficit [4–10]. Adolescents and women with

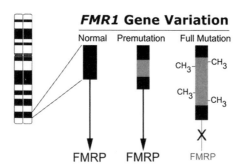

Fig. 1. FMR1 gene variations in FraX. Methylation of the gene in the full mutation leads to a significant reduction in FMRP levels.

the FraX full mutation are at high risk for major depression as well as anxiety and manifest abnormalities in social interaction and communication [11–16].

Individuals with FraX also are predisposed to manifesting a particular profile of intellectual strengths and weaknesses. This profile is similar in quality for both genders, although girls/women typically function at a much higher overall intellectual level and manifest less severe deficits than do boys/men. The characteristic cognitive profile includes weaknesses in attentional/executive function, visual memory and perception, mental manipulation of visual–spatial relationships among objects, visual–motor coordination, processing of arithmetical stimuli, and theory of mind and relative strengths in verbal-based skills.

Until recently, our understanding of cognitive and behavioral development in individuals with FraX was based primarily on cross-sectional studies [17–19] or a small number of longitudinal investigations that were limited by small sample size, broad age range, widely varying time intervals between assessments, or retrospective design [20–23]. These early studies suggested that, with respect to same aged peers, individuals with FraX showed a slowed developmental trajectory, a phenomenon believed to contribute to the observation of declining standardized IQ and adaptive behavior scores in affected individuals.

More recently, data from large prospective longitudinal investigations of preschool and school-age children with FraX have begun to appear [24–29]. Results from these studies have begun to elucidate the progression of cognitive function, academic skills, and adaptive and autistic behaviors in children with FraX ranging in age from 12 months to 14 years. Overall, results from these studies support the hypothesis that children with FraX are not losing skills over time, but rather have difficulty maintaining a developmental trajectory similar to age-matched peers [29]. These studies also have begun to clarify the effects of FMRP levels and autistic behavior on cognitive, academic, and adaptive behavioral development [27–29]. Overall, the presence of autistic behavior is related to poorer outcome. Developmental strengths in young children with FraX occur in domains related to general knowledge and daily living skills, whereas weaknesses are observed in socialization, communication, and visual–spatial processing.

Although increasing numbers of studies are emerging regarding development in young children with FraX, prospective, longitudinal and even cross-sectional data addressing issues of development in later adolescence and early adulthood are extremely limited. To the best of our knowledge, only two studies incorporating longitudinal design components have included subjects whose age extends into late adolescence or early adulthood. In one study, autistic and psychiatric symptoms were found to be stable over time in 18 boys/men aged 6 to 76 years with FraX; however, this study used nonconventional assessment instruments and retrospective chart review for some aspects of the investigation and did not include measures of cognitive ability [30]. In a second, multicenter study, the trajectory of adaptive behavior was examined in a broad age range of children, adolescents, and adults with FraX by aggregation of already collected Vineland data across several sites. Strengths in daily living skills were observed in several age groups, whereas weaknesses were observed for the communication domain [31].

Other investigations of FraX examining adolescence and adulthood have been cross-sectional in nature. Two recent studies examining language abilities [32,33] showed that individuals with a diagnosis of FraX and autism have a lower overall nonverbal IQ and do not perform as well on receptive language or theory of mind tasks compared with individuals with FraX without autism. The results of these investigations also suggest that cognitive impairments observed in childhood continue into adolescence and young adulthood [33].

Brain structure and function

Brain imaging studies establish an unambiguous link between FraX and abnormalities of brain morphology. Two recent comprehensive reviews of these findings are available and include a description of linkages among measures of anatomy, cognition, behavior, and FMRP [1,34]. In the context of overall normal brain size in individuals with FraX, disproportionate volume increases are seen in the caudate nucleus, whereas decreases are observed in the superior temporal gyrus, amygdala, and cerebellar vermis. These neuroanatomic variations in FraX are robust, particularly those observed in the caudate, and can be linked to variation in measures of *FMR1* expression, age, cognition, and behavior. Further, results from diffusion tensor imaging show reduced fractional anisotropy within prefrontal-caudate and parietal pathways in FraX. Abnormalities in white matter connectivity, putatively related to FMRP's function in regulating axonal pathfinding [35], may further disrupt the integrity of critical neurofunctional networks involved in executive function and visual–spatial processing in FraX.

Identifiable associations among measures of FMRP, neuroanatomy, cognition, and behavior in FraX suggest that the morphologic findings described above are clinically meaningful. For example, cerebellar vermis size (reduced in FraX) is positively correlated with measures of IQ and FMRP and negatively correlated with severity of autistic behavior [10,36]. Caudate nucleus volume (increased in FraX) is negatively correlated with measures of IQ and FMRP [37]. Thus, an increasing degree of aberrant brain morphology is associated with lower IQ and FMRP and higher levels of behavioral dysfunction. In contrast, larger caudate size is associated with higher IQ for controls [37]. This suggests that increases in caudate volume in individuals with FraX reflect aberrant neuronal organization.

Despite the high prevalence of FraX as a heritable genetic disorder, detailed postmortem studies of humans are rare. Early studies pointed to morphologic abnormalities of cortical dendritic processes [38], a finding similar to that reported in the *FMR1* knockout mouse [39,40]. More recent postmortem studies of four human brains revealed inconsistent results, with one study of two brothers with FraX reporting only mild ventricular enlargement [41]. Observations reported in the second study of two unrelated men with FraX included cellular abnormalities of the cerebellum and hippocampus, in addition to dilated lateral ventricles [42]. Quantitative histologic analyses of samples from areas shown to be morphologically abnormal in imaging studies, such as the caudate nucleus, amygdala, and superior temporal gyrus (STG), have not been performed.

Our understanding of the functional neuroanatomy of FraX has increased substantially in the last several years. Consistent with the cognitive and behavioral manifestations associated with FraX, functional MRI studies found aberrant neural patterns associated with tasks that assess visual–spatial and declarative memory [43–45], arithmetic reasoning [46], cognitive interference [47], response inhibition [48–50] (note that Ref. [48] examined response inhibition and set-shifting conditions together), gaze and face processing [51], and emotion processing. A synthesis of these fMRI results strongly support the hypothesis that the following key brain systems are particularly impaired in FraX: the fronto-striatal network underlying executive function and the STG and limbic system underlying gaze and emotion processing, with hyperactivation of the insula reflecting hyperarousal [52].

Pharmacologic interventions

Few medication trials have been conducted to specifically target cognitive and behavioral problems in FraX. Early case reports indicating that concentration span and attention problems in FraX could be alleviated by administration of high doses of folic acid [53,54] were not proved in double-blind placebo-controlled trials [55–58]. Antidepressant and stimulant medication seem to be the most frequently prescribed classes of drug administered to children and adults with FraX [59]. In the only double-blind placebo-controlled cross-over trial of stimulant medication conducted to date, 15 children with FraX (13 boys, 2 girls), aged 3 to 11 years, received methylphenidate (0.3 mg/kg twice daily) or dextroamphetamine (0.2 mg/kg daily) for 1 week [60]. Ten of the 15 children were judged to be clinical responders on methylphenidate; however, improvements could not be demonstrated for most of the outcome measures, with only teacher ratings indicating improvement in sociability and attention. In a single-case study of a 6-year-old boy with FraX, behavior problems seemed to improve during treatment with the tricyclic antidepressant medication imipramine, but worsened when the child was administered methylphenidate [61]. Large doses of the β-blocker propranolol administered to a 32-year old man with FraX indicated some improvement in aggression and stereotypic behavior [62]. Finally, L-acetylcarnitine, administered at dosages of 50 mg/kg twice daily, also was reported to be effective in reducing behavior problems in boys with FraX [63]. The low numbers of subjects treated in these studies indicate that larger double-blinded trials should be conducted before these medications can be evaluated judiciously.

More recent pharmacologic interventions have begun to target neurochemical and synaptic deficits specifically generated by the absence of FMRP. An excellent example of this new generation of study is the recent trial of the ampakine (AMPA) compound CX516, a medication that potentiates AMPA receptors in the brain [64]. These receptors play an important role in synaptic transmission; recent studies in the FMR1 knock-out mouse indicated that AMPA receptors are reduced significantly in number and activity. In a randomized, double-blind placebo-controlled trial, 24 adults with FraX (17 men and 7 women, aged 18 to 49 years) received 600 mg daily of CX516 for 1 week, and then the dosage was increased to 900 mg daily for 3 weeks. Side effects were minimal, although three individuals experienced an allergic rash to the compound and one subject did not complete the trial because of a severe rash. Although no clear improvement in cognitive or behavioral measures could be demonstrated, nine individuals who were treated with CX516 in combination with risperidone showed some improvement, suggesting that cotreatment with antipsychotics may be beneficial in some cases.

An open-label pilot study of the antiglucocorticoid medication mifepristone (RU-486) was conducted recently in our laboratory. Glucocorticoid type II (GR-II) receptors are reduced significantly in hippocampal neurons in the FMR1 knockout mouse. In addition, boys/men with FraX have elevated levels of cortisol, suggesting that some of the behavioral features observed in FraX (eg, hyperarousal, hyperactivity) may result from dysfunction of the hypothalamic-pituitary-adrenal (HPA) axis [34,65]. At high dosages (600 mg daily), mifepristone actively blocks GR-II receptors in the prefrontal cortex, causing a rapid increase in circulating cortisol by blocking the feedback loop of the HPA axis. We speculated that mifepristone could help to "reset" the normal rhythm of the HPA axis, and, thereby, cause improvements in behavioral functioning associated with HPA axis dysfunction. In an open-label trial, we administered 600 mg daily of mifepristone to eight boys and men with FraX aged 12 to 21 years. Outcome measures included the Aberrant Behavior Checklist, which parents filled out at baseline, day 7, day 14, and 2 weeks following discontinuation of the medication. Four participants developed a mild to moderate skin rash, and, as a precautionary measure, we recommended that they discontinue the medication before the scheduled 14 days (one participant on day 2 and three participants on day 10). Of the seven participants who completed at least 10 days of the trial, behavior problems improved in two participants (as evidenced by decreasing total scores on the Aberrant Behavior Checklist for child 2 and child 4; Fig. 2); however, behavior problems seemed to worsen in one participant (child 5). Therefore, it is unclear at

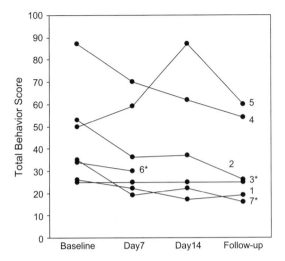

Fig. 2. Scores obtained on the Aberrant Behavior Checklist for seven children (numbered 1–7) at baseline, day 7 of mifepristone, day 14 of mifepristone, and 14 days following discontinuation of mifepristone. Children who discontinued the mediation after day 10 are indicated by an asterisk.

this time whether mifepristone may be clinically useful for children with FraX. We plan to titrate the medication in a double-blind trial of mifepristone in a larger group of participants.

In summary, medication trials to specifically target symptoms of FraX are extremely limited. Although mild reduction of symptoms can be obtained in individuals with FraX who are treated with antidepressants or stimulants, there is a pressing need for new, more effective, disease-specific treatments in young children with this condition.

Behavioral interventions

A large body of literature has emerged documenting the influence of environmental factors on behavior disorders shown by individuals with developmental disabilities [66–69]. These studies showed that many behavior disorders (eg, aggression, self-injury, and stereotypic behaviors) are influenced by antecedent and consequent social-environmental events. These environmental events include antecedent task or social demands, contingent removal of task or social demands, low levels of antecedent attention, contingent presentation of attention, changes in routines, and low levels of sensory stimulation. Manipulation of these environmental events can dramatically reduce the occurrence of these problem behaviors [70–72]. In a large sample of 152 individuals with developmental disabilities who showed self-injurious behavior (SIB), for example, Iwata and colleagues [68] found that in 64% of cases, problem behaviors were maintained by social-environmental reinforcement contingencies (eg, removal of task demands, delivery of attention); in an additional 25% of cases, SIB was evoked by antecedent nonsocial environmental events (eg, low levels of environmental stimulation). Treatments that were matched to the function of the behavior disorder (eg, ignoring behaviors that were maintained by attention, not allowing the child to escape from social or task demands, or providing alternate forms of sensory stimulation for those behaviors maintained by sensory stimulation) were highly successful.

In a postal survey of 55 boys with FraX, aged 1 to 12 years, parents reported that 58% of the children had shown SIB at some point during their lifetime [73] and that SIB was most likely to occur following changes in routine (87%), the presentation of difficult commands (65%), or difficult tasks (61%) or to gain adult attention (3%). In our laboratory, we systematically manipulated levels of antecedent social and task demands in 114 children with FraX (74 boys and 40 girls) to determine the specific conditions under which problem behaviors in FraX were more likely to occur [74]. By comparing levels of problem behaviors observed during a face-to-face interview, silent reading, oral reading, and a singing task, we showed that problem behaviors were significantly more likely to occur in the interview and singing conditions and were significantly less likely to occur in the silent and oral reading conditions. Therefore, in children with FraX, it seems that behavior problems are maintained predominantly by social escape. Systematic exposure to social interaction (escape extinction) combined with social skills training may be an effective treatment for problem behaviors in FraX [74].

To target eye contact aversion in FraX, we recently piloted a behavioral shaping technique to increase eye contact duration [75]. To aid the shaping process, we used a percentile reinforcement schedule, a method that allows the therapist to carefully track the student's performance and progress. Six boys with FraX, aged 8 to 17 years, underwent the training in two 1-hour sessions. Three of the children required the implementation of an overcorrection procedure (ie, maintaining the child's head in an upright position) to augment the shaping process and eliminate the appearance of problem behaviors. Results showed that even in time-limited, 1-hour sessions, eye contact duration improved significantly in four of the six boys without concomitant increases in hyperarousal or behavioral problems. These data suggest that eye contact aversion, although often believed to be unamenable to change in FraX, can be improved significantly using basic behavioral shaping techniques. We did not set out to resolve this problem in the children permanently, only to show that treatment was possible. Further studies are needed to determine whether these gains can be generalized and maintained.

Thus far, interventions for individuals with FraX have not been targeted to FraX-specific skill deficits, and to date, behavioral interventions have been conducted using heterogeneous strategies, without outcome data to support their efficacy. In the behavior analytic literature, several behavioral techniques were shown to help children with developmental disabilities improve social and educational skills. These included modeling, coaching, physical guidance, shaping, chaining, fading, matching-to-sample, and errorless learning techniques [76]. Surprisingly, we know of no published studies that have used these techniques to teach children with FraX. In our laboratory, we recently demonstrated the feasibility of teaching basic math and geography concepts to children with FraX using matching-to-sample and errorless learning techniques [77]. Five children (four boys and one girl) were taught to match decimals to fractions and states to capitals using a computerized training program. The children received hundreds of training trials conducted over 1 to 2 days in time-limited sessions on the computer. Results indicated that three of the five children successfully demonstrated knowledge of the geography relations at posttest, and four of the children successfully learned the math relations. These results suggest that some children with FraX may benefit from intensive behavioral training programs similar to those conducted for children with autism [78–80].

Summary

Many avenues of research on FraX have flourished over the past 25 years. For example, knowledge of the molecular genetic basis of FraX has grown at a rapid pace, and animal models have been created that promise to bring new insight into the effects of FMRP on brain development [81]. Much new information about the neurobehavioral phenotype and developmental trajectory of young children with FraX also has been reported.

Although it is clear that mutations of the *FMR1* gene increase the risk for neuropsychiatric dysfunction, there remains a relative lack of knowledge of how specific neural factors mediate this risk. Information of this nature is vital to understanding the neural basis of brain dysfunction in FraX as well as being required for the judicious design and testing of new disease-specific treatments. Finally, most treatment trials in FraX have been symptom-based or derived from other disorders as opposed to being informed by FraX-specific research data.

Over the past decade, clinical neuroscience research increasingly has begun to interrogate and merge multiple levels of scientific inquiry. A particularly good example is "imaging genomics," where data derived from assessment of genotype, neural systems, and phenotype are combined to better understand variation in human behavior [82]. Investigators also are increasingly undertaking the study of more homogenous groups in an attempt to map fundamental molecular events to specific changes in brain structure and function, and, ultimately, to cognitive-behavioral outcome. Examples include velo-cardio-facial syndrome [83], Williams syndrome [84], and Turner syndrome [85]. Behavioral neurogenetic research provides a glimpse of the future of neuropsychiatric, and more broadly, clinical neuroscience investigation—where the complex interplay between genetic risk and environment can be appreciated, described, and elucidated more fully. Thus, although the information gained in this area will have specific benefit to persons with FraX, it also will have broader relevance to understanding how genetic-neurobiologic pathways and environmental factors modify the risk for cognitive, emotional, and behavioral dysfunction.

References

[1] Reiss AL, Dant CC. The behavioral neurogenetics of fragile X syndrome: analyzing gene-brain-behavior relationships in child developmental psychopathologies. Dev Psychopathol 2003;15(4):927–68.
[2] Reiss A. Childhood developmental disorders. Presented at the Convergence of Neuroscience, Behavioral Science, Neurology, and Psychiatry. Scottsdale, AZ, January 2005.
[3] Verkerk AJ, Pieretti M, Sutcliffe JS, et al. Identification of a gene (FMR-1) containing a CGG repeat coincident with a breakpoint cluster region exhibiting length variation in fragile X syndrome. Cell 1991;65(5):905–14.
[4] Freund LS, Reiss AL, Abrams MT. Psychiatric disorders associated with fragile X in the young female. Pediatrics 1993;91(2):321–9.
[5] Hagerman RJ, Jackson C, Amiri K, et al. Girls with fragile X syndrome: physical and neuro-cognitive status and outcome. Pediatrics 1992;89(3):395–400.
[6] Lachiewicz AM. Abnormal behaviors of young girls with fragile X syndrome. Am J Med Genet 1992;43(1–2):72–7.
[7] Lachiewicz AM, Dawson DV. Behavior problems of young girls with fragile X syndrome: factor scores on the Conners' parent's questionnaire. Am J Med Genet 1994;51(4): 364–9.
[8] Lesniak-Karpiak K, Mazzocco MM, Ross JL. Behavioral assessment of social anxiety in females with Turner or fragile X syndrome. J Autism Dev Disord 2003;33(1):55–67.
[9] Mazzocco MM, Baumgardner T, Freund LS, et al. Social functioning among girls with fragile X or Turner syndrome and their sisters. J Autism Dev Disord 1998;28(6):509–17.
[10] Mazzocco MM, Kates WR, Baumgardner TL, et al. Autistic behaviors among girls with fragile X syndrome. J Autism Dev Disord 1997;27(4):415–35.
[11] Freund LS, Reiss AL, Hagerman R, et al. Chromosome fragility and psychopathology in obligate female carriers of the fragile X chromosome. Arch Gen Psychiatry 1992;49(1): 54–60.
[12] Hagerman RJ, Sobesky WE. Psychopathology in fragile X syndrome. Am J Orthopsychiatry 1989;59(1):142–52.
[13] Sobesky WE, Hull CE, Hagerman RJ. Symptoms of schizotypal personality disorder in fragile X women. J Am Acad Child Adolesc Psychiatry 1994;33(2):247–55.
[14] Sobesky WE, Taylor AK, Pennington BF, et al. Molecular/clinical correlations in females with fragile X. Am J Med Genet 1996;64(2):340–5.
[15] Thompson NM, Gulley ML, Rogeness GA, et al. Neurobehavioral characteristics of CGG amplification status in fragile X females. Am J Med Genet 1994;54(4):378–83.
[16] Thompson NM, Rogeness GA, McClure E, et al. Influence of depression on cognitive functioning in fragile X females. Psychiatry Res 1996;64(2):97–104.
[17] Dykens E, Leckman J, Paul R, et al. Cognitive, behavioral, and adaptive functioning in fragile X and non- fragile X retarded men. J Autism Dev Disord 1988;18(1):41–52.
[18] Dykens EM, Hodapp RM, Leckman JF. Adaptive and maladaptive functioning of institutionalized and noninstitutionalized fragile X males. J Am Acad Child Adolesc Psychiatry 1989;28(3):427–30.
[19] Wiegers AM, Curfs LM, Vermeer EL, et al. Adaptive behavior in the fragile X syndrome: profile and development. Am J Med Genet 1993;47(2):216–20.

[20] Dykens EM, Hodapp RM, Ort S, et al. The trajectory of cognitive development in males with fragile X syndrome. J Am Acad Child Adolesc Psychiatry 1989;28(3):422–6.

[21] Fisch GS, Carpenter NJ, Holden JJ, et al. Longitudinal assessment of adaptive and maladaptive behaviors in fragile X males: growth, development, and profiles. Am J Med Genet 1999;83(4):257–63.

[22] Fisch GS, Carpenter NJ, Simensen R, et al. Longitudinal changes in cognitive-behavioral levels in three children with FRAXE. Am J Med Genet 1999;84(3):291–2.

[23] Wright-Talamante C, Cheema A, Riddle JE, et al. A controlled study of longitudinal IQ changes in females and males with fragile X syndrome. Am J Med Genet 1996;64(2):350–5.

[24] Bailey DB Jr, Hatton DD, Skinner M, et al. Autistic behavior, FMR1 protein, and developmental trajectories in young males with fragile X syndrome. J Autism Dev Disord 2001;31(2): 165–74.

[25] Fisch GS, Simensen RJ, Schroer RJ. Longitudinal changes in cognitive and adaptive behavior scores in children and adolescents with the fragile X mutation or autism. J Autism Dev Disord 2002;32(2):107–14.

[26] Hatton DD, Sideris J, Skinner M, et al. Autistic behavior in children with fragile X syndrome: prevalence, stability, and the impact of FMRP. Am J Med Genet A 2006;140: 1804–13.

[27] Hatton DD, Wheeler AC, Skinner ML, et al. Adaptive behavior in children with fragile X syndrome. Am J Ment Retard 2003;108(6):373–90.

[28] Roberts JE, Schaaf JM, Skinner M, et al. Academic skills of boys with fragile X syndrome: profiles and predictors. Am J Ment Retard 2005;110(2):107–20.

[29] Skinner M, Hooper S, Hatton DD, et al. Mapping nonverbal IQ in young boys with fragile X syndrome. Am J Med Genet A 2005;132(1):25–32.

[30] Sabaratnam M, Murthy NV, Wijeratne A, et al. Autistic-like behaviour profile and psychiatric morbidity in fragile X syndrome: a prospective ten-year follow-up study. Eur Child Adolesc Psychiatry 2003;12(4):172–7.

[31] Dykens E, Ort S, Cohen I, et al. Trajectories and profiles of adaptive behavior in males with fragile X syndrome: multicenter studies. J Autism Dev Disord 1996;26(3):287–301.

[32] Abbeduto L, Murphy MM, Cawthon SW, et al. Receptive language skills of adolescents and young adults with Down or fragile X syndrome. Am J Ment Retard 2003;108(3):149–60.

[33] Lewis P, Abbeduto L, Murphy M, et al. Cognitive, language and social-cognitive skills of individuals with fragile X syndrome with and without autism. J Intellect Disabil Res 2006; 50(Pt 7):532–45.

[34] Hessl D, Rivera SM, Reiss AL. The neuroanatomy and neuroendocrinology of fragile X syndrome. Ment Retard Dev Disabil Res Rev 2004;10(1):17–24.

[35] Brown V, Jin P, Ceman S, et al. Microarray identification of FMRP-associated brain mRNAs and altered mRNA translational profiles in fragile X syndrome. Cell 2001;107(4): 477–87.

[36] Mostofsky SH, Mazzocco MM, Aakalu G, et al. Decreased cerebellar posterior vermis size in fragile X syndrome: correlation with neurocognitive performance. Neurology 1998;50(1): 121–30.

[37] Reiss AL, Abrams MT, Greenlaw R, et al. Neurodevelopmental effects of the FMR-1 full mutation in humans. Nat Med 1995;1(2):159–67.

[38] Hinton VJ, Brown WT, Wisniewski K, et al. Analysis of neocortex in three males with the fragile X syndrome. Am J Med Genet 1991;41(3):289–94.

[39] Grossman AW, Elisseou NM, McKinney BC, et al. Hippocampal pyramidal cells in adult Fmr1 knockout mice exhibit an immature-appearing profile of dendritic spines. Brain Res 2006;1084(1):158–64.

[40] Nimchinsky EA, Oberlander AM, Svoboda K. Abnormal development of dendritic spines in FMR1 knock-out mice. J Neurosci 2001;21(14):5139–46.

[41] Reyniers E, Martin JJ, Cras P, et al. Postmortem examination of two fragile X brothers with an FMR1 full mutation. Am J Med Genet 1999;84(3):245–9.

[42] Sabaratnam M. Pathological and neuropathological findings in two males with fragile-X syndrome. J Intellect Disabil Res 2000;44(Pt 1):81–5.

[43] Greicius MD, Boyett-Anderson JM, Menon V, et al. Reduced basal forebrain and hippocampal activation during memory encoding in girls with fragile X syndrome. Neuroreport 2004;15(10):1579–83.

[44] Kwon H, Menon V, Eliez S, et al. Functional neuroanatomy of visuospatial working memory in fragile X syndrome: relation to behavioral and molecular measures. Am J Psychiatry 2001;158(7):1040–51.

[45] Menon V, Kwon H, Eliez S, et al. Functional brain activation during cognition is related to FMR1 gene expression. Brain Res 2000;877(2):367–70.

[46] Rivera SM, Menon V, White CD, et al. Functional brain activation during arithmetic processing in females with fragile X syndrome is related to FMR1 protein expression. Hum Brain Mapp 2002;16(4):206–18.

[47] Tamm L, Menon V, Johnston CK, et al. fMRI study of cognitive interference processing in females with fragile X syndrome. J Cogn Neurosci 2002;14(2):160–71.

[48] Cornish K, Swainson R, Cunnington R, et al. Do women with fragile X syndrome have problems in switching attention: preliminary findings from ERP and fMRI. Brain Cogn 2004; 54(3):235–9.

[49] Hoeft F, Hernandez A, Parthasarathy S, et al. Fronto-striatal dysfunction and compensatory mechanisms in male adolescents with fragile X syndrome. Human Brain Mapping, in press.

[50] Menon V, Leroux J, White CD, et al. Frontostriatal deficits in fragile X syndrome: relation to FMR1 gene expression. Proc Natl Acad Sci USA 2004;101(10):3615–20.

[51] Garrett AS, Menon V, MacKenzie K, et al. Here's looking at you, kid: neural systems underlying face and gaze processing in fragile X syndrome. Arch Gen Psychiatry 2004;61(3): 281–8.

[52] Critchley HD. Neural mechanisms of autonomic, affective, and cognitive integration. J Comp Neurol 2005;493(1):154–66.

[53] Brown WT, Jenkins EC, Friedman E, et al. Folic acid therapy in the fragile X syndrome. Am J Med Genet 1984;17(1):289–97.

[54] Gustavson KH, Dahlbom K, Flood A, et al. Effect of folic acid treatment in the fragile X syndrome. Clin Genet 1985;27(5):463–7.

[55] Fisch GS, Cohen IL, Gross AC, et al. Folic acid treatment of fragile X males: a further study. Am J Med Genet 1988;30(1–2):393–9.

[56] Froster-Iskenius U, Bodeker K, Oepen T, et al. Folic acid treatment in males and females with fragile-(X)-syndrome. Am J Med Genet 1986;23(1–2):273–89.

[57] Hagerman RJ, Jackson AW, Levitas A, et al. Oral folic acid versus placebo in the treatment of males with the fragile X syndrome. Am J Med Genet 1986;23(1–2):241–62.

[58] Strom CM, Brusca RM, Pizzi WJ. Double-blind, placebo-controlled crossover study of folinic acid (Leucovorin) for the treatment of fragile X syndrome. Am J Med Genet 1992;44(5): 676–82.

[59] Berry-Kravis E, Potanos K. Psychopharmacology in fragile X syndrome–present and future. Ment Retard Dev Disabil Res Rev 2004;10(1):42–8.

[60] Hagerman RJ, Murphy MA, Wittenberger MD. A controlled trial of stimulant medication in children with fragile X syndrome. Am J Med Genet 1988;30:377–92.

[61] Hilton DK, Martin CA, Heffron WM, et al. Imipramine treatment of ADHD in a fragile X child. J Am Acad Child Adolesc Psychiatry 1991;30:831–4.

[62] Cohen IL, Tsiouris JA, Pfadt A. Effects of long-acting propanolol on agonistic and stereotyped behaviors in a man with pervasive developmental disorder and fragile X syndrome: a double-blind, placebo-controlled study. J Clin Psychopharmacol 1991;11(6):398–9.

[63] Torrioli MG, Vernacotola S, Mariotti P, et al. Double-blind, placebo-controlled study of L-acetylcarnitine for the treatment of hyperactive behavior in fragile X syndrome. Am J Med Genet 1999;87(4):366–8.

[64] Berry-Kravis E, Krause SE, Block SS, et al. Effect of CX516, an AMPA-modulating compound, on cognition and behavior in fragile X syndrome: a controlled trial. J Child Adolesc Psychopharmacol 2006;16(5):525–40.

[65] Hessl D, Glaser B, Dyer-Friedman J, et al. Cortisol and behavior in fragile X syndrome. Psychoneuroendocrinology 2002;27(7):855–72.

[66] Carr EG, Durand VM. The social-communicative basis of severe behavior problems in children. In: Reiss S, Bootzin R, editors. Theoretical issues in behavior therapy. New York: Academic Press; 1985.

[67] Durand VM, Carr EG. Social influences on "self-stimulatory" behavior: analysis and treatment application. J Appl Behav Anal 1987;20:119–32.

[68] Iwata BA, Pace GM, Dorsey MF, et al. The functions of self-injurious behavior: an experimental epidemiological analysis. J Appl Behav Anal 1994;27:215–40.

[69] Hanley GP, Iwata BA, McCord BE. Functional analysis of problem behavior: a review. J Appl Behav Anal 2003;36:147–85.

[70] Taylor JC, Carr EG. Severe problem behaviors related to social interaction: I. Attention seeking and social avoidance. Behav Modif 1992;16:305–35.

[71] Pelios L, Morren J, Tesch D, et al. The impact of functional analysis methodology on treatment choice for self-injurious and aggressive behavior. J Appl Behav Anal 1999;32:185–95.

[72] Call NA, Wacker DP, Ringdahl JE, et al. An assessment of antecedent events influencing noncompliance in an outpatient clinic. J Appl Behav Anal 2004;37:145–58.

[73] Symons FJ, Clark RD, Hatton DD, et al. Self-injurious behavior in young boys with fragile X syndrome. Am J Med Genet A 2003;118(2):115–21.

[74] Hall S, DeBernardis M, Reiss A. Social escape behaviors in children with fragile X syndrome. J Autism Dev Disord 2006;36(7):935–47.

[75] Hall SS, Maynes NP, Reiss AL. Using percentile schedules to increase eye contact in children with fragile X syndrome. J Appl Behav Anal, in press.

[76] Elliott SN, Gresham FM. Social skills intervention guide: practical strategies for social skills training. Circle Pines (MN): American Guidance Service; 1991.

[77] Hall SS, DeBernardis GM, Reiss AL. The acquisition of stimulus equivalence in individuals with fragile X syndrome. J Intellect Disabil Res 2006;50:643–51.

[78] Cohen H, Amerine-Dickens M, Smith T. Early intensive behavioral treatment: replication of the UCLA model in a community setting. J Dev Behav Pediatr 2006;27(2 Suppl):S145–55.

[79] Lovaas OI. Behavioral treatment and normal educational and intellectual functioning in young autistic children. J Consult Clin Psychol 1987;55(1):3–9.

[80] McEachin JJ, Smith T, Lovaas OI. Long-term outcome for children with autism who received early intensive behavioral treatment. Am J Ment Retard 1993;97:359–372.

[81] Bagni C, Greenough WT. From mRNP trafficking to spine dysmorphogenesis: the roots of fragile X syndrome. Nat Rev Neurosci 2005;6(5):376–87.

[82] Hariri AR, Weinberger DR. Imaging genomics. Br Med Bull 2003;65:259–70.

[83] Gothelf D, Eliez S, Thompson T, et al. COMT genotype predicts longitudinal cognitive decline and psychosis in 22q11.2 deletion syndrome. Nat Neurosci 2005;8(11):1500–2.

[84] Meyer-Lindenberg A, Mervis CB, Faith Berman K. Neural mechanisms in Williams syndrome: a unique window to genetic influences on cognition and behaviour. Nat Rev Neurosci 2006;7(5):380–93.

[85] Hart SJ, Davenport ML, Hooper SR, et al. Visuospatial executive function in Turner syndrome: functional MRI and neurocognitive findings. Brain 2006;129(Pt 5):1125–36.

ELSEVIER
SAUNDERS

Child Adolesc Psychiatry Clin N Am
16 (2007) 677–693

CHILD AND
ADOLESCENT
PSYCHIATRIC CLINICS
OF NORTH AMERICA

Velocardiofacial Syndrome

Doron Gothelf, MD[a,b,*]

[a]*Department of Child Psychiatry, Behavioral Neurogenetics Center, Schneider Children's*
Medical Center of Israel, 14 Kaplan Street, Petah Tiqwa, Israel 49202
[b]*Sackler Faculty of Medicine, Tel Aviv University, 14 Kaplan Street, Tel Aviv, Israel 49202*

One syndrome, multiple names

What is known today as velocardiofacial syndrome (VCFS) was described first clinically by Kirkpatrick and DiGeorge [1] in the 1960s and by Shprintzen and colleagues [2] in the 1970s. DiGeorge syndrome was defined as a constellation of immunologic deficiencies secondary to thymus hypoplasia, hypocalcemia secondary to hypoparathyroidism, and congenital cardiac anomalies [1]. Shprintzen syndrome, later renamed VCFS, was characterized by palate anomalies ("velo"), congenital cardiovascular defects ("cardio"), and mild facial dysmorphism ("facial") [2]. In the early 1990s, researchers discovered that DiGeorge syndrome and VCFS were caused by a microdeletion in the long arm of chromosome 22 at band 22q11.2 [3–5]. Today, the clinical diagnosis of the syndrome may be verified by a cytogenetic test, fluorescence in situ hybridization (FISH) [6]. It also has been established that, in addition to the above-mentioned signs and symptoms, the phenotypic spectrum of VCFS is extremely wide and includes more than 180 possible congenital anomalies, learning disabilities, and psychiatric manifestations. Therefore, some clinicians and scientists suggested renaming the syndrome 22q11.2 deletion syndrome. In this article, the author uses the name that is most widely known to clinicians, VCFS.

Prevalence

To determine the exact prevalence of VCFS, all live-born infants would need to be screened for the 22q11.2 deletion. Because the high cost of the FISH test precludes population-based screening, only minimum-prevalence

---

* The Behavioral Neurogenetics Center, Department of Child Psychiatry, Schneider Children's Medical Center of Israel, 14 Kaplan St., Petah Tiqwa, Israel 49202.
E-mail address: gothelf@post.tau.ac.il

1056-4993/07/$ - see front matter © 2007 Elsevier Inc. All rights reserved.
doi:10.1016/j.chc.2007.03.005
childpsych.theclinics.com

estimates are available, based on cases referred to cardiology and genetics clinics or included in registries of congenital defects. A recent review reported a minimum prevalence of between 1 in 5900 to 1 in 9700 live births [7]. The actual prevalence probably is much higher; cases may be missed because of the frequently mild phenotypic expression of the syndrome and the low awareness by clinicians of the full spectrum of its manifestations.

Clinical manifestations

The physical phenotype of VCFS is highly heterogeneous, with 180 possible clinical manifestations. The most common ones are described below.

Congenital anomalies are present in about 75% of patients who have VCFS [8]. The most prevalent are tetralogy of Fallot, ventricular septal defect with pulmonary atresia, persistent truncus arteriosus, and interrupted aortic arch. On screening of patients with cardiac anomalies, 3% to 15% had the chromosomal deletion indicative of VCFS. The frequency of the deletion was especially high in the subgroups with the specific anomalies listed above [8].

Abnormal facies are common in VCFS and are characterized by hypoplastic alae nasi, prominent nasal root, long narrow face with flat cheeks, narrow eye opening, small mouth and retruded chin, and small-cupped ears (Fig. 1).

Palatal abnormalities are present in up to 75% of patients. Most affected patients have insufficiency of the palate, with cleft palate being less common and cleft lip being rare. Clinically, the cleft anomalies in VCFS cause hypernasal speech [9].

Hypocalcemia and T-cell immunodeficiency, described in the DiGeorge syndrome phenotype, are caused by a hypoplastic parathyroid and thymus gland, respectively.

Other physical features of VCFS include tortuous retinal vessels, growth retardation, juvenile rheumatoid arthritis, and urinary system anomalies.

Besides the physical abnormalities, cognitive deficits and psychiatric disorders, including schizophrenia, are common in VCFS. The type and evolution of cognitive deficits and psychiatric symptoms in VCFS are described in detail in the second half of this article.

Suspected diagnosis of velocardiofacial syndrome: clinical guidelines

The question of utmost relevance to psychiatrists is when to suspect the presence of the 22q11 microdeletion in the differential diagnosis of a patient who has a psychiatric disorder. Schizophrenia and VCFS are highly associated, and about 25% of individuals who have VCFS develop schizophrenia

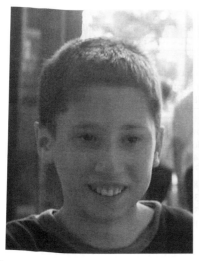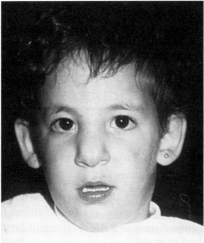

Fig. 1. Facial features in individuals with VCFS. Note the narrow eye opening and the long narrow face with flat cheeks (*left panel*) and the prominent nasal root and retruded chin (*right panel*).

(Table 1) [10]. Conversely, the rate of the 22q11.2 deletion in adults with schizophrenia is only 0.3% to 2% [11,12]. Rates are higher in patients who have childhood-onset schizophrenia (5.7%) [13], and in patients who have schizophrenia and additional major manifestation of VCFS, namely, cardiac and palate anomalies, typical facies, hypocalcemia, or learning disabilities (from 20% for one manifestation to 53% for two) [14,15]. The prevalence of the 22q11 deletion in other psychiatric disorders associated with VCFS probably is much lower. For example, no cases of 22q11 deletion were found in a group of 100 children who had attention deficit hyperactivity disorder (ADHD) [16].

The likelihood of the 22q11 deletion accompanying a typical physical manifestation of VCFS depends on its specific type. For example, the rate of 22q11 deletion is high in patients with tetralogy of Fallot, persistent truncus arteriosus, and interrupted arch [8]. It also should be borne in mind that the palatal anomalies often are covert and identifiable only by the presence of hypernasal speech; nasoendoscopic evaluation is necessary for their confirmation [17]. Referring patients for FISH analysis on the basis of a single sign/symptom probably is not cost-effective, and the author recommends cytogenetic testing only in the presence of at least two major signs/symptoms (see Table 1; e.g., schizophrenia + hypernasal speech; mental retardation or borderline IQ + tetralogy of Fallot).

Etiology and pathophysiology

VCFS is caused by a microdeletion in chromosome 22q11.2. About 90% of patients with VCFS have a deletion of 3 million base pairs, and most of

developmental disabilities, such as autism spectrum disorders [37,38]. Because they are not the common symptoms that are seen in typically developing children with OCD, some clinicians define them separately as perservative or stereotypic behaviors.

Recent studies that focused on autism spectrum symptoms in children who had VCFS reported rates of 14% to 45%; in 5% to 11% of patients, the symptoms met the DSM-IV-TR criteria for autistic disorders [28,39–41]. Whether they represent forme frust autism remains controversial, however. It could be argued that the social deficits in children who have VCFS reflect poor social skills secondary to the cognitive deficits and mental retardation. Language delays and communication abnormalities, another aspect of autism, are also common in VCFS, and relate, at least in part, to the general developmental delay and cleft anomalies. In support of a nonspecific association between VCFS and autism are the high reported rates of autism in many other neurogenetic syndromes (see the article by Feinstein and Singh elsewhere in this issue).

Late adolescence and adulthood

The increased rate of psychiatric disorders in children who have VCFS is similar to that in children with other developmental disabilities [27]; however, by late adolescence and early adulthood, this picture seems to change. On 5-year follow up, the VCFS group still showed high levels of anxiety and externalizing symptoms and aggressive behavior that were apparent at age 12.5 years, but the age- and cognitively-matched controls, who had had comparable findings in childhood, now showed considerable improvement in psychiatric behaviors [42]. In addition, by the second evaluation, 32% of the patients who had VCFS had acquired psychotic disorders—mostly schizophrenia and schizoaffective disorder—as opposed to only 4% of the controls.

Other studies also reported that 25% of subjects who had VCFS had schizophrenia-like psychotic disorder by early adulthood [10]. The average age of onset varied from 11 to 26 years [10,43,44]. The clinical characteristics of the psychotic disorder in VCFS are similar to those in the general population of patients who have schizophrenia [43]; however, the 25-fold higher rate of schizophrenia in VCFS compared with the general population and the 10-fold higher rate compared with patients with other developmental disabilities indicate that schizophrenia-like psychosis probably is specific to VCFS [45]. The rate of psychosis in VCSF is even higher than in offspring of a schizophrenic parent [46]. These findings make VCFS the most common known genetic risk factor for schizophrenia.

Cognitive deficits in velocardiofacial syndrome

The average full-scale IQ score in individuals with VCFS is in the mid-70s, within the borderline-intelligence range [47]. In 25% to 40% of subjects, intelligence is in the mental retardation range. When present, mental retardation usually is mild. The cognitive profile of subjects who have VCFS is characterized by relative strengths in the areas of reading, spelling, and rote memory and relative weaknesses in the areas of visuospatial memory and arithmetic [48]; it seems to change with development: Cross-sectional studies in children who had VCFS indicated an 8- to 10-point higher verbal IQ (VIQ) than performance IQ (PIQ) [49], whereas in adults, VIQ was 3.6 points lower than PIQ [50]. A recent longitudinal study confirmed that during adolescence there is a decline in VIQ scores of individuals who have VCFS [51].

Cognitive and neuroimaging studies of children who had VCFS conducted in the last decade provided information on the specific cognitive deficits and their possible underlying neural circuits [48] (for a comprehensive review of brain development and anatomy, see the article by Schaer and Eliez elsewhere in this issue). The frontostriatal and frontoparietal neural networks seem to be particularly affected. Children perform worse than would be expected by their cognitive level on tasks requiring shifts of attention, cognitive flexibility, and working memory (frontal cortex and caudate nucleus) [52,53] and on tasks involving visuospatial and numerical abilities (posterior parietal cortex) [54]. Compatible findings were reported in neuroimaging studies showing morphologic changes in the frontal cortex [55,56] and reduced parietal gray matter and white matter volumes, even after controlling for their reduced cortical volumes [57–59]. In addition, children who had VCFS had abnormal activation of the parietal cortex on functional MRI during performance of mathematical [60] and response-inhibition tasks. In a preliminary study, the author's team showed that adolescents who had VCSF performed equally well to controls on the Go/No Go response inhibition task; however, to do so, they had to activate more superior and inferior parietal regions [61]. In line with this finding, researchers recently proposed that a parietal dysfunction in individuals who have VCFS may impair their ability to orient visual cues and contribute to an overall executive dysfunction [62].

Risk factors for psychosis and cognitive impairment in velocardiofacial syndrome

Schizophrenia-like psychotic disorder occurs in up to one third of individuals who have VCFS and is a relatively specific debilitating developmental process of the syndrome. Thus, a major goal for researchers and clinicians is to identify early risk factors for psychosis in VCFS.

Several cross-sectional studies reported mild, subthreshold psychotic symptoms in one third to one half of children who had VCFS [27,34,63]; however, their methodology was of limited sensitivity, relying mainly on parental reports and not direct clinical interviews. In a more recent longitudinal study of 28 children who had VCFS evaluated during late childhood–early adolescence and again 5 years later [42], the presence of subthreshold psychotic symptoms, anxiety and depression symptoms, and lower VIQ during childhood significantly predicted the onset of psychotic disorders at follow-up. OCD was the strongest predictor among the anxiety disorders; all four subjects who had OCD at baseline exhibited psychotic disorders in early adulthood. Although ADHD is recognized as the most common psychiatric disorder in VCFS (40% to 50% of subjects), its presence did not seem to place the children at a greater risk for later psychotic disorder [42].

Together, these studies suggest a prolonged gradual evolution of the psychotic disorders in VCSF. Longitudinal studies of non-VCFS schizophrenia reported a similar drawn-out process [64], wherein neurologic, cognitive, and behavioral manifestations were already present from early childhood [65]. These findings negate the original assumption of a short prodrome of weeks to months between the appearance of neuropsychiatric symptoms and the onset of schizophrenia.

In addition to neuropsychiatric risk factors, the longitudinal study also suggested possible genetic risk factors in the emergence of psychosis in VCFS [42]. The *COMT* gene is located within the 1.5-million base pair microdeletion region implicated in VCSF. Therefore, all subjects who have VCFS have only one copy of the gene. The longitudinal study showed that the children carrying the low-activity (Met) allele of the *COMT* gene had a more significant decline in VIQ and language scores than those carrying the high-activity (Val) allele. The Met subgroup also had more severe psychotic symptoms, as manifested by their scores on the Brief Psychiatric Rating Scale, than the Val subgroup. Therefore, it seems that subjects who have VCFS who are hemizygous for the *COMT* Met allele are at particularly high risk for cognitive decline and psychotic symptoms during adolescence and young adulthood. A functional MRI study of individuals who had VCFS reported less efficient cingulate activity during performance of a response inhibition task in those carrying the Met allele than in those with the Val allele [61]. Further support for the critical role of Met hemizygosity in the pathogenesis of neuropsychiatric symptoms in VCFS was provided by an Israeli study [66], wherein the Met subgroup had a significantly higher prevalence of ADHD and OCD than did the Val subgroup.

In healthy individuals and individuals who have schizophrenia but not VCSF [67,68], the Val allele is associated with worse prefrontal cognitive function. This discrepancy may be understood using the Goldman-Rakic model of the inverted U–shaped relationship between cortical dopamine signaling and cognitive functioning [69]. The model, based on animal and human studies, shows that intermediate levels of the D1 dopamine cortical receptor "tone" are required for optimal cognitive performance. Too little and too much D1 receptor stimulation yielded less than optimal cognitive functioning [70–72].

Nevertheless, the role of the *COMT* gene in the pathogenesis of psychosis in VCFS is not certain. For example, some subjects in the longitudinal study [27] who had the Val allele showed a decrease in VIQ and later psychosis. This finding is supported by some other studies showing conflicting results [73,74]. The discrepancy may be attributable to the use of a cross-sectional versus a longitudinal design and to differences in sample ages. It is also possible that the cognitive deficiencies and susceptibility to psychosis of individuals who have VCFS are a consequence of a synergistic interaction between *COMT* and additional genes from the 22q11.2 deletion region. One candidate for such interaction is the highly polymorphic *PRODH* gene, which codes for proline oxidase, a mitochondrial enzyme that catalyzes the first step in the proline degradation pathway. In studies in the general population, several variants of the gene were associated with increased susceptibility to schizophrenia [75]. Hyperprolinemia also has been associated with mental retardation and psychotic disorders [76]. In an animal model, *PRODH*-deficient mice showed a robust up-regulation of *COMT* mRNA and protein expression, which was interpreted as a homeostatic response to enhanced dopaminergic signaling in the frontal cortex secondary to the gene deficiency [77]. In line with the animal findings, a recent study reported that within the overall 22q11.2DS population, subjects who had hyperprolinemia and the *COMT* Met allele were three times more likely to have a psychotic disorder [78].

Psychiatric treatment

The physical and psychiatric morbidity and cognitive deficits in VCFS vary widely in scope and severity. Because multiple developmental trajectories are affected in psychitatric treatments for individuals with VCFS, a multimodal treatment approach is required, including behavioral interventions for anxiety disorders and abnormal behaviors (eg, repetitive behaviors, stereotypes), social skills training, parental guidance, and psychiatric medications. This section focuses on a few pivotal aspects of psychitatric treatments for individuals with VCFS. In the almost total absence of publications on psychosocial or psychiatric treatment in VCFS and the paucity of empiric data, this section is based largely on the author's clinical experience.

Psychiatric evaluation

The high rate of psychiatric disorders in VCFS, and their evolutionary nature, warrants a routine psychiatric evaluation annually or biannually during childhood and more frequently during adolescence. Screening for mild and even subthreshold psychotic and internalizing symptoms is of utmost importance, because they predict the later onset of full-blown schizophrenia-like psychotic disorder [42]. Because these symptoms usually are not disruptive, as opposed for example to hyperactivity and oppositional symptoms, they can be overlooked easily.

Psychiatric medications

Antipsychotics

Preliminary data indicate that the administration of atypical antipsychotic agents to adolescents/young adults with prodromal symptoms of schizophrenia, in the absence of VCFS, may delay or prevent the appearance of the full-blown syndrome [79–81]. Thus, strong consideration should be given to their use in children who have VCFS who exhibit even mild (ie, subsyndromal) psychotic symptoms. Given that individuals who have VCFS and severe cardiac anomalies are at an increased risk for arrhythmias, psychiatrists should choose antipsychotic drugs that are less likely to increase the Q-T interval on the electrocardiogram and should monitor treated patients closely at each dosage titration and thereafter. Although the psychotic symptoms associated with VCFS improve with antipsychotic medication, they tend to be more treatment-resistant than are those in patients who have schizophrenia but not VCFS [82].

Stimulants

Because ADHD is the most common psychiatric disorder in VCFS, the question of whether to prescribe stimulant medication, such as methylphenidate, is raised frequently. There are several concerns regarding the use of stimulants in subjects who have VCFS because of their increased risk for psychosis and depression—both are possible side effects of these medications—and the frequent presence of congenital cardiac anomalies, which can increase the risk for hypertension and tachycardia. In the only open-label study of stimulant use in VCFS, the author and colleagues [29] found that a low dosage of methylphenidate (0.3 mg/kg) administered for 1 month to children and adolescents effectively and safely reduced ADHD symptoms in 75% of cases (9/12). The average duration of the methylphenidate effect was 3.2 hours. Side effects were similar to those described in typical children (ie, poor appetite, irritability, sadness, and stomachaches), but they were always mild and in no case were the reason for discontinuation of treatment. None of the children developed psychotic or manic symptoms. Longer-term, placebo-controlled trails are needed to confirm these findings.

Other psychiatric medications

Although mood stabilizers, such as valproic acid and antidepressants, and in particular, serotonin-specific reuptake inhibitors, are prescribed frequently to patients who have VCFS, there are no studies on their efficacy and safety in this setting. In one study of five patients who had VCFS and OCD and were treated with fluoxetine (dosage range: 30–60 mg/d), four showed significant improvement in OCD symptoms [30]. The only side effect was transient abdominal discomfort in one patient.

Pathophysiologically based medications

All subjects who have VCFS miss one copy of the *COMT* gene, which codes for the COMT enzyme that is responsible for degrading dopamine. There are a few case series reporting the effect of medications that lower synaptic dopamine levels on psychiatric symptoms [83,84]. In one of them, five subjects who had VCFS and carried *COMT* Met allele were treated with metyrosine, a tyrosine hydroxylase inhibitor [83]. Psychiatric symptoms were alleviated in these cases, and clinical improvement was associated with a decline in cerebrospinal fluid levels of homovalinic acid, the metabolite of dopamine. Metyrosine is not a registered antipsychotic medication, however, and it may cause hypotension.

Mentoring program

For several years, the author's Behavioral Neurogenetics Center in Israel has been running a mentoring program for children and adolescence who have VCFS, which is staffed by undergraduate psychology students. The major goal of the program is to provide the children with a meaningful relationship that provides them emotional support and encouragement and strengthens their self-confidence. The mentors meet the children in their homes for "one-on-one" interaction. Initially, they serve simply as "good listeners," empathizing with the children and providing support and advice. Once a bond has been formed and the child develops trust in the mentor, the groundwork is laid. Within this framework, structured therapeutic interventions are established, such as involving the mentor in the child's behavioral modification program, which are targeted to the specific difficulties of each child [85].

Acknowledgments

This work was funded in part by the National Alliance for Research on Schizophrenia and Depression (NARSAD) Young Investigator Award and the Basil O'Connor Starter Scholar Research Award of the March of Dimes (Grant No. 5-FY06-590).

References

[1] Kirkpatrick JA Jr, DiGeorge AM. Congenital absence of the thymus. Am J Roentgenol Radium Ther Nucl Med 1968;103:32–7.
[2] Shprintzen RJ, Goldberg RB, Lewin ML, et al. A new syndrome involving cleft palate, cardiac anomalies, typical facies, and learning disabilities: velo-cardio-facial syndrome. Cleft Palate J 1978;15:56–62.
[3] Carey AH, Kelly D, Halford S, et al. Molecular genetic study of the frequency of monosomy 22q11 in DiGeorge syndrome. Am J Hum Genet 1992;51:964–70.
[4] Driscoll DA, Budarf ML, Emanuel BS. A genetic etiology for DiGeorge syndrome: consistent deletions and microdeletions of 22q11. Am J Hum Genet 1992;50:924–33.

[5] Driscoll DA, Spinner NB, Budarf ML, et al. Deletions and microdeletions of 22q11.2 in velo-cardio-facial syndrome. Am J Med Genet 1992;44:261–8.

[6] Driscoll DA, Salvin J, Sellinger B, et al. Prevalence of 22q11 microdeletions in DiGeorge and velocardiofacial syndromes: implications for genetic counselling and prenatal diagnosis. J Med Genet 1993;30:813–7.

[7] Botto LD, May K, Fernhoff PM, et al. A population-based study of the 22q11.2 deletion: phenotype, incidence, and contribution to major birth defects in the population. Pediatrics 2003;112:101–7.

[8] Marino B, Mileto F, Digilio MC, et al. Congenital cardiovascular disease and velo-cardio-facial syndrome. In: Murphy KC, Scambler PJ, editors. Velo-cardio-facial syndrome: a model for understanding microdeletion disorders. Cambridge (MA): Cambridge University Press; 2005. p. 47–82.

[9] Kirscher RE. Palatal anomalies and velopharyngeal dysfunction associated with velo-cardio-facial syndrome. In: Velo-cardio-facial syndrome: a model for understanding microdeletion disorders. Cambridge (MA): Cambridge University Press; 2005. p. 83–104.

[10] Murphy KC, Jones LA, Owen MJ. High rates of schizophrenia in adults with velo-cardio-facial syndrome. Arch Gen Psychiatry 1999;56:940–5.

[11] Arinami T, Ohtsuki T, Takase K, et al. Screening for 22q11 deletions in a schizophrenia population. Schizophr Res 2001;52:167–70.

[12] Karayiorgou M, Morris MA, Morrow B, et al. Schizophrenia susceptibility associated with interstitial deletions of chromosome 22q11. Proc Natl Acad Sci U S A 1995;92: 7612–6.

[13] Sporn A, Addington A, Reiss AL, et al. 22q11 deletion syndrome in childhood onset schizophrenia: an update. Mol Psychiatry 2004;9:225–6.

[14] Bassett AS, Hodgkinson K, Chow EW, et al. 22q11 deletion syndrome in adults with schizophrenia. Am J Med Genet 1998;81:328–37.

[15] Gothelf D, Frisch A, Munitz H, et al. Velocardiofacial manifestations and microdeletions in schizophrenic inpatients. Am J Med Genet 1997;72:455–61.

[16] Bastain TM, Lewczyk CM, Sharp WS, et al. Cytogenetic abnormalities in attention-deficit/hyperactivity disorder. J Am Acad Child Adolesc Psychiatry 2002;41:806–10.

[17] Shprintzen RJ, Golding-Kushner KJ. Evaluation of velopharyngeal insufficiency. Otolaryngol Clin North Am 1989;22:519–36.

[18] Morrow B, Goldberg R, Carlson C, et al. Molecular definition of the 22q11 deletions in velo-cardio-facial syndrome. Am J Hum Genet 1995;56:1391–403.

[19] McDonald-McGinn DM, Tonnesen MK, Laufer-Cahana A, et al. Phenotype of the 22q11.2 deletion in individuals identified through an affected relative: cast a wide FISHing net! Genet Med 2001;3:23–9.

[20] Ryan AK, Goodship JA, Wilson DI, et al. Spectrum of clinical features associated with interstitial chromosome 22q11 deletions: a European collaborative study. J Med Genet 1997; 34:798–804.

[21] Prescott K, Ivins S, Hubank M, et al. Microarray analysis of the Df1 mouse model of the 22q11 deletion syndrome. Hum Genet 2005;116:486–96.

[22] Funke B, Pandita RK, Morrow BE. Isolation and characterization of a novel gene containing WD40 repeats from the region deleted in velo-cardio-facial/DiGeorge syndrome on chromosome 22q11. Genomics 2001;73:264–71.

[23] McDermid HE, Morrow BE. Genomic disorders on 22q11. Am J Hum Genet 2002;70: 1077–88.

[24] Paylor R, Glaser B, Mupo A, et al. Tbx1 haploinsufficiency is linked to behavioral disorders in mice and humans: implications for 22q11 deletion syndrome. Proc Natl Acad Sci U S A 2006;103:7729–34.

[25] Shprintzen RJ. Velo-cardio-facial syndrome: a distinct behavioral phenotype. Ment Retard Dev Disabil Res Rev 2000;6:142–7.

[26] Arnold PD, Siegel-Bartelt J, Cytrynbaum C, et al. Velo-cardio-facial syndrome: implications of microdeletion 22q11 for schizophrenia and mood disorders. Am J Med Genet 2001;105: 354–62.
[27] Feinstein C, Eliez S, Blasey C, et al. Psychiatric disorders and behavioral problems in children with velocardiofacial syndrome: usefulness as phenotypic indicators of schizophrenia risk. Biol Psychiatry 2002;51:312–8.
[28] Fine SE, Weissman A, Gerdes M, et al. Autism spectrum disorders and symptoms in children with molecularly confirmed 22q11.2 deletion syndrome. J Autism Dev Disord 2005;35: 461–70.
[29] Gothelf D, Gruber R, Presburger G, et al. Methylphenidate treatment for attention-deficit/ hyperactivity disorder in children and adolescents with velocardiofacial syndrome: an open-label study. J Clin Psychiatry 2003;64:1163–9.
[30] Gothelf D, Presburger G, Zohar AH, et al. Obsessive-compulsive disorder in patients with velocardiofacial (22q11 deletion) syndrome. Am J Med Genet Neuropsychiatr Genet 2004;126:99–105.
[31] Papolos DF, Faedda GL, Veit S, et al. Bipolar spectrum disorders in patients diagnosed with velo-cardio- facial syndrome: does a hemizygous deletion of chromosome 22q11 result in bipolar affective disorder? Am J Psychiatry 1996;153:1541–7.
[32] Prinzie P, Swillen A, Vogels A, et al. Personality profiles of youngsters with velo-cardio-facial syndrome. Genet Couns 2002;13:265–80.
[33] Swillen A, Devriendt K, Ghesquiere P, et al. Children with a 22q11 deletion versus children with a speech-language impairment and learning disability: behavior during primary school age. Genet Couns 2001;12:309–17.
[34] Baker KD, Skuse DH. Adolescents and young adults with 22q11 deletion syndrome: psychopathology in an at-risk group. Br J Psychiatry 2005;186:115–20.
[35] Antshel KM, Fremont W, Roizen NJ, et al. ADHD, major depressive disorder, and simple phobias are prevalent psychiatric conditions in youth with velocardiofacial syndrome. J Am Acad Child Adolesc Psychiatry 2006;45:596–603.
[36] Debbane M, Glaser B, Gex-Fabry M, et al. Temporal perception in velo-cardio-facial syndrome. Neuropsychologia 2005;43:1754–62.
[37] Dykens EM, Leckman JF, Cassidy SB. Obsessions and compulsions in Prader-Willi syndrome. J Child Psychol Psychiatry 1996;37:995–1002.
[38] Mervis CB, Klein-Tasman BP. Williams syndrome: cognition, personality, and adaptive behavior. Ment Retard Dev Disabil Res Rev 2000;6:148–58.
[39] Antshel KM, Aneja A, Strunge L, et al. Autistic spectrum disorders in velo-cardio facial syndrome (22q11.2 deletion). J Autism Dev Disord 2007, in press.
[40] Niklasson L, Rasmussen P, Oskarsdottir S, et al. Neuropsychiatric disorders in the 22q11 deletion syndrome. Genet Med 2001;3:79–84.
[41] Vorstman JA, Morcus ME, Duijff SN, et al. The 22q11.2 deletion in children: high rate of autistic disorders and early onset of psychotic symptoms. J Am Acad Child Adolesc Psychiatry 2006;45:1104–13.
[42] Gothelf D, Feinstein C, Thompson T, et al. Risk factors for the emergence of psychotic disorders in adolescents with 22q11.2 deletion syndrome. Am J Psychiatry 2007;164(4):663–9.
[43] Bassett AS, Chow EW, AbdelMalik P, et al. The schizophrenia phenotype in 22q11 deletion syndrome. Am J Psychiatry 2003;160:1580–6.
[44] Usiskin SI, Nicolson R, Krasnewich DM, et al. Velocardiofacial syndrome in childhood-onset schizophrenia. J Am Acad Child Adolesc Psychiatry 1999;38:1536–43.
[45] Turner TH. Schizophrenia and mental handicap: an historical review, with implications for further research. Psychol Med 1989;19:301–14.
[46] Murphy KC. Schizophrenia and velo-cardio-facial syndrome. Lancet 2002;359:426–30.
[47] Swillen A, Devriendt K, Legius E, et al. Intelligence and psychosocial adjustment in velocardiofacial syndrome: a study of 37 children and adolescents with VCFS. J Med Genet 1997;34:453–8.

692   GOTHELF

[48] Simon TJ, Bish JP, Bearden CE, et al. A multilevel analysis of cognitive dysfunction and psychopathology associated with chromosome 22q11.2 deletion syndrome in children. Dev Psychopathol 2005;17:753–84.
[49] Campbell LE, Swillen A. The cognitive spectrum in velo-cardio-facial syndrome. In: Velo-cardio-facial syndrome: a model for understanding microdeletion disorders. Cambridge (MA): Cambridge University Press; 2005. p. 147–64.
[50] Henry JC, van Amelsvoort T, Morris RG, et al. An investigation of the neuropsychological profile in adults with velo-cardio-facial syndrome (VCFS). Neuropsychologia 2002;40: 471–8.
[51] Gothelf D, Eliez S, Thompson T, et al. COMT genotype predicts longitudinal cognitive decline and psychosis in 22q11.2 deletion syndrome. Nat Neurosci 2005;8:1500–2.
[52] Sobin C, Kiley-Brabeck K, Daniels S, et al. Networks of attention in children with the 22q11 deletion syndrome. Dev Neuropsychol 2004;26:611–26.
[53] Woodin M, Wang PP, Aleman D, et al. Neuropsychological profile of children and adolescents with the 22q11.2 microdeletion. Genet Med 2001;3:34–9.
[54] Kates WR, Burnette CP, Bessette BA, et al. Frontal and caudate alterations in velocardiofacial syndrome (deletion at chromosome 22q11.2). J Child Neurol 2004;19:337–42.
[55] Eliez S, Barnea-Goraly N, Schmitt JE, et al. Increased basal ganglia volumes in velo-cardio-facial syndrome (deletion 22q11.2). Biol Psychiatry 2002;52:68–70.
[56] Simon TJ, Bearden CE, Mc-Ginn DM, et al. Visuospatial and numerical cognitive deficits in children with chromosome 22q11.2 deletion syndrome. Cortex 2005;41:145–55.
[57] Campbell LE, Daly E, Toal F, et al. Brain and behaviour in children with 22q11.2 deletion syndrome: a volumetric and voxel-based morphometry MRI study. Brain 2006;129(pt 5): 1218–28.
[58] Eliez S, Schmitt JE, White CD, et al. Children and adolescents with velocardiofacial syndrome: a volumetric MRI study. Am J Psychiatry 2000;157:409–15.
[59] Kates WR, Burnette CP, Jabs EW, et al. Regional cortical white matter reductions in velocardiofacial syndrome: a volumetric MRI analysis. Biol Psychiatry 2001;49:677–84.
[60] Eliez S, Blasey CM, Menon V, et al. Functional brain imaging study of mathematical reasoning abilities in velocardiofacial syndrome (del22q11.2). Genet Med 2001;3:49–55.
[61] Gothelf D, Hoeft F, Hinard C, et al. Abnormal cortical activation during response inhibition in 22q11.2 deletion syndrome. Hum Brain Mapp 2007, in press.
[62] Bish JP, Ferrante SM, McDonald-McGinn D, et al. Maladaptive conflict monitoring as evidence for executive dysfunction in children with chromosome 22q11.2 deletion syndrome. Dev Sci 2005;8:36–43.
[63] Debbane M, Glaser B, David MK, et al. Psychotic symptoms in children and adolescents with 22q11.2 deletion syndrome: neuropsychological and behavioral implications. Schizophr Res 2006;84:187–93.
[64] Poulton R, Caspi A, Moffitt TE, et al. Children's self-reported psychotic symptoms and adult schizophreniform disorder: a 15-year longitudinal study. Arch Gen Psychiatry 2000;57: 1053–8.
[65] Niemi LT, Suvisaari JM, Tuulio-Henriksson A, et al. Childhood developmental abnormalities in schizophrenia: evidence from high-risk studies. Schizophr Res 2003;60:239–58.
[66] Gothelf D, Michaelovsky E, Frisch A, et al. Association of the low-activity COMT 158 Met allele with ADHD and OCD in subjects with velocardiofacial syndrome. Int J Neuropsychopharmacol 2006;31:1–8.
[67] Egan MF, Goldberg TE, Kolachana BS, et al. Effect of COMT Val108/158 Met genotype on frontal lobe function and risk for schizophrenia. Proc Natl Acad Sci U S A 2001;98:6917–22.
[68] Mattay VS, Goldberg TE, Fera F, et al. Catechol O-methyltransferase val158-met genotype and individual variation in the brain response to amphetamine. Proc Natl Acad Sci U S A 2003;100:6186–91.
[69] Goldman-Rakic PS, Muly EC 3rd, Williams GV. D(1) receptors in prefrontal cells and circuits. Brain Res Brain Res Rev 2000;31:295–301.

[70] Zahrt J, Taylor JR, Mathew RG, et al. Supranormal stimulation of D1 dopamine receptors in the rodent prefrontal cortex impairs spatial working memory performance. J Neurosci 1997;17:8528–35.

[71] Cai JX, Arnsten AF. Dose-dependent effects of the dopamine D1 receptor agonists A77636 or SKF81297 on spatial working memory in aged monkeys. J Pharmacol Exp Ther 1997;283: 183–9.

[72] Seamans JK, Yang CR. The principal features and mechanisms of dopamine modulation in the prefrontal cortex. Prog Neurobiol 2004;74:1–57.

[73] Bearden CE, Jawad AF, Lynch DR, et al. Effects of a functional COMT polymorphism on prefrontal cognitive function in patients with 22q11.2 deletion syndrome. Am J Psychiatry 2004;161:1700–2.

[74] Glaser B, Debbane M, Hinard C, et al. No evidence for an effect of COMT Val158Met genotype on executive function in patients with 22q11 deletion syndrome. Am J Psychiatry 2006;163:537–9.

[75] Bender HU, Almashanu S, Steel G, et al. Functional consequences of PRODH missense mutations. Am J Hum Genet 2005;76:409–20.

[76] Paterlini M, Zakharenko SS, Lai WS, et al. Transcriptional and behavioral interaction between 22q11.2 orthologs modulates schizophrenia-related phenotypes in mice. Nat Neurosci 2005;8:1586–94.

[77] Liu H, Heath SC, Sobin C, et al. Genetic variation at the 22q11 PRODH2/DGCR6 locus presents an unusual pattern and increases susceptibility to schizophrenia. Proc Natl Acad Sci U S A 2002;99:3717–22.

[78] Raux G, Bumsel E, Hecketsweiler B, et al. Involvement of hyperprolinemia in cognitive and psychiatric features of the 22q11 deletion syndrome. Hum Mol Genet 2007;16: 83–91.

[79] McGlashan TH, Zipursky RB, Perkins D, et al. Randomized, double-blind trial of olanzapine versus placebo in patients prodromally symptomatic for psychosis. Am J Psychiatry 2006;163:790–9.

[80] McGorry PD, Yung AR, Phillips LJ, et al. Randomized controlled trial of interventions designed to reduce the risk of progression to first-episode psychosis in a clinical sample with subthreshold symptoms. Arch Gen Psychiatry 2002;59:921–8.

[81] Thomas LE, Woods SW. The schizophrenia prodrome: a developmentally informed review and update for psychopharmacologic treatment. Child Adolesc Psychiatr Clin N Am 2006; 15:109–33.

[82] Gothelf D, Frisch A, Munitz H, et al. Clinical characteristics of schizophrenia associated with velo-cardio-facial syndrome. Schizophr Res 1999;35:105–12.

[83] Graf WD, Unis AS, Yates CM, et al. Catecholamines in patients with 22q11.2 deletion syndrome and the low-activity COMT polymorphism. Neurology 2001;57:410–6.

[84] O'Hanlon JF, Ritchie RC, Smith EA, et al. Replacement of antipsychotic and antiepileptic medication by L-alpha-methyldopa in a woman with velocardiofacial syndrome. Int Clin Psychopharmacol 2003;18:117–9.

[85] DuBois DL, Holloway BE, Valentine JC, et al. Effectiveness of mentoring programs for youth: a meta-analytic review. Am J Community Psychol 2002;30:157–97.

[86] Shprintzen RJ, Goldberg R, Golding-Kushner KJ, et al. Late-onset psychosis in the velo-cardio-facial syndrome. Am J Med Genet 1992;42:141–2.

[87] Pulver AE, Nestadt G, Goldberg R, et al. Psychotic illness in patients diagnosed with velo-cardio-facial syndrome and their relatives. J Nerv Ment Dis 1994;182:476–8.

ELSEVIER
SAUNDERS

Child Adolesc Psychiatric Clin N Am
16 (2007) 695–708

CHILD AND
ADOLESCENT
PSYCHIATRIC CLINICS
OF NORTH AMERICA

Prader-Willi Syndrome: Medical Prevention and Behavioral Challenges

Fortu Benarroch, MD[a],*, Harry J. Hirsch, MD[b],
Larry Genstil, PhD[b], Yael E. Landau, MA[b],
Varda Gross-Tsur, MD[b]

[a]Child and Adolescent Psychiatry, Hadassah Hospital, Mount Scopus,
POB 24035, Jerusalem 91240, Israel
[b]Neuropediatric Unit, Shaare Zedek Medical Center, POB 3235,
Jerusalem 91301, Israel

Prader-Willi syndrome (PWS), first described by Prader, Labhart, and Willi in 1956, is a genetic disorder caused by deletion or impaired expression of paternal genes in a critical area of chromosome 15. The incidence ranges from 1:10,000 to 1:20,000 births, with equal distribution in both sexes and all ethnic groups [1]. This neurogenetic multisystemic disorder is characterized by infantile hypotonia, mental retardation, feeding difficulty in infancy that evolves to an extreme drive to eat in childhood, dysmorphic features, short stature, hypogonadism, sleep apnea, diabetes, and severe maladaptive behaviors, including obsessive, compulsive, and oppositional behaviors. There is a widely accepted view that the neurologic underpinnings of PWS involve hypothalamic dysregulation; however, brain imaging techniques suggest that other brain regions are also involved [2,3].

We begin this article with a brief discussion of the genetic basis of PWS followed by a description of the characteristic medical features, the comorbidity associated with this syndrome, a review of endocrine abnormalities, and hormonal treatment. We present the profile of intellectual impairment and the characteristic pattern of maladaptive behavior, with emphasis on the psychiatric aspects of PWS, and conclude with a discussion of behavioral and institutional treatment issues.

This study was supported in part by grants from the Peretz Naftali Foundation and the Mirsky Foundation.

* Corresponding author. Hadassah-Hebrew University Medical Center, Jerusalem, Israel.
E-mail address: fortuben@hadassah.org.il (F. Benarroch).

1056-4993/07/$ - see front matter © 2007 Elsevier Inc. All rights reserved.
doi:10.1016/j.chc.2007.03.007

Genetics

Deletion or abnormal expression of paternal genes in chromosome 15q11-13 can result in the Prader-Willi phenotype. Complete or partial deletion of paternal 15q11-q13 accounts for 70% of affected patients, whereas approximately 25% have uniparental maternal disomy (UPD). In normal chromosome pairs, each chromosome is derived from a different parent. The term "uniparental disomy" indicates that both copies of a particular chromosome derive from only one of the parents. Inheriting both copies of chromosome 15 from the mother results in PWS. Older maternal age seems to be a more common factor in patients who have UPD and is associated with meiotic nondisjunctive events that result in uniparental disomic zygotes [4,5]. An estimated 1% to 5% of patients who have PWS have a mutation in the imprinting center, which causes abnormal gene expression despite the presence of anatomically intact paternal and maternal chromosomes 15 [4–6]. Imprinting refers to the differential expression of genetic material depending on whether the gene is derived from the mother or father. If a gene is paternally imprinted, the gene derived from the father is inactive and only the gene derived from the mother is expressed. Microdeletions, detected by sequence analysis, have been reported in only 15% of patients with proven imprinting defects.

The inheritance of PWS is almost always sporadic. The risk to siblings and other first-degree relatives is less than 1% when the molecular defect is a deletion or UPD. A mutation in the imprinting center, found in 1% to 5% of patients, carries a 50% risk of family recurrence. Determination of the specific type of genetic defect is essential for counseling parents regarding risk to future offspring.

Fluorescent in situ hybridization detects nearly all patients with deletions in the 15q11-q13 region. A technique using microsatellite markers can determine if all of the alleles are of maternal origin (UPD). The most sensitive method for detecting nearly all cases of PWS, however, is DNA methylation analysis. The diagnosis of PWS is confirmed by finding a methylation pattern characteristic of exclusively maternal alleles. Patients who are suspected of having PWS should first undergo methylation analysis. If the methylation test result is positive, fluorescent in situ hybridization or microsatellite studies can be applied subsequently to determine the exact type of molecular defect present.

Although PWS is not included in routine prenatal screening, the severity of this syndrome may justify inclusion of PWS in routine prenatal genetic disease screening.

Medical considerations

Medical problems are inherent within the clinical diagnostic criteria of PWS and differ according to the stage of life [7]. Perinatally, the manifestations are difficult delivery, central hypotonia, poor sucking, motor delay, and failure to thrive, which often necessitate special feeding techniques such as nasogas-tric tubes. The characteristic dysmorphic features include dolichocephaly and almond-shaped eyes. Small mouth, hands, and feet, speech articulation defects, and a distinct prosody become apparent in childhood. In adulthood, mild hypotonia with decreased muscle bulk and tone is present [8].

The resting metabolic rate is lower than expected for age. This rate, in combination with a low level of general motor activity and overeating, leads quickly to severe morbid obesity. The obesity is central in distribution and is the major cause of morbidity and mortality: cardiopulmonary compromise, type 2 diabetes mellitus, hypertension, thrombophlebitis, leg edema, and sleep apnea [8]. The abnormal metabolic rate may account for the prolonged and exaggerated responses to standard dosages of medications and anes-thetic agents [9,10].

Sleep and breathing disorders are attributed to central dysfunction al-though exacerbated by obesity. The manifestations of nocturnal breathing ab-normalities are excessive daytime sleepiness, abnormal ventilatory responses to hypoxia, and hypercapnia. Treatment includes adenotonsillectomy, noc-turnal ventilation, weight control, and behavioral interventions [11]. Orthope-dic problems, such as scoliosis/kyphosis and osteoporosis, are frequent [7].

Thick, viscous saliva may predispose to dental caries and contribute to articulation problems and can complicate airway management. Products for increasing saliva production have proved beneficial in treating dry mouth and improving dental hygiene [8].

High pain threshold, decreased vomiting, and altered homeostatic hypo-thalamic control of body temperature characterize PWS. As a result, subtle signs or symptoms can be the harbinger of serious underlying disease. Phy-sicians should be alert to changes in behavior, temperature, mood, or minor complaints in individuals who have PWS [12]. In light of hyperphagia and possible ingestion of spoiled food, lack of or the presence of vomiting may signal a life-threatening illness. Controversy exists as to whether sudden, unexpected death is a feature of PWS and if the life expectancy is decreased compared with the general population [13].

In conclusion, the medical picture of individuals who have PWS involves multiple systems: central nervous, respiratory, gastrointestinal, cardiovascu-lar, dermatologic, and urogenital. Medical treatment demands prevention and treatment of weight gain because most of the serious medical problems are a direct consequence of morbid obesity. A multidisciplinary approach with anticipatory care and appropriate attention to medical problems as they occur can improve the quality of life of patients who have PWS.

Endocrine disorders and hormonal treatment

Children who have PWS show variable degrees of impaired growth hormone (GH) secretion along with low levels of serum insulin and insu-lin-like growth factors. If untreated, 50% of individuals who have PWS fail to reach a normal adult height. GH treatment of these children results in a significant and persistent increase in height velocity and height standard deviation scores [14].

Beyond increasing final height, GH has other important beneficial effects in patients who have PWS. Infants in whom GH treatment was started before age 18 months show significantly increased mobility skill acquisition. In children who were treated before 3 years, there is decreased percent body fat mass and increased lean body mass. Older children and adolescents maintain a sustained decrease in body fat mass and increased lean body mass and bone mineral density [15]. Resting energy expenditure is also increased [15]. Pulmonary function, measured by peak flow rate, vital capacity, and forced expiratory flow, improved during 6 months of GH treatment [16].

Although side effects of GH treatment in children are rare, there are concerns that children who have PWS may be at increased risk for worsening of scoliosis, development of diabetes mellitus, and death from obstructive sleep apnea or central hypoventilation. Among 328 children who have PWS who were treated with GH for 1 to 2 years, 5 developed type 2 diabetes mellitus and one case of type 1 diabetes was observed [17]. Monitoring for scoliosis is recommended during treatment because scoliosis is common in PWS and may worsen as linear growth increases.

Reports of sudden death in children who have PWS receiving GH raised concerns of increased mortality in these patients. To date, however, there is no convincing evidence that children treated with GH have a higher mortality rate than nontreated patients [17,18]. Although GH may stimulate growth of lymphoid tissue, including tonsils and adenoids, and exacerbate any pre-existing obstructive sleep apnea, GH exerts beneficial effects on respiratory function by decreasing body fat mass while increasing lean body mass. Additional risk factors for mortality include severe obesity and concurrent upper respiratory tract infections. A strict dietary and behavioral program of weight control should be initiated before starting GH treatment, and a sleep study should be conducted to evaluate oxygen saturations or sleep apnea. We also recommend repeating the sleep study 1 month after onset of treatment. If there is an increase in sleep apnea or hypoxia, GH treatment may need to be stopped until the factors contributing to impaired respiratory function are corrected. It may be prudent to withdraw GH treatment during acute upper respiratory or other intercurrent infections.

Hypogonadism is a consistent feature of PWS; cryptorchidism and micropenis are common—although not universal—findings. Boys undergo some pubertal development, but midpubertal arrest generally occurs. Most girls undergo spontaneous development of breast tissue during adolescence, probably because of estrogen production from peripheral aromatization in adipose tissue. Spontaneous menarche has been described in 44% of girls older than age 15 years, but menses are often limited to periodic spotting [19]. Pregnancy was reported in two women with genetically documented PWS. Fertility has not been reported in men who have PWS.

It has generally been assumed that hypogonadism in PWS is explained by gonadotropin deficiency caused by hypothalamic dysfunction. Recently, Eiholzer and colleagues [20] found that boys who have PWS may have a combined central and peripheral hypogonadism that consists of low leutinizing hormone levels along with low inhibin B and high follicle-stimulating hormone levels. These findings suggest that boys who have PWS have a primary Sertoli and/or germ cell defect or early germ cell loss.

The medical rationale for sex hormone replacement therapy includes prevention or treatment of osteoporosis, improvement of muscle mass and function by androgen replacement in male patients, and prevention of the albeit rare possibility of pregnancy by use of oral contraceptives. Testosterone may be administered as an intramuscular depot preparation (testosterone enanthate in oil) at intervals of 2 to 4 weeks, starting with a low dose of 50 mg every 4 weeks and gradually increasing to full adult replacement of 200 mg every 2 weeks. Peak and trough testosterone levels on the intramuscular regimen may result in aggressive behavior and emotional lability. Testosterone patches may be preferable because they provide stabile levels of testosterone. Oral contraceptives that contain a low dose of estrogen are usually adequate to maintain regular menses and prevent deterioration in bone density. In addition to sex hormone replacement, calcium and vitamin supplements should be recommended when low bone density is found.

Cognition

Mental retardation is a major characteristic of PWS. In a meta-analysis of 575 people who have PWS, only 5% were of normal intelligence, one third were found to be moderately retarded, and most were in the borderline mildly retarded range. No IQ decline was seen with age [21]. Unfortunately, their immature social behavior often masks their intellectual abilities [22].

A pattern of cognitive strengths and weaknesses is apparent, although not all individuals who have PWS show this profile [21]. As a group, their main strengths are in the domains of visuospatial performance, reading and decoding, long-term memory, and exceptional skills with jigsaw puzzles [23,24]. Areas of disability are short-term memory, auditory processing, socialization, and mathematical skills. They also show low performance in sequential as opposed to simultaneous processing [23].

Individuals who have the UPD genetic type may display slightly higher cognitive skills than individuals with deletions. The differences reported are that individuals who have UPD have a higher average verbal intelligence and impaired coding ability. One hypothesis is that these differences are a manifestation of the influences of gender-specific imprinted genes on cerebral lateralization, a hypothesis that needs further investigation [25].

To date no comprehensive study has assessed executive functions in children who have PWS. Even attention deficit hyperactivity disorder, in which executive functions are typically impaired, only recently has been documented in PWS [26,27]. The severe medical problems may divert attention from the impaired executive functions and attention deficit hyperactivity disorder. In persons with relatively high IQ, impaired executive functions may be a partial explanation for the apparent discrepancy between their intelligence and their overall low level of academic, neuropsychological, and social functioning [26].

In a pilot study on adults who have PWS, beneficial effects in mental speed, flexibility, and motor performance during GH treatment have been reported [28]. It is essential to recognize and address the specific cognitive characteristics of persons who have PWS and their areas of strength and disabilities, which will enable therapists to tailor educational interventions to achieve optimal expression of intellectual abilities.

Behavioral characteristics and psychiatric issues in Prader-Willi syndrome

Behavioral patterns are remarkably consistent among persons who have PWS, albeit with a wide spectrum of intensity and frequency. The characteristic symptom complex is often termed "the behavioral phenotype of PWS," which qualifies persons who have PWS for an Axis I diagnosis of "personality change due to a medical condition" [29]. Forster and Gourash [30] suggested a useful classification in domains that we have modified in accordance with our clinical experience.

Food-seeking related behaviors

The endless pursuit for food starts around the age of 6 years. The core abnormality is not an increased appetite but an impaired satiety response [31]. If unrestricted, persons who have PWS can eat enormous quantities of food, and when regular food is unavailable, they eat frozen, raw, or even pet food. One of our patients left his sheltered group house for 13 hours without any supervision and gained 29 pounds during that short period. Common techniques for obtaining food are night raids to the kitchen, manipulating well-meaning adults, and taking food from the garbage or other children's bags, but may also include begging, lying, stealing, and breaking locks. The pursuit for food may culminate in dangerous behaviors, such as providing sex services in exchange for food. To date, there is no effective medication to ameliorate this problem [32]; its management requires 24-hour-a-day supervision, restrictive measures, planned physical activity, and a strict diet (≤ 1200 cal/d) divided into consistently scheduled meals. Every person in the immediate environ must be cognizant of the deleterious effect food has for the person who has PWS.

Traits indicating lack of flexibility

Children who have PWS sometimes can be described as stubborn, insisting on sameness, and unable to adjust to changes already at the age of 5 years. They tend to get stuck on certain issues, perseverating in their speech or repeatedly asking the same question. They need a predictable and unchanging daily schedule, because slight deviations from the usual routine can result in severe temper tantrums. This reaction may be caused, at least in part, by impaired executive functions and low performance in sequential processing (see the section on cognition), which render them dependent on learned routines and acquired patterns.

A second aspect of the inflexibility in individuals who have PWS is the development of rituals, which range from simply collecting useless items or hair pulling to bizarre rituals, such as playing with feces. Compulsive behaviors, examples of which are skin picking, hoarding, ordering, and "just right" phenomena, are more frequent in patients who have PWS than among patients who have other developmental disorders, with the exception of pervasive developmental disorder [33,34]. Skin picking is seen in at least one third of the patients and may cause severe skin infections. Anal and vaginal digging are more common than reported by patients, and the resulting bleeding can lead to unnecessary medical investigations [35,36]. Although the exact prevalence of full-blown obsessive-compulsive disorder in PWS is unknown, symptoms cause significant impairment in more than 45% of individuals who have PWS [33].

Oppositional behaviors and interpersonal problems

Children who have PWS challenge the caregivers' consistency and will for maintaining limits, not only in food-related issues. These children are egocentric and argue, lie, manipulate, and confabulate to change rules, obtain their wishes, or justify misbehavior. Their social judgment is poor, even considering their intellectual ability, and interpretation of visually presented social information is on a level with that of children who have pervasive developmental disorder [37]. When these interpersonal disabilities are compounded to the repetitive behaviors in PWS, overlapping many seen in pervasive developmental disorder [33], it is not surprising that the prevalence of pervasive developmental disorder among persons who have PWS is high [38].

Traits indicating abnormal emotional regulation

Children who have PWS have little tolerance for uncertainty, to which they respond with explosive behavior, and they react to minor frustrations with temper tantrums. Their affective regulation is also disturbed, manifested by mood swings from joy to irritability. The impaired satiety response, skin picking, and high pain threshold also can be viewed as the consequence of impaired regulatory mechanisms. Gourash and Forster [39] have suggested that these traits may represent a failure in modifying feedback pathways.

Several studies have found that most maladaptive behaviors, including self-injury, stealing, and obsessive-compulsive symptoms, are significantly more severe in persons who have PWS whose genetic defect is deletion (compared to individuals who have UPD) [40,41]. IQ, family environment, and parenting styles also impact on the behavioral traits, however, and result in a great variability among individuals who have PWS. It is essential to have an accurate record of the behavioral baseline of each patient at each developmental stage, including frequency and intensity of each symptom, for at least two important reasons:

- In persons who have PWS, the main reaction to any stressor is exacerbation of these symptoms. Changes in the behavioral baseline can be the first cue to uncover a psychological cause of distress (eg, secret abuse, traumatic stress) or a physical illness.
- Accurate monitoring of these symptoms is essential for a differential diagnosis between the characteristic behavioral profile and the comorbid psychiatric disorders in individuals who have PWS.

Comorbid psychiatric disorders

Levels of psychopathology are found to be higher among persons who have PWS than among persons with intellectual disability of other origins [42]. Attention deficit hyperactivity disorder and obsessive-compulsive disorder already have been discussed, and this section focuses on mood and psychotic disorders.

Sudden bursts of disturbed mood, as part of the "normal" behavioral pattern in PWS, are generally trigger-dependent and short lived. During adolescence, prolonged waves of restlessness and dysphoric or anxious mood may appear. Preoccupations that cause severe distress tend to dominate the thought content but either resolve spontaneously within a few days or evolve into clinical depression. In some cases there is a rapid change into a hypomanic episode, with confusion, restlessness, and increased goal-directed behavior that lasts a few days to a few weeks. In 15% to 17% of persons who have PWS, these two latter clinical developments are sufficiently prolonged and profound to justify a diagnosis of mood disorder [43].

During late adolescence and adulthood, delusions, most often of paranoid type, may appear in the course of one of these waves of disturbed mood. Hallucinations are not common in individuals who have PWS. This high risk for psychotic episodes is almost exclusively associated with the UPD or imprinting genetic types [44]. The combination of cyclic mood disturbance and delusions is consistent with the European diagnostic category of "cycloid psychosis," which is frequently used in publications on PWS. Boer and colleagues [44] reported a prevalence of 28% for severe affective disorders with psychotic features in this age group.

Psychopharmacology

The therapeutic and side effects of medications in patients who have PWS often can be greater than expected, even in severely obese patients who receive low dosages when considering their body weight. For many patients, one fourth to one half of the normally prescribed dose is sufficient, whereas usual dosage levels may cause toxic reactions or exacerbation of behavior problems [9]. Severely reduced metabolism by some components of cytochrome 450, a metabolic abnormality documented in one third of individuals who have PWS, may partly explain this sensitivity to medications [10].

There is no specific pharmacologic treatment for the behavioral disturbances typical of PWS. No safe drug has been found to be effective against hyperphagia. The only candidate found to justify a controlled study was fenfluramine [45]. Although the trial was successful, this medication is currently considered unsafe because of cardiopulmonary adverse effects. Anecdotal reports and a few open-label trials suggested the effectiveness of some symptomatic psychopharmacologic interventions [32]. Selective serotonin reuptake inhibitor drugs may result in some improvement in compulsions, anxiety, and mood, although they may trigger severe mood switches and require careful monitoring of mood response. Carbamazepine has reduced violent outbursts in two case reports [32]. Recently, two open-label studies (12 patients in total) showed positive effects of topiramate on mood and skin picking [35,36]. From our experience, methylphenidate is effective in treating symptoms of attention deficit hyperactivity disorder in PWS but does not decrease appetite. Atypical antipsychotic drugs in low doses can be helpful during psychotic episodes. It is important to keep in mind that some of these episodes are reactive to an environmental stress, such as grief, so in these cases it is justified to consider withdrawal of medications [30]. Neuroleptics can be used when behavior and emotional control become dangerously impaired despite satisfactory environmental treatment. Low doses of risperidone in seven patients resulted in notable improvement in maladaptive behaviors during a 37-week follow-up, and patients did not experience weight gain [46].

In periods of severely disturbed behavior, a wise combination of psychiatric medication and behavioral measures seems to be the best option. Professionals who treat persons who have PWS are sometimes challenged by such severe and continued behavioral disruptions that they may be tempted to consider medications or psychiatric hospitalizations as "quick fixes" for these individuals. It is essential to keep in mind that most

physicians who are familiar with PWS are obtained as needed. Patients from all parts of the country are seen in our clinic at least once a year for a routine follow-up or at times of crisis, when the therapists in charge of the daily management in the community request additional assistance.

Epilogue

Preventing morbid obesity and managing the maladaptive behaviors in persons who have PWS are the most important goals that require lifelong commitment of the therapists. When the person is an adult and capable of making informed decisions, restrictive supervision raises serious legal and ethical dilemmas that demand balance among quality of life, life-saving cohesive measures, and free will [49]. Food is not the only treatment issue that needs confrontation; sexual behaviors, diabetes mellitus, scoliosis, and devices for the treatment of nocturnal respiratory disorders are additional therapeutic fronts that need consent and compliance from the maturing individual who has PWS. Although these issues are beyond the scope of this article, they highlight the treatment dilemmas involved in managing this multisystemic disorder that only becomes more complex with increasing age. We can only emphasize the need to approach each person who has PWS as an individual, be sensitive to traits and strengths (related to and especially unrelated to PWS), and choose among the therapeutic approaches most appropriate.

Acknowledgments

The authors are deeply grateful to Professor Ruth Shalev for her thoughtful comments and suggestions in revising the manuscript.

References

[1] Whittington JE, Holland AJ, Webb T, et al. Population prevalence and estimated birth incidence and mortality rate for people with Prader-Willi syndrome in one UK health region. J Med Genet 2001;38:792–8.
[2] Yamada K, Matsuzawa H, Uchiyama M, et al. Brain developmental abnormalities in Prader-Willi syndrome detected by diffusion tensor imaging. Pediatrics 2006;118(2):e442–8.
[3] Kim SE, Jin DK, Cho SS, et al. Regional cerebral glucose metabolic abnormality in Prader-Willi syndrome: an 18F-FDG PET study under sedation. J Nucl Med 2006;47(7): 1088–92.
[4] Glaser B, Hirsch HJ. Genetics for endocrinologists. London: Remedica Publishing; 2003. p. 70–3.
[5] Driscoll DJ. The genetics of Prader-Willi syndrome. Pharmacia International Growth Database Report No. 20. Stockholm (Sweden), International Board/Pharmacia Corporation; 2002. p. 5–10.
[6] Fridman C, Varela MC, Kok F, et al. Prader-Willi syndrome: genetic tests and clinical findings. Genet Test 2000;4:387–92.
[7] Holm VA, Cassidy SB, Butler MG, et al. Prader- Willi syndrome: consensus diagnostic criteria. Pediatrics 1993;91:398–402.

[8] Cassidy SB. Prader-Willi syndrome. J Med Genet 1997;34:917–23.

[9] Whitman BY, Greenswag LR. Psychological and behavioral management. In: Greenswag LR, Alexander RC, editors. Management of Prader-Willi syndrome. 2nd edition. New York: Springer-Verlag; 1995. p. 125–41.

[10] Roof E, Shelton R, Wilkinson G, et al. The use of psychotropic medications in Prader-Willi syndrome. Presented at the 20th Annual PWSA (USA) National Conference. Orlando (FL); July 27, 2005.

[11] Nixon GM, Brouillette RT. Sleep and breathing in Prader-Willi syndrome. Pediatr Pulmonol 2002;34:209–17.

[12] Zipf WB. Prader-Willi syndrome: the care and treatment of infants, children, and adults. Adv Pediatr 2004;51:409–34.

[13] Nagai T, Obata K, Tonoki H, et al. Cause of sudden, unexpected death of Prader-Willi syndrome patients with or without growth hormone treatment. Am J Med Genet 2005; 136(1):45–8.

[14] Burman P, Ritzen EM, Lindgren AC. Endocrine dysfunction in Prader-Willi syndrome: a review with special reference to GH. Endocr Rev 2001;22:787–99.

[15] Carrel AL, Moerchen V, Myers SE, et al. Growth hormone improves mobility and body composition in infants and toddlers with Prader-Willi syndrome. J Pediatr 2004;145:744–9.

[16] Haqq AM, Stadler DD, Jackson RH, et al. Effects of growth hormone on pulmonary function, sleep quality, behavior, cognition, growth velocity, body composition, and resting energy expenditure in Prader-Willi syndrome. J Clin Endocrinol Metab 2003;88:2206–12.

[17] Craig ME, Cowell CT, Larsson P, et al. Growth hormone treatment and adverse events in Prader-Willi syndrome: data from KIGS (the Pfizer International Growth Database). Clin Endocrinol (Oxf) 2006;65:178–85.

[18] Lee PDK. Growth hormone and mortality in Prader-Willi syndrome. Growth, Genetics, and Hormones 2006;22:17–23.

[19] Crino A, Schiaffini R, Ciampalini P, et al. Hypogonadism and pubertal development in Prader-Willi syndrome. Eur J Pediatr 2003;162:327–33.

[20] Eiholzer U, l'Allemand D, Rousson V, et al. Hypothalamic and gonadal components of hypogonadism in boys with Prader-Labhart-Willi syndrome. J Clin Endocrinol Metab 2006; 91:892–8.

[21] Curfs LMG, Fryns JP. Prader-Willi syndrome: a review with special attention to the cognitive and behavioral profile. Birth Defects Orig Artic Ser 1992;28(1):99–104.

[22] Whittington J, Holland A, Webb T, et al. Academic underachievement by people with Prader-Willi syndrome. J Intellect Disabil Res 2004;48(2):188–200.

[23] Dykens EM, Hodapp RM, Walsh K, et al. Profiles, correlates, and trajectories of intelligence in Prader-Willi syndrome. J Am Acad Child Adolesc Psychiatry 1992;31(6): 1125–30.

[24] Dykens EM, Hodapp RM, Finucane BM. Genetics and mental retardation syndromes. Baltimore: Paul H. Brookes; 2000.

[25] Whittington J, Holland A, Webb T, et al. Cognitive abilities and genotype in a population-based sample of people with Prader-Willi syndrome. J Intellect Disabil Res 2004;48(2): 172–87.

[26] Gross-Tsur V, Landau YE, Benarroch F, et al. Cognition, attention and behavior in Prader-Willi syndrome. J Child Neurol 2001;16:288–90.

[27] Wigren M, Hansen S. ADHD symptoms and insistence on sameness in Prader-Willi syndrome. J Intellect Disabil Res 2005;49(6):449–56.

[28] Hoybye C, Thoren M, Bohm B. Cognitive, emotional, physical and social effects of growth hormone treatment in adults with Prader-Willi syndrome. J Intellect Disabil Res 2005;49(4): 245–52.

[29] Holland AJ, Whittington JE, Butler J, et al. Behavioural phenotypes associated with specific genetic disorders: evidence from a population-based study of people with Prader-Willi syndrome. Psychol Med 2003;33(1):141–53.

[30] Forster JL, Gourash LM. Managing Prader-Willi syndrome: a primer for psychiatrists. Available at: www.pwsausa.org. Accessed November 4, 2006.

[31] Lindgren AC, Barkeling B, Hagg A, et al. Eating behavior in Prader-Willi syndrome, normal weight, and obese control groups. J Pediatr 2000;137:50–5.

[32] Dykens E, Shah B. Psychiatric disorders in Prader-Willi syndrome: epidemiology and management. CNS Drugs 2003;17:167–78.

[33] Greaves N, Prince E, Evans DW, et al. Repetitive and ritualistic behaviour in children with Prader-Willi syndrome and children with autism. J Intellect Disabil Res 2006;50(Pt 2): 92–100.

[34] Dykens EM, Leckman JF, Cassidy SB. Obsessions and compulsions in Prader-Willi syndrome. J Child Psychol Psychiatry 1996;37(8):995–1002.

[35] Shapira NA, Lessig MC, Lewis MH, et al. Effects of topiramate in adults with Prader-Willi syndrome. Am J Ment Retard 2004;109:301–9.

[36] Smathers SA, Wilson JG, Nigro MA. Topiramate effectiveness in Prader-Willi syndrome. Pediatr Neurol 2003;28(2):130–3.

[37] Koenig K, Klin A, Schultz R. Deficits in social attribution ability in Prader-Willi syndrome. J Autism Dev Disord 2004;34(5):573–82.

[38] Veltman MW, Craig EE, Bolton PF. Autism spectrum disorders in Prader-Willi and Angelman syndromes: a systematic review. Psychiatr Genet 2005;15(4):243–54.

[39] Gourash L, Forster J. Lack of satiety: it is not just about food. Presented at the 20th Annual PWSA (USA) National Conference. Orlando (FL); July 27, 2005.

[40] Gillessen-Kaesbach G, Robinson W, Lohmann D, et al. Genotype-phenotype correlation in a series of 167 deletion and non-deletion patients with Prader-Willi syndrome. Hum Genet 1995;96(6):638–43.

[41] Hartley SL, Maclean WE Jr, Butler MG, et al. Maladaptive behaviors and risk factors among the genetic subtypes of Prader-Willi syndrome. Am J Med Genet A 2005;136(2): 140–5.

[42] Reddy LA, Pfeiffer SI. Behavioral and emotional symptoms of children and adolescents with Prader-Willi Syndrome. J Autism Dev Disord 2006 [Epub ahead of print].

[43] Vogels A, De Hert M, Descheemaeker MJ, et al. Psychotic disorders in Prader-Willi syndrome. Am J Med Genet 2004;127(3):238–43.

[44] Boer H, Holland A, Whittington J, et al. Psychotic illness in people with Prader-Willi syndrome due to chromosome 15 maternal uniparental disomy. Lancet 2002;359(9301): 135–6.

[45] Selikowitz M, Sunman J, Pendergast A, et al. Fenfluramine in Prader-Willi syndrome: a double-blind, placebo-controlled trial. Arch Dis Child 1990;65:112–4.

[46] Durst R, Rubin-Jabotinsky K, Raskin S, et al. Risperidone in treating behavioural disturbances of Prader-Willi syndrome. Acta Psychiatr Scand 2000;102(6):461–5.

[47] Whitman BY, Jackson K. Tools for psychological and behavioral management. In: Butler MG, Lee PDK, Whitman BY, editors. Management of Prader-Willi syndrome. 3rd edition. New York: Springer; 2006. p. 317–43.

[48] Genstil L, Nabulsi Y. Social skills training through video feedback. Presented at the 17th Annual PWSA (USA) National Conference. Salt Lake City (UT); July 11, 2002.

[49] Holland AJ, Wong J. Genetically determined obesity in Prader-Willi syndrome: the ethics and legality of treatment. J Med Ethics 1999;25:230–6.

ELSEVIER
SAUNDERS

Child Adolesc Psychiatric Clin N Am
16 (2007) 709–722

CHILD AND
ADOLESCENT
PSYCHIATRIC CLINICS
OF NORTH AMERICA

Turner Syndrome

Shelli R. Kesler, PhD

Department of Psychiatry and Behavioral Sciences, Stanford University,
401 Quarry Road, MC5795, Stanford, CA 94305-5795, USA

Turner syndrome (TS) is a complex phenotype associated with complete or partial monosomy of the X chromosome, usually the result of a sporadic chromosomal nondisjunction. TS is one of the most common sex chromosome abnormalities, affecting approximately 1 in 2000 live-born girls [1–3]. The physical phenotype associated with TS includes short stature, ovarian failure, webbed neck, cardiac abnormalities, impaired glucose tolerance, thyroid disease, and hearing loss [1,4–7]. There is considerable heterogeneity of phenotypic features, with short stature and gonadal dysgenesis being the most consistent [3]. Most girls who have TS are treated with growth hormone (GH) and estrogen replacement therapies (ERT) [1].

Genetics

Karyotypes

TS is defined by a partially or completely absent X chromosome. Most (approximately 50%) girls who have TS have a 45,X or nonmosaic karyotype [8,9]. Several karyotype variations exist, including short or long arm deletion, ring X, isochromosome of the long arm (resulting in a fusion of chromosome arms), and mosaicism, a combination of cell lines such as 45,X and 46,XX [10]. Many reports indicate that mosaicism tends to moderate outcome [3,7], and studies show that physical features, such as cardiovascular symptoms and gonadal dysfunction, tend to vary in frequency across the different karyotypes [10]. It is currently unclear exactly how these various karyotypes differ in terms of cognitive-behavioral function.

Genotype-phenotype associations

In a typically developing girl with a normal complement of 46 chromosomes, one of the X chromosomes is inactivated during early embryonic

E-mail address: skesler@stanford.edu

1056-4993/07/$ - see front matter © 2007 Elsevier Inc. All rights reserved.
doi:10.1016/j.chc.2007.02.004   *childpsych.theclinics.com*

development, a phenomenon known as dosage compensation or lyonization [11,12]. This epigenetic mechanism functions to equalize the dosage of X-linked genes between girls and boys. Several genes on the "inactive" X chromosome in girls actually escape inactivation to at least some degree, however [13,14]. TS might be considered the result of partial or complete absence of these genes that escape inactivation.

Genes that are potentially associated with aspects of the TS phenotype are likely to be the ones that escape X inactivation and have functional homologs on the Y chromosome. One such gene is the short stature homeobox gene located on the pseudoautosomal region of the X chromosome. The short stature homeobox gene has been identified as a candidate gene for short stature [15,16] and skeletal abnormalities associated with TS, including high arched palate, abnormal auricular development, cubitus valgus, genu valgum, Madelung deformity, and short metacarpals [17]. Other candidate genes are currently under investigation.

Genomic imprinting

Differential outcome stemming from genomic imprinting is another genetic factor of interest in TS [18]. Whether an imprinted gene is expressed depends on its parental origin [19,20]. Although the issue remains controversial, a limited number of studies investigating imprinting effects in TS has demonstrated a possible influence on cognitive-behavioral phenotype. Individuals who retain the maternal X chromosome (Xm) may demonstrate greater impairments compared with persons with the paternal X chromosome (Xp) [21–25]. Our laboratory demonstrated altered neurodevelopment in temporal and occipital regions in individuals with Xm compared with controls, whereas individuals with Xp were not significantly different from controls [21,22]. Others have demonstrated no imprinting effects in cognitive performance [26] or neurodevelopment [27,28]. Some researchers have observed individuals with Xp rather than Xm to have poorer outcome [29]. The results of another study suggested that each parent-of-origin TS subgroup might be associated with a particular profile of deficits [30].

Physical abnormalities

The most common (ie, frequency of $\geq 50\%$) physical abnormalities affecting girls who have TS include short stature, infertility, estrogen deficiency, hypertension, elevated hepatic enzymes, middle ear infection, micrognathia, bone age retardation, decreased bone mineral content, cubitus valgus, and poor thriving during the first postnatal year [1]. Girls who have TS also have significantly higher risks for certain diseases compared with the general population, including hypothyroidism, diabetes, heart disease, osteoporosis, congenital malformations (eg, heart, urinary system, face, neck, ears), neurovascular disease, cirrhosis of the liver, and colon and rectal cancers [1].

Cardiac abnormalities are considered the most serious medical problems associated with TS. A high rate of morbidity exists among the TS population, primarily because of congenital and acquired heart conditions, such as coarctation of the aorta, biscuspid aortic valves, mitral valve prolapse, hypertension, ischemic heart disease, and arteriosclerosis [1,4,31–33].

Cognitive phenotype

Visuospatial skills

Individuals who have TS typically demonstrate normal global intellectual functioning; however, nonverbal abilities are often significantly impaired [7,34,35]. An uneven cognitive profile, with verbal skills tending to be significantly higher than nonverbal skills, is often considered to be the hallmark of cognitive ability in TS. Girls who have TS have been shown to demonstrate intact— if not superior—language development compared with controls. For example, studies have shown higher reading levels, accuracy, and comprehension in participants who have TS compared with age-matched typically developing controls [36]. Individuals who have TS also have been shown to have better receptive vocabulary skills and understand significantly more low-frequency (less common) words than controls [37]. One study of girls who have TS indicated poorer ability in word retrieval and nonlexical reading in conjunction with preserved performance in irregular word reading, phoneme analysis, and letter fluency compared with controls, however [38].

In contrast, girls who have TS are at high risk for developing deficits in visuospatial, visual-perceptual, and visual-constructional abilities [39–42]. Specifically, girls who have TS tend to demonstrate significant deficits on tests of mental rotation, object assembly, and face recognition but perform comparably to controls on visual sequential memory and block span tests [38]. Deficits on visuospatial tasks often include right-left disorientation and difficulty with design copying and an executive function component with poor planning and organization [43–48]. Cornoldi and colleagues [49] suggested that although TS may be associated with general visuospatial deficits, individual differences in specific performance patterns may exist. Visuospatial impairments tend to be resistant to estrogen and androgen-replacement therapies, which suggests that this characteristic may be independent of hormone effects and require a more precise intervention [35,40].

Visuospatial skills are known to be associated primarily with parietal-occipital pathways [50–52]. Neuroimaging studies suggest that parietal-occipital metabolism and morphology are abnormal in individuals who have TS compared with healthy controls [21,53–59]. We also showed that these volumetric differences may be specific to the superior parietal lobule and the postcentral gyrus, regions associated with visuospatial function, visuomotor learning, and spatial working memory [53].

Executive skills

Although not reported as frequently as visuospatial deficits, impaired executive function also has been observed in individuals who have TS. Problems with executive skills associated with TS may include impaired attention and concentration, problem-solving ability, organization, working memory, behavioral control and use of goal-directed strategies, and increased impulsivity and slower processing speed [29,35,46,60–62]. TS also may be associated with increased risk for attention deficit hyperactivity disorder [63]. Russell and colleagues [26] reported an 18-fold increased prevalence in TS compared with controls. Several studies have demonstrated abnormal brain activation patterns in prefrontal-striatal pathways associated with executive task performance in girls who have TS [43,64,65].

Connectivity of visuospatial and executive functions

We have illustrated that participants who have TS tend to perform comparably to controls during easier tasks but fail when task demands are increased. Brain activation in frontal-parietal regions tends to be increased compared with controls during easier tasks but reduced during more difficult tasks [43,66]. When there is no spatial component, girls who have TS perform similarly to controls on executive tasks and tend to show increased prefrontal activation [67].

These data suggest that although executive tasks in general may require more effort for individuals who have TS, they may be able to compensate for this weakness to some degree by recruiting additional prefrontal resources. They seem to be unable to successfully engage alternate or additional systems when there is a spatial component, however, particularly during more difficult tasks. This profile of spatial executive deficits could be explained by several factors, including aberrant neurodevelopment in the parietal and frontal lobes or an impairment in frontal-parietal connectivity. Supporting this possibility, we demonstrated significantly reduced white matter integrity in parietal-frontal pathways [68].

We also examined functional connectivity in girls who have TS using functional MRI results from three tasks that are known to engage frontal-parietal systems. Functional connectivity analyses provide insight into regions that are likely connected within functional networks [69]. We found that activation in the parietal regions was negatively correlated with frontal activation in girls who have TS during all three tasks. On the other hand, controls demonstrated positive correlations between parietal and frontal regions during the three tasks (Kesler SR, AL Reiss, unpublished data, 2006). These findings suggested that the interaction between parietal and frontal lobe systems may provide a more precise explanation for spatial-executive deficits in TS than independent parietal or frontal lobe impairments.

Many of the cognitive impairments noted among individuals who have TS may reflect similar problems with integrating relevant neural systems.

For example, TS has been associated with difficulties in integration of details into a gestalt and global versus local deficits [70]. Individuals who have TS also seem to be at risk for difficulties with arithmetic [56,57,71,72] and spatial memory [30,35,73,74]. These abilities rely partly on integration of visuospatial and executive functioning. Focusing on the integration of cognitive systems in TS might suggest directions for intervention. For example, cognitive remediation programs should include exercises that strengthen connection of systems (eg, visuospatial-executive) rather than independent functions (visuospatial only).

Psychosocial functioning

Impairments in social functioning have been noted among individuals who have TS. Adolescent girls who have TS are at greater risk for having problems related to lower social activity, poor social coping skills, and increased immaturity, hyperactivity, and impulsivity compared with their peers [63]. Girls who have TS may have more difficulties maintaining relationships and relating to others, have fewer friends, and tend to be more socially isolated than controls [75]. Social difficulties in girls who have TS may stem partially from impairments in face and emotion processing and interpreting gaze in individuals who have TS [76–80]. Some researchers have suggested that a diagnosis of autism, a neurodevelopmental disorder characterized by social deficits, is more common among girls who have TS, but this suggestion remains controversial [25,81,82].

Because the amygdala is known to be involved in recognition of facial emotion and social judgment [83], neuroimaging studies have investigated amygdala development associated with TS. Good and colleagues [27] showed that girls who have TS have significantly enlarged amygdala volumes compared with female and male control participants. Our laboratory confirmed enlarged amygdala volumes associated with TS using a different but complementary neuroimaging method [28].

A functional MRI study demonstrated enhanced right amygdala activation to fearful faces in individuals who have TS compared with controls. Amygdala activation in controls tended to peak initially and then decrease over time, whereas in girls who have TS, activation persisted with little change in magnitude. Performance on a facial emotion recognition task also was correlated with amygdala and fusiform activation in the control but not the TS group. Functional coactivation between the amygdala and fusiform was decreased in the TS group compared with controls. The authors suggested that impaired appraisal of facial affect and habituation to fearful stimuli may stem from impaired functional connectivity between these structures in the TS group [84].

Studies of TS also have shown aberrant neurodevelopment in the orbitofrontal cortex and superior temporal sulcus, additional regions involved in social cognition and face processing [27,55,57]. Some researchers believe that social skills deficits in TS stem largely from visuospatial, nonverbal impairments similar to the cognitive-behavioral profile associated with nonverbal learning disorder [70,85]. The neuroimaging studies suggested that psychosocial functioning in TS may be independent of visuospatial skills deficits. Specifically, deficits in amygdala function but not posterior visuospatial processing systems were observed in association with facial emotion processing tasks. Skuse and colleagues [24] argued that social cognition performance in TS does not correlate strongly with visuospatial ability and that nonverbal deficits cannot adequately explain the findings that individuals who have TS tend to show greater impairment for fearful stimuli [76,77]. A primary nonverbal deficit would seem to affect appraisal of all facial emotions similarly. This is an area of functioning in TS that requires further investigation.

Psychiatric disorders

Shyness, anxiety, low self-esteem, and depression, frequently linked to self-consciousness over physical appearance or infertility, have been described in studies of TS. Psychiatric functioning remains an area of limited and conflicting information in TS, however, and requires further study. In a study of 100 individuals aged 16 to 61 who have TS, Schmidt and colleagues [86] used four rating scales and noted significantly higher anxiety, shyness, and depression and lower self-esteem compared with controls. These findings were irrespective of factors such as age, education, and marital status. Girls aged 9 to 17 who have TS demonstrated lower self-esteem and higher levels of state anxiety than controls using different self-report measures [87]. Keysor and colleagues [88] reported that individuals aged 12 to 22 who have TS showed heightened physiologic arousal, including skin conductance, heart rate, and gastrocnemius electromyography, during certain cognitive tasks. A recent study indicated that low self-esteem and poor social adjustment are associated with delayed or absent sexual relationship experiences [89]. Whereas many reports have suggested height, physical appearance, or infertility as underlying factors in low self-esteem, Carel and colleagues [89] demonstrated that hearing loss, socioeconomic status, and cardiac problems also may contribute to impaired social adjustment.

Another group noted lower self-perception and bodily attitude but no evidence of depression in 50 young women who have TS (mean age 18+0.3) who completed self-report scales [90]. One study that included self-report and parental ratings indicated that girls aged 6 to 22 who have TS were not significantly more anxious than controls [91]. A large study that involved 100 women aged 16 to 61 who have TS using a structured diagnostic interview indicated that lifetime incidence of mood disorders, but not anxiety, was twice as high as community-based samples. Current and lifetime prevalence of psychiatric syndromes, including mood and anxiety disorders, was not substantially higher in individuals who have TS than individuals in medical outpatient or gynecologic clinics. This finding suggested that mood disturbance in TS is not likely specific to TS but is increased because of medical problems in general [92].

Treatment

Growth hormone

One of the most common clinical features among individuals who have TS is short stature, which can affect peer relationships and social adjustment. GH is typically prescribed to children who have TS to increase final height. Girls who have TS who were treated with GH for 1 year were significantly taller than girls who did not receive GH [93]. Studies suggest that GH treatment can result in achievement of normal adult height, and starting GH at an early age (4–6 years) seems to be a factor in the success of the treatment [1,94,95]. The effects of GH on height can diminish after the first 1 to 2 years of administration, and an escalating dosage schedule is often required, with higher doses in adolescence [1,96].

Some clinicians have expressed concerns that GH treatment may result in undesirable changes to body proportions, such as enlarged feet and hands in adolescents [1]. Further research is needed in this area. Researchers also warn treatment providers to be wary of psychosocial problems related to weight management issues in TS [97]. GH treatment may result in increased lean body mass and decreased body fat, however, improving physical health associated with body composition [93,95].

GH does not affect bone mineral density [93] but may increase the risk of otitis media and certain joint disorders [1]. There also some concerns regarding increased risk of colon and lymphatic cancers [96]. GH decreases insulin sensitivity, which, in combination with a tendency toward greater adiposity in TS, may contribute to development of type 2 diabetes [98]. Insulin resistance tends to decrease after approximately 7 to 8 years of GH therapy, however, and returns to normal after GH therapy is discontinued [99].

It is unclear whether GH therapy affects cognitive function in girls who have TS. Few studies examining this relationship have been conducted. One small ($n = 20$) but well-designed study indicated no influence of GH on cognitive function in girls who have TS [100]. A follow-up study that used an expanded cognitive testing battery confirmed these findings [14].

Estrogen replacement therapy

One of the key features of TS is estrogen deficiency [101], which occurs secondary to ovarian dysgenesis or degeneration associated with early follicular apoptosis [1]. Despite ovarian abnormality being one of the most common features of TS [1], approximately 5% to 10% of girls who have TS demonstrate some degree of spontaneous puberty, and 2% to 7% of women experience spontaneous pregnancy [102]. These pregnancies tend to be at high risk for miscarriages, genetic abnormalities, stillbirths, and malformations [102]. There have been some rare reports of successful, uneventful pregnancies in women who have TS, however [102,103].

ERT is currently the standard treatment for estrogen deficiency/insufficiency. ERT ideally should be started around the age of 12 or at an age consistent with pubertal development in the patient's peers to decrease psychosocial distress [1]. ERT should be initiated also with consideration of GH therapy. Some reports have indicated that ERT can reduce final adult height in patients being treated with GH [104,105]. More recent studies have indicated that the use of transdermal or intramuscular estradiol administration [105] or initial use of a low-dose parenteral estradiol with an increasing dosage schedule [90,106,107] may reduce ERT's affect on height attainment, however.

Research has suggested that some features of cognitive impairment associated with TS may be related to estrogen function [100,108]. Certain cognitive deficits, such as motor speed, nonverbal processing time, and verbal and nonverbal memory, may improve after ERT [62,109]. Many other areas of cognitive function, particularly those associated with visuospatial and visual-motor processing and attention, seem to persist despite ERT [35]. ERT has been shown to have several beneficial effects, including age-appropriate development of secondary sexual characteristics, improved psychosocial functioning, increased bone mineral density, and better uterine development [110].

Girls who have TS also demonstrate androgen deficiency [101]. Androgens are believed to play a significant role in cognitive function, potentially enhancing cognitive performance and emotional state [111]. One study showed that oxandrolone (synthesized testosterone) may help improve certain cognitive functions, such as working memory performance in girls who have TS [40]. Further studies are required to determine if androgen replacement is an efficacious treatment for cognitive impairments associated with TS.

Psychosocial

Limited studies have been conducted regarding psychosocial treatment efficacy in TS. Existing studies are outdated and tend to involve case studies rather than randomized clinical trials or other more robust methods [112–114]. The paucity of literature in this area reflects our currently limited understanding of psychiatric functioning in TS. Emotional difficulties may stem primarily from chronic medical problems and social isolation rather than X monosomy.

It is hoped that continuing to more precisely define the cognitive, psychosocial, neurobiologic, endocrinologic, genetic, and other relevant aspects of TS will aid in developing more syndrome-specific psychosocial interventions. Based on our understanding of TS thus far, such interventions ideally should include a combination of the following based on individual strengths and weaknesses: (1) general coping and adaptive skills training and a specific focus on dealing with chronic medical problems, such as cardiovascular disease, hearing impairment, and infertility, (2) social skills training, including self-monitoring, social perspective taking, facial affect and body language recognition and interpretation, and group social skills therapy, (3) stress management training to help prevent and treat anxiety and mood disturbances, (4) emphasis on improving self-esteem and self-perception, and (5) internal and external strategies to compensate for cognitive weaknesses, such as using self-talk to pay attention and remain on task, focusing on doing one task correctly rather than doing several things at once, and paraphrasing what others have said to ensure comprehension.

Treatment plans should consider the individual's cognitive profile. Neuropsychological assessments can be vitally helpful in informing education and special education services and psychotherapy parameters. For example, a girl who has TS and has executive function deficits, such as abstract reasoning or attention impairments, is more likely to benefit from concrete, behaviorally oriented therapies rather than psychoanalytic ones.

Summary

Significant progress has been made in describing the cognitive-behavioral, neurobiologic, endocrinologic, physical, and genetic factors associated with Turner syndrome. Many questions remain, however. Existing studies have typically involved relatively small sample sizes, large age ranges, and mixed genotypes. Smaller sample sizes present potential difficulties in terms of power and generalizability. Large age ranges limit the ability to determine how hormone replacement therapies, particularly estrogen treatments, impact outcome in TS. There also have been no studies on gene expression patterns of girls with X monosomy and TS. Studies involving genetic analyses, such as microarray technology, are necessary to examine gene expression profiles in girls who have TS and identify potential candidate genes underlying the cognitive-behavioral impairments associated with TS. Continued studies of X-linked genes that escape inactivation and have Y chromosome homologs also are essential in identifying candidate genes involved in the cognitive-behavioral and physical phenotypes of TS.

Genetic profiles of participants, including genotype, karyotype, and genomic parental origin, are of particular interest for future studies of TS. Because individuals with the maternal X chromosome outnumber individuals who have the paternal X by approximately 2:1 [115,116], further studies are required that oversample for participants with Xp. Many studies tend to include only female subjects with a monosomic 45,X genotype (nonmosaic). To date, there has been no comprehensive study of the cognitive-behavioral features associated with various karyotypes in TS. The analyses involved in interpreting cognitive-behavioral outcome associated with cytogenetic variants are complex because of the large number of variants that exist. These studies would offer a unique opportunity to investigate the relationship between X chromosome gene function and cognitive-behavioral phenotype. Future studies could begin including individuals with mosaic TS genotypes and compare their outcome to persons with a nonmosaic genotype.

Finally, cross-modal, longitudinal, randomized clinical trials and other such comprehensive study designs are needed to start examining the relationships between aspects of TS, such as neurodevelopment, endocrine function, medical status, and cognitive outcome. These studies hopefully will aid us in developing syndrome-specific interventions that improve functioning and quality of life in individuals who have TS.

References

[1] Gravholt CH. Clinical practice in Turner syndrome. Nat Clin Pract Endocrinol Metab 2005;1(1):41–52.

[2] Jacobs PA. The chromosome complement of human gametes. In: Milligan SR, editor. Oxford reviews of reproductive biology. New York: Oxford University Press; 1992. p. 47–72.

[3] Jones KL. Smith's recognizable patterns of human malformations. 5th edition. New York: W.B. Saunders Company; 1997.

[4] Bondy CA, Bakalov VK. Investigation of cardiac status and bone mineral density in Turner syndrome. Growth Horm IGF Res 2006;(16 Suppl A):S103–8.

[5] Dhooge IJ, De Vel E, Verhoye C, et al. Otologic disease in Turner syndrome. Otol Neurotol 2005;26(2):145–50.

[6] Gungor N, et al. High frequency hearing loss in Ullrich-Turner syndrome. Eur J Pediatr 2000;159(10):740–4.

[7] Zinn AR, et al. Evidence for a Turner syndrome locus or loci at Xp11.2-p22.1. Am J Hum Genet 1998;63(6):1757–66.

[8] Kleczkowska A, et al. Cytogenetic findings in a consecutive series of 478 patients with Turner syndrome: the Leuven experience 1965–1989. Genet Couns 1990;1(3–4):227–33.

[9] Suri M, et al. A clinical and cytogenetic study of Turner syndrome. Indian Pediatr 1995; 32(4):433–42.

[10] Ogata T, Matsuo N. Turner syndrome and female sex chromosome aberrations: deduction of the principal factors involved in the development of clinical features. Hum Genet 1995; 95(6):607–29.

[11] Chang SC, et al. Mechanisms of X-chromosome inactivation. Front Biosci 2006;11:852–66.

[12] Lyon MF. X-chromosome inactivation and human genetic disease. Acta Paediatr Suppl 2002;91(439):107–12.

[13] Carrel L, Willard HF. X-inactivation profile reveals extensive variability in X-linked gene expression in females. Nature 2005;434(7031):400–4.

[14] Ross MT, et al. The DNA sequence of the human X chromosome. Nature 2005;434(7031): 325–37.

[15] Ellison JW, et al. PHOG, a candidate gene for involvement in the short stature of Turner syndrome. Hum Mol Genet 1997;6(8):1341–7.

[16] Rao E, et al. Pseudoautosomal deletions encompassing a novel homeobox gene cause growth failure in idiopathic short stature and Turner syndrome. Nat Genet 1997;16(1):54–63.

[17] Clement-Jones M, et al. The short stature homeobox gene SHOX is involved in skeletal abnormalities in Turner syndrome. Hum Mol Genet 2000;9(5):695–702.

[18] Hall JG. Genomic imprinting. Arch Dis Child 1990;65(10 Spec No):1013–5.

[19] Constancia M, et al. Imprinting mechanisms. Genome Res 1998;8(9):881–900.

[20] Nicholls RD. The impact of genomic imprinting for neurobehavioral and developmental disorders. J Clin Invest 2000;105(4):413–8.

[21] Brown WE, et al. Brain development in Turner syndrome: a magnetic resonance imaging study. Psychiatry Res 2002;116:187–96.

[22] Kesler SR, et al. Effects of X-monosomy and X-linked imprinting on superior temporal gyrus morphology in Turner syndrome. Biol Psychiatry 2003;54(6):636–46.

[23] Larizza D, et al. Two sisters with 45,X karyotype: influence of genomic imprinting on phenotype and cognitive profile. Eur J Pediatr 2002;161(4):224–5.

[24] Skuse DH. X-linked genes and mental functioning. Hum Mol Genet 2005;14(Spec No 1): R27–32.

[25] Skuse DH, et al. Evidence from Turner's syndrome of an imprinted X-linked locus affecting cognitive function [see comments]. Nature 1997;387(6634):705–8.

[26] Russell HF, et al. Increased prevalence of ADHD in Turner syndrome with no evidence of imprinting effects. J Pediatr Psychol 2006;31(9):945–55.

[27] Good CD, et al. Dosage-sensitive X-linked locus influences the development of amygdala and orbitofrontal cortex and fear recognition in humans. Brain 2003;126(Pt 11):2431–46.

[28] Kesler SR, et al. Amygdala and hippocampal volumes in Turner syndrome: a high-resolution MRI study of X-monosomy. Neuropsychologia 2004;42:1971–8.

[29] Loesch DZ, et al. Effect of Turner's syndrome and X-linked imprinting on cognitive status: analysis based on pedigree data. Brain Dev 2005;27(7):494–503.

[30] Bishop DV, et al. Distinctive patterns of memory function in subgroups of females with Turner syndrome: evidence for imprinted loci on the X-chromosome affecting neurodevelopment. Neuropsychologia 2000;38(5):712–21.

[31] Andersen NH, et al. Subclinical left ventricular dysfunction in normotensive women with Turner's syndrome. Heart 2006;92(10):1516–7.

[32] Bondy CA, et al. Prolonged rate-corrected QT interval and other electrocardiogram abnormalities in girls with Turner syndrome. Pediatrics 2006;118(4):e1220–5.

[33] Noe JA, Pittman HC, Burton EM. Congenital absence of the portal vein in a child with Turner syndrome. Pediatr Radiol 2006;36(6):566–8.

[34] Ross JL, et al. The effect of genetic differences and ovarian failure: intact cognitive function in adult women with premature ovarian failure versus Turner syndrome. J Clin Endocrinol Metab 2004;89(4):1817–22.

[35] Ross JL, et al. Persistent cognitive deficits in adult women with Turner syndrome. Neurology 2002;58(2):218–25.

[36] Temple CM, Carney R. Reading skills in children with Turner's syndrome: an analysis of hyperplexia. Cortex 1996;32(2):335–45.

[37] Temple CM. Oral fluency and narrative production in children with Turner's syndrome. Neuropsychologia 2002;40(8):1419–27.

[38] Rae C, et al. Enlarged temporal lobes in Turner syndrome: an X-chromosome effect? Cereb Cortex 2004;14(2):156–64.

[39] Nijhuis–van der Sanden MW, Eling PA, Otten BJ. A review of neuropsychological and motor studies in Turner syndrome. Neurosci Biobehav Rev 2003;27(4):329–38.

[40] Ross JL, et al. Androgen-responsive aspects of cognition in girls with Turner syndrome. J Clin Endocrinol Metab 2003;88(1):292–6.

[41] Rovet J. The cognitive and neuropsychological characteristics of females with Turner syndrome. In: Berch DB, Bender BG, editors. Sex chromosome abnormalities and human behavior: psychological studies. Boulder (CO): AAAS/Westview Press; 1990. p. 38–77.

[42] Temple CM, Carney RA. Patterns of spatial functioning in Turner's syndrome. Cortex 1995;31(1):109–18.

[43] Kesler SR, et al. Functional neuroanatomy of spatial orientation processing in Turner syndrome. Cereb Cortex 2004;14(2):174–80.

[44] LaHood BJ, Bacon GE. Cognitive abilities of adolescent Turner's syndrome patients. J Adolesc Health Care 1985;6(5):358–64.

[45] Reiss AL, et al. Contribution of the FMR1 gene mutation to human intellectual dysfunction. Nat Genet 1995;11(3):331–4.

[46] Romans SM, et al. Transition to young adulthood in Ullrich-Turner syndrome: neurodevelopmental changes. Am J Med Genet 1998;79(2):140–7.

[47] Rovet J, Szekely C, Hockenberry MN. Specific arithmetic calculation deficits in children with Turner syndrome. J Clin Exp Neuropsychol 1994;16(6):820–39.

[48] Rovet JF. The psychoeducational characteristics of children with Turner syndrome. J Learn Disabil 1993;26(5):333–41.

[49] Cornoldi C, Marconi F, Vecchi T. Visuospatial working memory in Turner's syndrome. Brain Cogn 2001;46(1–2):90–4.

[50] Culham JC, Kanwisher NG. Neuroimaging of cognitive functions in human parietal cortex. Curr Opin Neurobiol 2001;11(2):157–63.

[51] Podzebenko K, Egan GF, Watson JD. Widespread dorsal stream activation during a parametric mental rotation task, revealed with functional magnetic resonance imaging. Neuroimage 2002;15(3):547–58.

[52] Sack AT, et al. The experimental combination of rTMS and fMRI reveals the functional relevance of parietal cortex for visuospatial functions. Brain Res Cogn Brain Res 2002; 13(1):85–93.

[53] Brown WE, et al. A volumetric study of parietal lobe subregions in Turner syndrome. Dev Med Child Neurol 2004;46(9):607–9.

[54] Clark C, Klonoff H, Hayden M. Regional cerebral glucose metabolism in Turner syndrome. Can J Neurol Sci 1990;17(2):140–4.

[55] Cutter WJ, et al. Influence of X chromosome and hormones on human brain development: a magnetic resonance imaging and proton magnetic resonance spectroscopy study of Turner syndrome. Biol Psychiatry 2006;59(3):273–83.

[56] Molko N, et al. Functional and structural alterations of the intraparietal sulcus in a developmental dyscalculia of genetic origin. Neuron 2003;40(4):847–58.

[57] Molko N, et al. Brain anatomy in Turner syndrome: evidence for impaired social and spatial-numerical networks. Cereb Cortex 2004;14(8):840–50.

[58] Murphy DG, et al. A PET study of Turner's syndrome: effects of sex steroids and the X chromosome on brain. Biol Psychiatry 1997;41(3):285–98.

[59] Reiss AL, et al. Neurodevelopmental effects of X monosomy: a volumetric imaging study. Ann Neurol 1995;38(5):731–8.

[60] Kirk JW, Mazzocco MM, Kover ST. Assessing executive dysfunction in girls with fragile X or Turner syndrome using the Contingency Naming Test (CNT). Dev Neuropsychol 2005; 28(3):755–77.

[61] Romans SM, et al. Executive function in females with Turner syndrome. Dev Neuropsychol 1997;13:23–40.

[62] Ross J, Zinn A, McCauley E. Neurodevelopmental and psychosocial aspects of Turner syndrome. Ment Retard Dev Disabil Res Rev 2000;6(2):135–41.

[63] McCauley E, et al. Psychosocial development in adolescents with Turner syndrome. J Dev Behav Pediatr 2001;22(6):360–5.

[64] Haberecht MF, et al. Functional neuroanatomy of visuo-spatial working memory in Turner syndrome. Hum Brain Mapp 2001;14(2):96–107.

[65] Hart SJ, et al. Visuospatial executive function in Turner syndrome: functional MRI and neurocognitive findings. Brain 2006;129(Pt 5):1125–36.

[66] Kesler SR, Menon V, Reiss AL. Neuro-functional differences associated with arithmetic processing in Turner syndrome. Cereb Cortex 2006;16(6):849–56.

[67] Tamm L, Menon V, Reiss AL. Abnormal prefrontal cortex function during response inhibition in Turner syndrome: functional magnetic resonance imaging evidence. Biol Psychiatry 2003;53(2):107–11.

[68] Holzapfel M, et al. Selective alterations of white matter associated with visuospatial and sensorimotor dysfunction in Turner syndrome. J Neurosci 2006;26(26):7007–13.

[69] Horwitz B, Braun AR. Brain network interactions in auditory, visual and linguistic processing. Brain Lang 2004;89(2):377–84.

[70] Hepworth SL, Rovet JF. Visual integration difficulties in a 9-year-old girl with Turner syndrome: parallel verbal disabilities? Child Neuropsychol 2000;6(4):262–73.

[71] Temple CM, Marriott AJ. Arithmetical ability and disability in Turner's syndrome: a cognitive neuropsychological analysis. Dev Neuropsychol 1998;(14):47–67.

[72] Temple CM, Sherwood S. Representation and retrieval of arithmetical facts: developmental difficulties. Q J Exp Psychol A 2002;55(3):733–52.

[73] Pennington BF, et al. The neuropsychological phenotype in Turner syndrome. Cortex 1985; 21(3):391–404.

[74] Williams J, Richman L, Yarbrough D. A comparison of memory and attention in Turner syndrome and learning disability. J Pediatr Psychol 1991;16(5):585–93.

[75] Siegel PT, Clopper R, Stabler B. The psychological consequences of Turner syndrome and review of the national cooperative growth study psychological substudy. Pediatrics 1998; 102:488–91.

[76] Lawrence K, et al. Interpreting gaze in Turner syndrome: impaired sensitivity to intention and emotion, but preservation of social cueing. Neuropsychologia 2003;41(8): 894–905.

[77] Lawrence K, et al. Face and emotion recognition deficits in Turner syndrome: a possible role for X-linked genes in amygdala development. Neuropsychology 2003;17(1):39–49.

[78] Reiss AL, et al. The effects of X monosomy on brain development: monozygotic twins discordant for Turner's syndrome. Ann Neurol 1993;34(1):95–107.

[79] Ross JL, Kushner H, Zinn AR. Discriminant analysis of the Ullrich-Turner syndrome neurocognitive profile. Am J Med Genet 1997;72(3):275–80.

[80] Ross JL, et al. Ullrich-Turner syndrome: neurodevelopmental changes from childhood through adolescence. Am J Med Genet 1995;58(1):74–82.

[81] Donnelly SL, et al. Female with autistic disorder and monosomy X (Turner syndrome): parent-of-origin effect of the X chromosome. Am J Med Genet 2000;96(3):312–6.

[82] Hou M, Wang MJ, Zhong N. Principal genetic syndromes and autism: from phenotypes, proteins to genes [Chinese]. Beijing Da Xue Xue Bao 2006;38(1):110–5.

[83] Adolphs R. Is the human amygdala specialized for processing social information? Ann N Y Acad Sci 2003;985:326–40.

[84] Skuse DH, Morris JS, Dolan RJ. Functional dissociation of amygdala-modulated arousal and cognitive appraisal, in Turner syndrome. Brain 2005;128(Pt 9):2084–96.

[85] Rourke BP, et al. Child clinical/pediatric neuropsychology: some recent advances. Annu Rev Psychol 2002;53:309–39.

[86] Schmidt PJ, et al. Shyness, social anxiety, and impaired self-esteem in Turner syndrome and premature ovarian failure. JAMA 2006;295(12):1374–6.

[87] Kilic BG, Ergur AT, Ocal G. Depression, levels of anxiety and self-concept in girls with Turner's syndrome. J Pediatr Endocrinol Metab 2005;18(11):1111–7.

[88] Keysor CS, et al. Physiological arousal in females with fragile X or Turner syndrome. Dev Psychobiol 2002;41(2):133–46.

[89] Carel JC, et al. Self-esteem and social adjustment in young women with Turner syndrome: influence of pubertal management and sexuality. Population-based cohort study. J Clin Endocrinol Metab 2006;91(8):2972–9.

[90] van Pareren YK, et al. Psychosocial functioning after discontinuation of long-term growth hormone treatment in girls with Turner syndrome. Horm Res 2005;63(5):238–44.

[91] Lesniak-Karpiak K, Mazzocco MM, Ross JL. Behavioral assessment of social anxiety in females with Turner or fragile X syndrome. J Autism Dev Disord 2003;33(1):55–67.

[92] Cardoso G, et al. Current and lifetime psychiatric illness in women with Turner syndrome. Gynecol Endocrinol 2004;19(6):313–9.

[93] Ari M, et al. The effects of growth hormone treatment on bone mineral density and body composition in girls with Turner syndrome. J Clin Endocrinol Metab 2006;91(11):4302–5.

[94] Bechtold S, et al. Pubertal height gain in Ullrich-Turner syndrome. J Pediatr Endocrinol Metab 2006;19(8):987–93.

[95] Ito Y, et al. Low-dose growth hormone treatment (0.175 mg/kg/week) for short stature in patients with Turner syndrome: data from KIGS Japan. Endocr J 2006;53(5):699–703.

[96] Hindmarsh PC, Dattani MT. Use of growth hormone in children. Nat Clin Pract Endocrinol Metab 2006;2(5):260–8.

[97] Lagrou K, et al. Psychosocial functioning, self-perception and body image and their auxologic correlates in growth hormone and oestrogen-treated young adult women with Turner syndrome. Horm Res 2006;66(6):277–84.

[98] Salgin B, et al. Insulin resistance is an intrinsic defect independent of fat mass in women with Turner's syndrome. Horm Res 2006;65(2):69–75.

[99] Mazzanti L, et al. Turner syndrome, insulin sensitivity and growth hormone treatment. Horm Res 2005;64(Suppl 3):51–7.

[100] Ross JL, et al. Absence of growth hormone effects on cognitive function in girls with Turner syndrome. J Clin Endocrinol Metab 1997;82(6):1814–7.

[101] Hojbjerg Gravholt C, et al. Reduced androgen levels in adult Turner syndrome: influence of female sex steroids and growth hormone status. Clin Endocrinol (Oxf) 1999;50(6):791–800.

[102] Livadas S, et al. Spontaneous pregnancy and birth of a normal female from a woman with Turner syndrome and elevated gonadotropins. Fertil Steril 2005;83(3):769–72.

[103] Rizk DE, Deb P. A spontaneous and uneventful pregnancy in a Turner mosaic with previous recurrent miscarriages. J Pediatr Adolesc Gynecol 2003;16(2):87–8.

[104] Chernausek SD, et al. Growth hormone therapy of Turner syndrome: the impact of age of estrogen replacement on final height. Genentech, Inc., Collaborative Study Group. J Clin Endocrinol Metab 2000;85(7):2439–45.

[105] Davenport ML. Evidence for early initiation of growth hormone and transdermal estradiol therapies in girls with Turner syndrome. Growth Horm IGF Res 2006;16(Suppl A):S91–7.

[106] Rosenfield RL, et al. Salutary effects of combining early very low-dose systemic estradiol with growth hormone therapy in girls with Turner syndrome. J Clin Endocrinol Metab 2005;90(12):6424–30.

[107] Stephure DK. Impact of growth hormone supplementation on adult height in Turner syndrome: results of the Canadian randomized controlled trial. J Clin Endocrinol Metab 2005; 90(6):3360–6.

[108] Sartorio A, Ferrero S, Molinari E. Different effects of GH treatment on cognitive function in girls with Turner's syndrome and in adults with GH deficiency. J Clin Endocrinol Metab 1998;83(4):1396.

[109] Ross JL, et al. Effects of estrogen on nonverbal processing speed and motor function in girls with Turner's syndrome. J Clin Endocrinol Metab 1998;83(9):3198–204.

[110] Livadas S, et al. Prevalence of thyroid dysfunction in Turner's syndrome: a long-term follow-up study and brief literature review. Thyroid 2005;15(9):1061–6.

[111] MacLusky NJ, et al. Androgen modulation of hippocampal synaptic plasticity. Neuroscience 2006;138(3):957–65.

[112] Hynes P, Phillips W. Turner's syndrome: assessment and treatment for adult psychiatric patients. Am J Psychother 1984;38(4):558–65.

[113] Money J. Turner's syndrome: principles of therapy. Curr Psychiatr Ther 1976;16:21–8.

[114] Watson MA, Money J. Behavior cytogenetics and Turner's syndrome: a new principle in counseling and psychotherapy. Am J Psychother 1975;29(2):166–78.

[115] Jacobs B, Scheibel AB. A quantitative dendritic analysis of Wernicke's area in humans. I. Lifespan changes. J Comp Neurol 1993;327(1):83–96.

[116] Jacobs P, et al. Turner syndrome: a cytogenetic and molecular study. Ann Hum Genet 1997; 61(Pt 6):471–83.

ELSEVIER
SAUNDERS

Child Adolesc Psychiatric Clin N Am
16 (2007) 723–743

CHILD AND
ADOLESCENT
PSYCHIATRIC CLINICS
OF NORTH AMERICA

Rett Syndrome

Bruria Ben Zeev Ghidoni, MD

*Pediatric Neurology Unit, Safra Pediatric Hospital, Sheba Medical Center,
Ramat-Gan, Israel*

Rett syndrome (RS) is an X-linked dominant severe neurodevelopmental disorder affecting postnatal brain growth. It is the second most common cause of genetic mental retardation (MR) in girls and the first pervasive developmental disorder with a known genetic basis. RS was described first by an Austrian pediatrician Andreas Rett [1] in 1966; however, the syndrome gained international interest after Hagberg and colleagues [2] described 35 girls with a similar profile and gave the syndrome its name. Its prevalence ranges between 1 in 10,000 and 1 in 22,000 in the general population [3].

Girls who have classic RS are born after a normal pregnancy and delivery with apparently normal development through the first 6 months of life, except for deceleration in head growth from around the fourth month that usually results in microcephaly. This period is followed by developmental regression that includes social withdrawal, loss of purposeful hand usage, coinciding with the appearance of stereotypic hand movements (Fig. 1), and loss of acquired speech and language abilities. Apraxia and ataxia of gait are common symptoms.

The clinical criteria (necessary and supportive, Box 1) for classic RS were defined first by Hagberg and colleagues [4,5] in 1985 and revised after the gene responsible for RS was found in 2001.

The evolution of RS usually follows four stages [6]. Stage 1 (early onset or stagnation period) starts between 6 and 18 months and lasts from a few months to more than a year. It is sometimes overlooked because symptoms are usually subtle. Decreased eye contact and reduced interest in toys are accompanied by delays in gross motor skills (sitting or crawling). Slowing of head growth appears as does occasional subtle hand-wringing.

Stage II (rapid destructive [regression] stage) usually begins between ages 1 and 4 years and lasts for weeks to months. Hallmarks are loss of language and motor skills and appearance of stereotypic hand movements, social withdrawal with autistic-like behavior accompanied by extreme irritability

E-mail address: benzeev4@netvision.net.il

1056-4993/07/$ - see front matter © 2007 Published by Elsevier Inc.
doi:10.1016/j.chc.2007.03.004

childpsych.theclinics.com

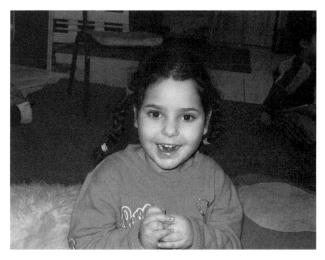

Fig. 1. A 3-year-old girl with classic Rett syndrome. Note the hand washing, the nondysmorphic facies, and the expressive eyes.

with screaming and crying episodes, disturbed sleep, and occasional feeding difficulties. Breathing abnormalities and vasomotor changes start to appear, accompanied by gait apraxia and evolving limb spasticity. Slowing of head growth continues.

Stage III (plateau or pseudostationary stage) starts between ages 2 and 10 years and lasts for years. Apraxia, motor problems, and seizures are prominent; however, there is usually improvement in behavior, less irritability and autistic-like features, better social and communication skills, improved alertness, and longer attention span. Many girls remain in this stage for most of their lives.

Stage IV (late motor deterioration stage) is characterized by reduced mobility related to increased rigidity, spasticity, and dystonic posturing accompanied by aggravation of scoliosis. Girls can lose their independent or partially dependent walking abilities. Part of these negative changes may be related to decreased motor interventions in educational and home setting environments; however, there is no decline in cognition, communication, or hand skills.

Major clinical features of Rett syndrome

Epilepsy

Epileptic seizures are reported in up to 90% of girls with RS. They usually start at around 2 to 4 years of age and include generalized tonic-clonic seizures, partial complex and simple partial seizures, and, less commonly,

---

Box 1. Criteria for the diagnosis of Rett syndrome

Necessary criteria
Apparently normal prenatal and perinatal history
Psychomotor development normal during the first 6 months
   (maybe delayed from birth)
Normal head circumference at birth
Postnatal deceleration of head growth (most individuals)
Loss of purposeful hand skills between 6 months and 2.5 years,
   temporarily associated with communication dysfunction and
   social withdrawal
Development of severely impaired expressive and receptive
   language and presence of apparent severe psychomotor
   retardation
Stereotypic hand movements, such as hand wringing/squeezing,
   clapping/tapping, mouthing and "washing"/rubbing
   automatism, appearing after hand skills are lost
Gait apraxia and truncal apraxia/ataxia appearing between
   ages 1 and 4 years
Diagnosis tentative until 2 to 5 years of age

Supportive criteria
Breathing dysfunction: periodic apnea during wakefulness,
   intermittent hyperventilation, breath-holding spells, forced
   expulsion of air or saliva
Electroencephalogram abnormalities: slow waking
   background and intermittent rhythmical slowing
Epileptiform discharges, with or without clinical seizures
Seizures
Spasticity, often with associated development of muscle
   wasting and dystonia
Impaired sleeping pattern from early infancy
Peripheral vasomotor disturbances
Progressive scoliosis or kyphosis
Growth retardation
Hypotrophic small and cold feet or hands

---

myoclonic and absence seizures [7]. Seizures may be provoked by fever, occur in clusters, especially early on, and tend to remit around adolescence, with only 20% to 30% of girls at this age suffering from significant epilepsy. Most girls respond to anticonvulsants. It is recommended to avoid barbiturates and benzodiazepines, which decrease alertness and responsiveness to the point of pseudodeterioration.

In addition, girls who have RS manifest many types of behaviors that imitate seizures clinically: vacant spells accompanied by apnea after a prolonged hyperventilation period or during prolonged breath holding, trembling, and opisthotonic posturing when waking from sleep or changing posture, and repetitive stereotypic movements resembling partial complex seizures. It is crucial to differentiate these behaviors from epileptic seizures to avoid the unnecessary and inappropriate use of anticonvulsants. Video electroencephalogram (EEG) recording of these behaviors is useful for clarifying the diagnosis [8].

Breathing abnormalities

Most individuals who have RS show some form of breathing abnormalities that usually appear at stages II and III during the awake state, including apnea, hyperventilation, breath holding, Valsalva breathing, and bloating. When frequent and severe, they interfere with the child's responsiveness and are "energy consuming." Breathing abnormalities relate to the immature autonomic regulatory brain stem systems [9] and can be resistant to pharmacologic interventions.

Stereotypic hand movements

Movements can precede, occur simultaneously, or follow the loss of hand skills. They are usually midline, chest level, asymmetric movements that include clasping, wringing, washing, tapping, and hand biting and sucking. They encompass 30% to 72% of waking hours; intensify when the child is excited, hungry, or tired; and subside partially with age. It is difficult for the child to stop these movements voluntarily, although some can do so for a short period of time on demand [10,11].

Sleep patterns

Patients who have RS have significant sleep problems especially in stages II and III, including difficulty falling asleep, frequent arousals accompanied by screaming or laughing spells, and imbalanced sleep cycle with nighttime alertness and frequent inappropriate naps during daytime. Sleep pattern analysis shows shorter than age-expected sleep cycles related to dysfunction of the serotonergic and dopaminergic pathways [12,13].

Communication

Most girls who have classic RS do not use verbal language. Between 50% and 69% have used several words in early development and 12% may have used short sentences; however, most lose the ability to speak by 40 months of age, although according to a recent Swedish survey, 19% continue to use some words [14,15]. The commonest way to express needs is by eye gazing and pointing [16], but they also communicate through pictures, written words (yes/no), gestures, facial expressions, and words or sounds with special meanings. According to the same survey, 39% of parents reported social interplay situations as the girls preferred activity and best contact situations as eating or being the "center of attention."

Seven girls with RS were tested using "eye gaze" technology. Length of fixation time was chosen to differentiate between "correct" and "incorrect" responses to verbal instructions, recognition, and matching objects and picture categorization using children 36 to 48 months of age-appropriate tasks. All girls responded consistently in all tasks and were right more often than wrong. The degree of motor and past speech history was related to performance [17].

Life expectancy

Females with RS usually survive into adulthood. Longevity is influenced by the severity of the overall disability; however, there is a higher risk for sudden death compared with controls of the same age. Some sudden deaths have been related to longer Q-T intervals and reduced heart rate variability as part of the autonomic dysfunction in RS [18,19].

Early symptoms and signs

The description of apparently normal development in the first months of life has been challenged by several investigators who commented that under close observation, girls who have RS show early hypotonia [20,21], motor problems [22], early jerking and lack of coordination [23], placidity, and perinatal difficulties requiring special nursery care [24]. One third of families in the Australian Rett Syndrome Database Population Registry reported difficulties in the first week of life, including feeding difficulties and assistance required to start breathing, followed by placidity in up to 58% of cases. Early symptoms were reported more commonly in girls who had RS with "severe" mutations [24].

Rett variants

Variants are described by the following "revised variant criteria" [5] (Box 2) or as specific entities. Girls of at least 10 years of age with MR of unexplained origin with at least 3 of the main criteria and at least 5 of 11 supportive criteria are diagnosed as Rett variants.

Variants defined as specific entities include [25]:

"Forme Fruste" - Milder variant; later regression, existing hand function, less stereotypic movements and occasional normocephaly

Preserved speech variant (PSV)

Congenital onset variant: significant delay in development from birth followed by typical clinical picture. No evidence of regression.

Early seizure onset variant: seizures, usually hypsarrhythmia, but other seizure types as the presenting symptom at first year of life, followed

---

Box 2. Diagnostic criteria for Rett variants

Main criteria
Loss of acquired fine finger skills in late infancy/early childhood
Loss of acquired single words/phrases/nuanced babble
Hand stereotypies/hands together or apart
Early deviant communicative ability
Deceleration of head growth of 2 standard deviation (even if
    within normal limits)
The RS disease profile: a regression period followed by a certain
    recovery of contact and communication in contrast to slow
    neuron-motor regression through school age and adolescence

Supportive criteria
Breathing irregularities: hyperventilation or breath holding
Bloating and marked air swallowing
Bruxism
Abnormal locomotion/gait dyspraxia
Scoliosis or kyphosis
Lower limb amyotrophy
Cold discolored feet, usually hypotrophic
Characteristic RS electroencephalographic development
Unprompted sudden laughing/screaming spells
Apparently diminished pain sensitivity
Intense eye contact or eye pointing

---

by RS like picture, usually of high severity. Most do not have methyl
CpG binding protein 2 *(MECP2)* mutations. Some of these cases have
recently been described as carrying CDKL5 mutations, which is
another X-linked gene [26].
Late regression variant: relatively late onset but typical phenotype
    evolving.
Male RS
Angelman-like: patients who have Angelman syndrome (AS) phenotype
    carrying MECP2 mutations

In all variants, except PSV and Angelman-like, *MECP2* mutations are
found in 25% to 40% of cases, which is a much lower frequency than
that found in classic cases [27,28].

Genetics

Linkage studies based on several familial cases of RS found linkage to the
Xq28 region [29], closely followed by identification of MECP2 as the

responsible gene for the syndrome. This gene is found to be mutated in up to 95% of the classic cases [30]. The gene product is made up of four exons and exists in two isoforms, created by alternative splicing of exon 2 [31]. MeCP2 is a nuclear protein that binds specifically to single methylated CG nucleotides on different genes and functions as a powerful transcription repressor. It contains three major functional domains: an 85–amino acid methyl binding domain (MBD) that binds to methylated DNA (CpG islands) on target genes; a 104–amino acid transcriptional repressor domain (TRD) interacting with histone deacetylase complex, together causing transcriptional repression of target genes by chromatin modifications; and a carboxy terminal domain containing a WW binding domain. Located within the TRD is a nuclear localization sequence (NLS) responsible for targeting MeCP2 into the cell nucleus [32–34]. MeCP2 also interacts with other transcription repressor factors besides histone deacetylase, making it a major heterochromatin inactivator [35,36].

Most *MECP2* mutations are de novo, a large proportion originating from the paternal germline, with a high spontaneous mutation rate. The paternal origin explains the high incidence of isolated cases and partially explains the few male cases [37]. Up to 70% of mutations occur in eight specific CpG hotspots along the gene, by deamination of methylated cytosine, creating C-T transitions [38,39]. The rest are less common mutations, including missense, nonsense, and small and large deletions mainly at exons 3 and 4 [40]. Large gene deletions detected only by multiple ligation dependant probe amplification (MLPA) technique (a polymerase chain reaction–based strategy) have been described recently, accounting for 6% of *MECP2* mutations [41]. Exon 1 mutations are rare (less than 0.5% of cases) [40]; however, lately, sequence variants within exon 1 have been detected in up to 1% of a nonspecific MR female group (N = 1410), whereas no variants were detected in an autistic sample (N = 410) [42].

Recently, Petel-Galil and colleagues [43] reported that, in several patients with clinically defined RS without a detectable coding sequence mutation, a change in *MECP2* RNA expression levels substantiated the clinical diagnosis.

Genotype–phenotype correlations

Symptom severity varies significantly in patients who have classic RS. Variations are described in stage II, such as age of onset, level of motor function, existence and severity of epilepsy, head circumference, and existence of autonomic dysfunction. Several studies have looked at genotype–phenotype correlations; in most studies, truncating mutations correlated with a more severe phenotype than missense mutations, and early truncation was more severe than late truncation [44,45]. Detailed relationships between clinical phenotype and mutation type and location were reported by Huppke and colleagues [46] as follows: (1) mutations affecting the NLS are more severe than mutations that do not affect the NLS; (2) carboxy-terminal deletion is less severe than other mutations; (3) truncation mutations are more severe than missense mutations, except in the carboxy-terminal region; and (4) missense mutations in MBD and TRD regions have the same impact on symptom severity.

X-inactivation (XCI) profile also affects the degree of severity. Ishii and colleagues [47] described differently affected identical twins with the R294X mutation; the milder case showed skewed XCI, whereas the more severely affected twin was randomly inactivated. Extreme skewed inactivation was found in some heterozygote carriers with mild phenotype (most likely protective), whereas their affected daughters had balanced XCI [28].

The XCI pattern in multiple brain regions, as well as in nonneuronal tissue of patients who had RS, was investigated. Individual variability was found across different brain regions in one patient, emphasizing that an XCI pattern in one particular tissue or cell type does not necessarily reflect its pattern in other tissues in the same individual [48].

Logistic regression applied to an RS mouse model proved that the level of skewing of XCI favoring the wild-type allele was inversely related to the severity of the observed phenotype, suggesting a skewing effect on phenotype even when the degree of scewing is not higher than 80% [49]. A statistically significant increase in clinical severity was linearly proportional to the increased expression of the active mutated allele in lymphocytes from girls who had RS with the two most common mutations: (R168X and T 158M) [50].

Three patients with pathogenic *MECP2* mutations with significant skewing (leukocytes), showed normal hand function, good motor skills, reading and writing abilities, reasonable language, and normal head circumference. All had episodes of hyperventilation and hand stereotypies under stress or anxiety. Two had undergone developmental regression in verbal, motor, or communication fields in the past, whereas the third, the least severely affected, had episodes of uncontrolled aggression [51].

Pathogenesis

The Mecp2 gene–deficient mouse models are excellent investigational tools for studying the pathogenesis and neurobiology of RS.

Null male mice develop neurologic symptoms at 4 to 6 weeks. Conditional deletion of *Mecp2* in postmitotic neurons results in a similar phenotype [52]. A mouse model with truncation mutation of MECP2 shows Rett-like features, including motor impairment, seizures, hypoactivity, scoliosis, and repetitive stereotyped forepaw clasping [53]. These mice also exhibit specific deficits in social behavior, making them a potential model for autism [54]. Null mice phenotypic abnormalities may be rescued by expression of transgenic Tau-Mecp2 fusion protein in postmitotic neurons [55]; however, two-fold expression of *MeCP2* in wild mice under its own

Table 1
Rett syndrome central nervous system proteins and neurotransmitters changes

CNS proteins and neurotransmitters	Change in RS compared with control
MAP2, MAP5, COX2	↓
CHAT and cholinergic vesicular transport	↓
CSF glutamate	↑
AMPA, NMDA receptors	↑ in young children ↓ in older children
Serotonin receptors in brainstem	↑
Dopamine	↓
NGF	↓
Substance P	↓
Biogenic amines	↕

Abbreviations: AMPA, α-amino-3-hydroxy-5-methylisoxazole-4- propionic acid receptor; CNS, central nervous system; COX2, cyclooxygenase 2; CHAT, choline acyltransferase; CSF, cerebrospinal fluid; MAP2, microtubule associated protein 2; MAP5, microtubule associated protein 5; NMDA, N-methyl d-aspartate; NGF, nerve growth factor.

Brain-derived neurotrophic factor *(BDNF)* was found to be a major target for MeCP2 by two separate laboratories. BDNF is a neurotrophin that is essential for adult neuronal plasticity, learning, and memory. MeCP2 is associated with methylated CpG sequences which upstream the *BDNF* promoter. Dissociation from the promoter, which is phosphorylation dependant, results in a switch to a transcriptionally permissive chromatin state. Mice that their BDNF gene was selectively knocked out in their forebrain shows an RS-like phenotype with similar brain pathology, whereas overexpressing BDNF in *Mecp2* mutant mice rescued a subset of RS-like features (mainly motor). These findings are consistent with reduced expression of BDNF in MECP2 mutant mice, while, basically, BDNF expression should be up-regulated. A disrupted response to activation related to higher BDNF basal levels in *Mecp2*-deficient mice might explain this paradox. Otherwise, low or absent BDNF levels and abnormally high levels produce aberrant maturation and reduced dendritic arborization [74–76].

DLX5, a gene encoding a homeobox transcription factor is involved in brain patterning. *DLX2* and Dlx5 directly regulate expression of glutamic acid decarboxylase, the key enzyme in γ-aminobutyric acid (GABA) production. By this mechanism they engage in specification and function of inhibitory GABAergic neurons in the mammalian forebrain—a subpopulation of neurons implicated in autism pathogenesis [77]. Dlx5 expression is doubled in *Mecp2*-deficient mice, most probably through the loss of normal Mecp2 interaction with a regulatory region of the DLX5 gene [78].

MeCP2 controls gene expression in the Prader-Willi syndrome/Angelman syndrome imprinted cluster at 15q11-13, affecting mainly *UBE3A* and *GABRB3* expression [79].

Recently, McGill and colleagues [80] demonstrated MeCP2 binding to methyl CpG dinucleotides on the corticotrophin-releasing hormone

promoter causes severe motor disability and death in adult mice
conclusions from these data are that *MECP2* expression in po
neurons is critical for brain function, and a delicate balance of M
required for proper neuronal maturation in the postnatal period [5]

At the last Rett Syndrome Research Foundation Conference (June
A. Bird (Cambridge University) showed that if the *Mecp2* gene of
mice is reversibly inactivated and then reactivated, symptoms disap
even after their obvious appearance. Although genetic manipulatio
this kind is not available in humans, this gives us a larger window of op
tunity for less sophisticated interventions [58].

MeCP2 was believed to be expressed ubiquitously in all tissues and stag
of development, but it is now accepted that its highest expression is in matu
neurons and its lowest expression is in glia. Expression in spinal cord an
hindbrain, which are early developing systems, precede expression in the hip
pocampus and cerebral cortex [59,60]. The gene expression develops progressively from deep cortical to superficial layers following cortical laminar
development ("inside-out"). This is consistent with the role of MeCP2 in post-
migrational neuronal development and synaptogenesis, making it a marker of
mature neurons in the postnatal brain [61]. The gradual increased expression
of MeCP2 in human brain continues during childhood [62]. It is becoming
clear that in mice and humans, MeCP2 has no significant role in early embryonic stages and is not involved significantly in cell fate decisions.

Gross brain tissue in girls and mice with RS appears to be relatively normal. Microcephaly is related to the decreased size of neuronal cell bodies,
whereas higher packing density is related to reduced pyramidal neurons,
dendritic spines, and arborization. These changes are most prominent in
layers 2/3 projection neurons of prefrontal, postfrontal, and anterior temporal regions and less prominent in the occipital regions, as has been shown in
autism [63–65]. Nonmutated (wild-type) neurons in individuals and heterozygote female mice with RS also show decreased expression of Mecp2 and
less than normal synaptogenesis related to the negative impact by the
"deprived environment" created by mutated neurons [66].

Using immunoblotting techniques, the RS brain shows reduction in all
dendritic proteins, but mainly in microtubule-associated protein (MAP)-5
(early dendritic differentiation marker) and MAP-2 (associated with dendritic branching) [67,68]. Minicolumn structures are arranged more tightly,
similar to autism brain [69], because of decreased MAP-2 cytoskeleton protein in the subplate neurons [67]. Synaptic development is impaired [70]. Abnormal levels of neurotrophic proteins, neurotransmitters, and their
receptors were described in several studies (Table 1) [71]. Some of the
data is less valid because the finding was described in only a few cases, at
various ages, by various techniques, and in postmortem samples. Presently,
researchers are looking for downstream targets for *MECP2* regulation.
General gene expression profile analysis reported that less than 5% of genes
are significantly altered, and, more commonly, are up-regulated [72,73].

(CRH) gene promoter. CRH is overexpressed in Mecp2[308] mutant mice, resulting in elevation of corticotropin and adrenal steroids causing increased anxiety-like behaviors and abnormal stress response. Frequently encountered anxiety-like behaviors in patients who have RS and increased urinary cortisol secretion are consistent with this mechanism of function. Repeated corticosteroid exposures and elevated CRH can affect dendritic branching and synaptic plasticity and cause memory impairment, making CRH regulation even more significant.

Rett syndrome and autism

Autism is a behavioral phenotypic end point for a wide variety of etiologic pathways. Autistic symptoms can exist separately or be combined with other cognitive and motor impairments.

RS and autism share several features, including loss of social and language skills coupled with a gain in repetitive stereotypic behaviors. These similarities led to the inclusion of RS as part of the autistic spectrum of disorders in the *Diagnostic and Statistical Manual of Mental Disorders, Revised Fourth Edition.* Many girls with RS are diagnosed as autistic until (if at all) more specific features surface.

An early study by Ollsen and Rett [81] compared the behavioral traits of 27 girls with RS with those of 18 children with idiopathic infantile autism and 18 children with autistic traits resulting from severe brain damage. Only the girls with RS showed nonautistic and social behaviors: approaching the examiner with a smile or laughing accompanied by long-lasting eye contact and sometimes with increased excitement (hyperventilation). In comparison with the other groups they hardly used any words. Their stereotypic hand movements were mainly midline, varying little in form or speed. There was little stereotypic playing with objects compared with the autistic group. The autistic group showed more "social defense reactions" and self-injurious activities. The investigators concluded that interest in social contact is stereotypic for girls with RS. Using the "14 behaviors" scale for Kanner autism, they claimed that girls who have RS and are older than 22 months of age do not have "infantile autism syndrome," and autistic-like behaviors observed in younger patients mainly result from severe general mental, emotional, and motor retardation, leading to "pseudoautistic abnormalities."

Gilberg [82] identified a considerable overlap between autism and RS in infancy through a retrospective questionnaire. Playing with hard objects, being in a world of one's own, and preference for being left alone was found only in the autistic group.

Mount and colleagues [83,84] conducted a study trying to evaluate the severity and specificity of autistic symptoms in patients who had RS compared with females who had nonspecific severe MR (SMR). The two groups were controlled for physical ability and developmental level. Using the Autism

Behavior Checklist scales, some autistic features rated higher in RS than in SMR, including sensory subscale (over- and undersensitivity to certain stimuli) and relating subscale (social relating of the individual). The scoring distribution pattern of all subscales differed from pure autism in both groups. From these studies, we can conclude that although girls who have classic RS have autistic features, especially during stage II, they do differ from those who have pure autism in their social interest and nature of stereotypies. This information should direct clinicians to better differentiate between the two groups and enable the diagnosis of RS at an earlier stage. It may influence the type of treatment interventions.

Despite all of the above, better investigated neuropathologic processes for RS may still be, at least in part, a model for autism. The underlying assumption is that, despite the differences, the pathologic development of particular brain systems at the structural, connectivity, or neurotransmitter level may be common to both.

Brain gross structure is preserved in RS and autism, although "autistic" brains are slightly larger than normal. No severe microscopic and ultrastructural changes are found in either disorder, but there is a decrease in neuronal size—accompanied by increased cell packing related to reduction of dendritic arborization—albeit in different brain regions [64,85].

Patients who have AS, who also show autistic features, have a lot in common with RS: loss or impairment of language, stereotyped behaviors, high seizure frequency, sleep abnormalities, and moderate to SMR. Up to 70% of the autistic population also is retarded [86].

One of the most commonly reported chromosomal alterations in autism is duplication of 15q11-q13 (1%), the region affected—although differently—in AS (by maternal deletion, paternal uniparental disomy, or specific UBE3A mutations). Two percent to 7% of patients with the clinical AS phenotype and no chromosome 15 abnormalities carry *MECP2* mutations [87].

As a connecting thread between all three entities, abnormally low Mecp2 expression at RNA and protein levels, compared with age-matched controls, were detected by quantitative immunofluorescence techniques in postmortem human cerebral cortex samples from subjects who had RS, autism, AS, and Prader-Willi syndrome [79].

The same researchers found decreased expression of *UBE3A* (AS-related gene) and *GABRB3* (β3 subunit of GABAa receptor gene), a nonimprinted gene from the same region, in *Mecp2*-deficient mice strains, RS human brain, AS brain, and autistic brain. These results suggest an overlapping pathway of gene dysregulation within the 15q11-q13 regions in RS, AS, and autism and implicate the role of MeCP2 in this regions' gene regulation in the postnatal mammalian brain [88].

MECP2 mutations in nonspecific autistic populations of children were investigated by several groups (Table 2) [89–94].

Looking at all of these studies, we can conclude that although there are phenotypic similarities and even common pathologic pathways between

Table 2
MECP2 alterations in autistic populations

Investigators	Investigated population	Technique and changes investigated	Findings
Vourch et al, 2001 [89]	59 pts (17 F/42 M) DSM-4 autism criteria + SMR	Direct sequencing; coding polymorphism, exon–intron boundaries	No mutations
Beyer et al, 2002 [90]	202 non-specific autistic pts	DHPLC, direct sequence	14 variations: 3 intron variations 5 silent mutations 3 known polymorphisms 4 new changes not cosegregating with phenotype
Carney et al, 2003 [91]	69 autistic girls	Direct sequencing	2 de novo mutations - no RS features, but 1 regressed at 18 months and 1 at 30 months; no extreme skewing
Zappella et al, 2003 [92]	19 autistic girls	Direct sequencing	2 previously described mutations: PSV phenotype early on prominent autism; one could draw, other could read and write
Lobo-Menendez et al, 2003 [93] South Carolina Autism project	99 pts (41 F/48 M)	Direct sequencing	3 polymorphisms (2 in UTRs)
Shibayama et al, 2004 [94]	214 psychiatric pts: 106 schizophrenia, 24 autism, 84 other	Direct sequencing; coding	One missense, 3 UTR variations intron exon areas in autistic group

Abbreviations: pts, patients; F, female; M, male; DSM-4, *Diagnostic and Statistical Manual of Mental Disorders, Fourth Edition*; DHPLC, denaturing high performance liquid chromatography; UTR, untranslated region.

idiopathic autism and RS, the number of *MECP2* mutations in nonselected autistic patients who do not have at least subtle "Rett-like" features is low.

Preserved speech variant

The girl who has "classic" RS is aphasic; however, it has been observed through the years that there is a subgroup of girls who, after the first regression, show gradual recovery of speech abilities in short or even more structured phrases, usually accompanied by improvement in hand usage. This subtype is called PSV [95].

Ten out of 18 girls with PSV harbored hot spot mutations, including C-terminal deletions (late deletion) and missense mutations (eg, T158 M, R133C, and R306C) [96].

XCI was sporadic in most. All fulfilled the criteria for infantile autism by the *Diagnostic and Statistical Manual of Mental Disorders, Fourth Edition* and Childhood Autism Rating Scale. Six were obese with kyphosis, genu valgum, flat feet, and normal or even large head circumference. Height was in the normal range except for one. None had seizures, although EEG was abnormal in most. Some started speaking only at an older age, using single words or short phrases with echolalia and repetitions. They functioned at the level of 1 to 3 years mentally [97].

According to the British Isles RS survey, 6% of girls with the *MECP2* mutation have the PSV variant. These patients showed a milder clinical picture with later regression (6 of 20 did not show regression), larger head circumference, less feeding difficulties, less epilepsy, and better general health than the girls who had classic RS. All could remember faces, places, and names. They were affectionate and preferred people to objects. Singing was their highest ranked leisure activity. They enjoyed slapstick infantile humor, and made choices on TV shows. They tended to get anxious in big crowds, noisy environments, at sadness or crying in others, and because of personal failure and changes in routines. Almost half could read and write and a few could draw. Although many could recite numbers, only one could do calculations. Conversational speech was recognized in most but it was fragmented with a soft breathless quality. Most had the R133C mutation or C-terminal deletions, usually without favorable XCI skewing.

Studying this interesting group of patients helps to understand the interests, likes, and dislikes of other girls who have RS [98].

Males with Mecp2 mutations

Although RS is an X-linked dominant disease, there is accumulating data on males with *MECP2* mutations, who can be grouped as follows:

Lethal or extremely severe neonatal encephalopathy with microcephaly, profound MR, severe hypotonia, severe feeding difficulties, occasional severe epilepsy, and early death—mainly identified in families with girls who have classic RS, usually with mild mutations [99,100].

Classic Rett-like picture: described in males with 47XXY karyotype or somatic mosaicism for MECP2 mutations causing a "female-like" clinical picture [101,102]. In the Israeli RS clinic, an XXY boy with classic RS features recently was found to have a large MECP2 deletion on one of his X chromosomes using the MLPA technique.

Nonlethal less severe and less specific forms with varied levels of MR and neurologic deficits: spasticity, ataxia, tremor, microcephaly to macrocephaly, and psychiatric disturbances. They usually carry mild *MECP2* mutations that do not cause an RS-like picture in females. Some were identified in families with several affected males termed "X-linked MR" (XLMR families) (syndromic or nonsyndromic).

Several Xq28-linked XLMR (nonsyndromic) families were investigated for *MECP2* mutations. Affected members of three families with variable male phenotypes carried mutations. In one family, patients had severe to mild nonprogressive MR with better motor than verbal skills. In the second family, they showed pyramidal features, essential tremor, and mild nonprogressive MR, with poor coordination and written language difficulties. Articulation difficulties and slightly lower IQ was found in the third family. All mutations were mild (in-frame deletions or missense mutations) [103–105].

Mecp2 mutations in mentally retarded children

Based on the finding of *MECP2* mutations in cases with XLMR, it was decided to extend the investigation to cases with nonspecific MR.

Klauck and colleagues [106] reported that the A140 V mutation was common in mentally retarded males. This finding has not been confirmed by others.

A Spanish group looked at 294 patients (males and females) with normal karyotype and no FMR-1 CGG abnormal repeats (Fragile X). Sixteen showed AS phenotype and 27 were Prader-Willi–like. Six different types of polymorphisms of the *MECP2* sequence were found in 10 patients (several had same polymorphism) - one novel silent change and one pathogenic missense MECP2 mutation in a girl with nonspecific MR (who on further observation showed some Rett-like features). They concluded that routine testing for MECP2 mutations is not warranted in the absence of good clinical indications, such as severe neonatal encephalopathy or Rett-like features [107]. To the contrary, in a female population with MR and even subtle Rett-like features, there is up to a 47% prevalence of *MECP2* mutations [108]. Recently, there have been several descriptions of males with nonsyndromic or syndromic MR, with or without microcephaly and cryptorchidism, with duplications or functional disomy of the Xq28 region. These clinical cases support the assumption, based on previous laboratory findings, that MeCP2 overexpression also is harmful [109,110].

Treatment

Throughout the last 20 years, in addition to symptomatic treatment, there have been several pharmacologic trials based on assumed RS-suspected pathophysiology:

L-Carnitine: suspected secondary mitochondrial deficiencies. Mild and short-lasting symptomatic improvement noticed [111].

Naltrexone - oral opiate antagonist: based on the finding of elevated cerebrospinal fluid (CSF) opioids in RS. Positive effect on breathing dysregulation was observed, followed by enhanced clinical deterioration that prevented further use [112].

Folinic acid: Ramaekers and colleagues [113] reported low CSF folic acid metabolites in four girls with RS, two (mutation negative) improved with oral folinic acid treatment. CSF findings and clinical changes with similar treatment were not confirmed on a larger-scale study and according to our RS clinic experience [114].

Dextromethorphan - an N-methyl-D-aspartic acid (NMDA) blocker: glutaminergic NMDA receptor abnormalities detected on functional brain mapping in patients who had RS; preliminary results showed benefits in epilepsy control and general well-being (S. Naidu, IRSA meeting, personal communication, 2006).

Betaine and folic acid: an effort to increase MeCP2 target genes methylation; no clinical improvement noticed [115].

Several theoretic interventions are suggested based on recent knowledge of pathogenesis, but they should be tried first on the RS mice models:
BDNF-increasing drugs: lithium and other antidepressants [116]
Semax (N-terminal fragment of corticotropin): devoid of hormonal activity, but can increase BDNF and central dopamine release [117]
CRH-blocking agents that reduce anxiety [80]

Until specific mechanism-related interventions can be developed further, treatment will continue to be based on core symptomatology, including epilepsy, spasticity, sleep problems, anxiety and other behavioral difficulties, drooling, gastrointestinal symptoms, and orthopedic interventions. These treatments are combined with a comprehensive nonmedical approach that includes special physiotherapy, and speech, occupational, and music therapy directed toward strengthening the abilities of girls who have RS [11].

References

[1] Rett A. On an unusual brain atrophy syndrome in hyperammonemia in childhood. Wein Med Wochenschr 1966;116(37):723–6.
[2] Hagberg B, Aicardi J, Dias K, et al. A progressive syndrome of autism, dementia, ataxia, and loss of purposeful hand use in girls: Rett syndrome: report of 35 cases. Ann Neurol 1983;14(4):471–9.
[3] Percy AK. Rett syndrome: current status and new vistas. Neurol Clin 2002;20(4):1125–41.

[4] Hagberg B, Goutieres F, Hanefeld F, et al. Rett syndrome: criteria for inclusion and exclusion. Brain Dev 1985;7(3):372–3.

[5] Hagberg B, Hanefeld F, Percy A, et al. An update on clinically applicable diagnostic criteria in Rett syndrome. Comments to RS clinical criteria consensus panel satellite to European Pediatric Neurology Society Meeting, Baden, Baden, Germany 2001. Eur J Ped Neurol 2002;6:293–7.

[6] Hagberg B. Rett syndrome: clinical and biological aspects. London: McKeith Press; 1992.

[7] Witt-Engerstrom I. Age related occurrence of signs and symptoms in the Rett syndrome. Brain Dev 1992;14:S11–20.

[8] Glase DG, Schultz RJ, Frost JD. Rett syndrome: characterization of seizures versus non-seizures. Electroencephalogr Clin Neurophisiol 1998;106:79–83.

[9] Julu PO, Kerr AM, Apartopoulos F, et al. Characterization of breathing and associated central autonomic dysfunction in the Rett disorder. Arch Dis Child 2001;85:29–37.

[10] Lotan M, Roth D. The effect of hand vibrators on the hand stereotypes and function in Rett syndrome– two case studies. Israel Physiotherapy 1996;52:23–6.

[11] Lotan M, Ben-Zeev B. Rett syndrome: a review with emphasis on clinical characteristics and intervention. Phram World Sci 2006;6:1517–41.

[12] Nomura Y. Early behavior characteristics and sleep disturbances in Rett syndrome. Brain Dev 2005;27:S35–42.

[13] Piazza CC, Fisher W, Kiesewetter BS, et al. Aberrant sleep patterns in children with Rett syndrome. Brain Dev 1990;2:488–93.

[14] Uchino J, Suzuki M, Hoshino K, et al. Development of language in Rett syndrome. Brain Dev 2001;23:S233–5.

[15] Lavas J, Slotte A, Jochym-Nygren M, et al. Communication and eating proficiency in 125 girls with Rett syndrome: the Swedish Rett Centre Survey. Disabil Rehabil 2006;28(20): 1267–79.

[16] Leonard H, Fyfe S, Leonard S, et al. Functional status, medical impairment and rehabilitation resources in 84 females with Rett syndrome: a snapshot across the world from a parental perspective. Disabil Rehabil 2001;23:107–17.

[17] Baptista PM, Mercadante MT, Macedo EC, et al. Cognitive performance in Rett syndrome girls: a pilot study using eye tracking technology. J Intellect Disabil Res 2006;50(9):662–6.

[18] Sekul EA, Moak JP, Scultz RJ, et al. Electrocardiographic findings in Rett syndrome; an explanation for sudden death? J Pediatr 1994;125:80–2.

[19] Byard RW. Forensic issues and possible mechanisms of sudden death in Rett syndrome. J Clin Forensic Med 2006;13(2):96–9.

[20] Kerr AM, Montague J, Stephenson JB. The hands and the mind—"pre—and post regression" in Rett syndrome. Brain Dev 1987;9(5):487–90.

[21] Heilstedt HA, Shabbazian MD, Lee B. Infantile hypotonia as a presentation of Rett syndrome. Am J Med Genet 2002;111:238–42.

[22] Kerr AM. Early clinical signs in the Rett disorder. Neuropediatrics 1995;26:67–71.

[23] Leonard H, Bower C. Is the girl with RS normal at birth? Dev Med Child Neurol 1998;40: 115–21.

[24] Leonard H, Moore H, Carey M, et al. Genotype and early development in Rett syndrome; the value of international data. Brain Dev 2005;27(Suppl 11):S59–68.

[25] Hagberg B, Gillberg C. Rett Variants– rettoid phenotypes. In: Hagberg B, Anvert M, Wahlstrom J, editors. Rett syndrome- clinical and biological aspects. London: MacKeith Press; 1993. p. 40–60.

[26] Evans JC, Archer HL, Colley JP, et al. Early onset seizures and Rett like features associated with mutations in CDKL5. Eur J Hum Genet 2005;13:1113–20.

[27] Auranen M, Vanahala R, Vosman M, et al. MECP2 gene analysis in classical RS and in patients with Rett like features. Neurology 2001;56:611–7.

[28] Hoffbuhr K, Devaney JM, La Fleur B, et al. MECP2 mutations in children with and without the phenotype of Rett syndrome. Neurology 2001;56:1486–95.

[29] Sirianni N, Naidu S, Pereira J. Rett syndrome: confirmation of X-linked dominant inheritance, and localization of the gene to Xq28. Am J Hum Genet 1998;63:1552–8.

[30] Amir RE, Van Den Veyver IB, Wan B, et al. Rett syndrome is caused by mutations in X-linked MECP2, encoding methyl CpG-binding protein 2. Nat Genet 1999;23:185–8.

[31] Mnatzakanian GN, Lohi H, Munteanu I, et al. A previously unidentified MECP2 open reading frame defines a new protein isoform relevant to Rett syndrome. Nat Genet 2004; 36:339–41.

[32] Nan X, Ng HH, Johnson C, et al. Transcriptional repression by the methyl CpG binding protein MeCP2 involved an histone deacetylase complex. Nature 2004;393:386–9.

[33] Nan X, Campoy FJ, Bird A. MeCP2 is a transcriptional repressor with abundant binding sites in genomic chromatin. Cell 1997;88:471–81.

[34] Nan X, Tate P, Li E, et al. DNA methylation specifies chromosomal localization of MECP2. Mol Cell Biol 1996;16(1):414–21.

[35] Kimura H, Shiota K. Methyl CpG binding protein MeCP2 is a target molecule for maintenance DNA methyltransferase, Dnmt1. J Biol Chem 2003;278:4806–12.

[36] Harikrishnan KN, Chow MZ, Baker EK, et al. Brahma links to SW1/SNF chromatin remodeling complex with MeCP2 dependant transcriptional silencing. Nat Genet 2005; 37:254–64.

[37] Girard M, Couvert P, Carric A, et al. Parental origin of de novo MECP2 mutations in Rett syndrome. Eur J Hum Genet 2001;9:231–6.

[38] Wam M, Lee SS, Zhang X. Rett syndrome and beyond: recurrent spontaneous and familial MECP2 mutations at CpG hotspots. Am J Hum Genet 1999;65:1520–9.

[39] Lee SS, Wam M, Francke U. Spectrum of MECP2 mutations in Rett syndrome. Brain Dev 2001;23(Suppl 11):S138–43.

[40] Philippe C, Villard L, De Roux N, et al. Spectrum and distribution of MECP2 mutations in 424 Rett syndrome patients: a molecular update. Eur J Med Genet 2006;49:9–18.

[41] Ravn K, Nielsen JB, Skjeldal OH, et al. Large genomic rearrangements in MECP2. Hum Mutat 2005;25(3):324–6.

[42] Harvey CG, Menon SD, Stacchowiak B, et al. Sequence variants within exon 1 of MECP2 occur in females with mental retardation. Am J Med Genet B Neuropsychiatr Genet 2005;144(3):355–60.

[43] Petel-Galil Y, Ben-Zeev B, Greenbaum I, et al. Comprehensive diagnosis of Rett syndrome relying on genetic, epigenetic and expression evidence of deficiency of the methyl—CpG-binding protein 2 gene: study of a cohort of Israeli patients. J Med Genet 2006;43(12): e56–63.

[44] Cheadle JO, Gill H, Fleming M, et al. Long reading sequence analysis of the MECP2 gene in Rett syndrome patients; correlation of disease severity with mutation type and location. Hum Mol Genet 2000;9(7):1119–29.

[45] Charman T, Neilson TCS, Mash V, et al. Dimensional phenotypic analysis and functional categorization of mutations reveal novel genotype-phenotype associations in Rett syndrome. Eur J Hum Genet 2005;13:1121–30.

[46] Huppke P, Held M, Hanefeld F, et al. Influence of mutation type and location on phenotype in 123 patients with Rett syndrome. Neuropediatrics 2002;33(2):63–8.

[47] Ishii T, Makita Y, Ogawa A, et al. The role of different X-inactivation pattern on the variable clinical phenotype with Rett syndrome. Brain Dev 2001;223:S161–4.

[48] Gibson JHY, Williamson SL, Arbuckle S, et al. X chromosome inactivation patterns in brain in Rett syndrome: implications for the disease phenotype. Brain Dev 2005;27: 266–70.

[49] Young JI, Zoghbi HY. X chromosome inactivation patterns are unbalanced and affect the phenotype outcome in a mouse model of Rett syndrome. Am J Hum Genet 2004;74:511–20.

[50] Archer H, Evans J, Leonard H, et al. Correlation between clinical severity in Rett syndrome patients with a R168X or T158 M MECP2 mutations and the direction and degree of skewing of X chromosome inactivation. J Med Genet 2006;44(2):148–52.

[51] Huppke P, Maier EM, Warnke A, et al. Very mild cases of Rett syndrome with skewed X inactivation. J Med Genet 2006;43:814–6.

[52] Chen RZ, Akbarian S, Tudor M, et al. Deficiency of methyl CpG binding protein-2 in CNS neurons results in Rett like phenotype in mice. Nat Genet 2001;27:327–31.

[53] Shabbazian M, Young J, Yuva-Paylor L, et al. Mice with truncated MECP2 recapitulate many Rett syndrome features and display hyperacetylation of histone H3. Neuron 2002; 35:243–54.

[54] Moretti P, Bouwknecht JA, Teague R, et al. Abnormalities of social interactions and home cage behavior in a mouse model of Rett syndrome. Hum Mol Genet 2005;14:205–20.

[55] Luikenhuis S, Giacometti E, Beard C, et al. Expression of MECP2 in post mitotic neurons rescues Rett syndrome in mice. Proc Natl Acad Sci U S A 2004;101:6033–8.

[56] Collins AL, Levenson JM, Vilaythong AP, et al. Mild overexpression of MECP2 causes a progressive neurological disorder in mice. Hum Mol Genet 2004;13:2679–89.

[57] LaSalle JM, Hogart A, Thatcher N. Rett syndrome: a Rosetta stone for understanding the molecular pathogenesis of autism. Int Rev Neurobiol 2005;7:131–65.

[58] Miller G. Getting a read on Rett syndrome. Science 2006;314:1536–7.

[59] Reichwald K, These J, Winches T, et al. Comparative sequence analysis of the MECP2 locus in human and mouse reveals new transcribed regions. Mamm Genome 2000;11: 182–90.

[60] Shahbazian MD, Antalffy B, Armstrong D, et al. Insights into Rett syndrome: MeCP2 levels display tissue and cell specific differences and correlate with neuronal maturation. Hum Mol Genet 2002;11:115–24.

[61] Kishi N, Macklis JD. MECP2 is progressively expressed in post-migratory neurons and is involved in neuronal maturation rather than cell fate decisions. Mol Cell Neurosci 2004;27: 306–21.

[62] Neul JL, Zoghbi HY. Rett syndrome: a prototypical neurodevelopmental disorder. Neuroscientist 2004;10(2):118–28.

[63] Subramaniam B, Naidu S, Reiss AL. Neuroanatomy in Rett syndrome: cerebral cortex and posterior fossa. Neurology 1997;48:399–407.

[64] Armstrong D, Dunn JK, Antalffy B, et al. Selective dendritic alterations in the cortex of Rett syndrome. J Neuropathol Exp Neurol 1995;54:195–201.

[65] Kishi N, Macklis JD. Dissecting MECP2 function in the central nervous system. J Child Neurol 2005;20:753–9.

[66] Braunschweig D, Simcox T, Samaco RC, et al. X-chromosome inactivation ratios affect MECP2 wild type expression within mosaic Rett syndrome and Mecp2-/+ mouse brain. Hum Mol Genet 2004;13:1275–86.

[67] Kaufmann WE, Naidu S, Budden S. Abnormal expression of microtubule associated protein 2 in the neo-cortex of Rett syndrome. Neuropediatrics 1995;26:109–13.

[68] Kaufmann WE, Worley PF, Taylor CV, et al. Cyclo-oxygenase 2 expression during rat neocortical development and in Rett syndrome. Brain Dev 1997;19:25–34.

[69] Casanova MF, Buxhocveden DP, Switala A, et al. Rett syndrome as a minicolumnopathy. Clin Neuropathol 2003;22:163–8.

[70] Kauffman WE. Cortical development in Rett syndrome: molecular, neurochemical and anatomical aspects. In: Kerr AM, Engerstrom W, editors. Rett disorder and the developing brain. England: Oxford University Press; 2001. p. 85–110.

[71] Armstrong DD. Neuropathology of Rett syndrome. Ment Retard Dev Disabil Res Rev 2002;8:72–6.

[72] Clanton C, Jean OH, Hyder K, et al. Gene expression profiling in post-mortem Rett syndrome brains: differential gene expression and patient classification. Neurobiol Dis 2001;8:847–65.

[73] Tudor M, Akbarian S, Chen RZ, et al. Transcriptional profiling of a mouse model for Rett syndrome reveals subtle transcriptional changes in the brain. Proc Natl Acad Sci U S A 2002;99:15536–41.

[74] Chen WG, Chang Q, Lin Y. Depression of BDNF transcription involves calcium dependant phosphorylation of MeCP2. Science 2003;202:885–9.
[75] Martinowich K, Hattori D, Wu H. DNA methylation related chromatin remodeling in activity dependant BDNF gene regulation. Science 2003;202:890–3.
[76] Kaufmann WE, Johnston MV, Blue ME. MeCP2 expression and function during brain development: implications for Rett syndrome's pathogenesis and clinical evolution. Brain Dev 2005;27:S77–87.
[77] Stuhmer T, Anderson SA, Ekker M, et al. Ectopic expression of the Dlx genes induced glutamic acid decarboxylase and Dlx expression. Development 2002;129:245–52.
[78] Horike S, Cai S, Myano M. Loss of silent chromatin looping and impaired imprinting of DLX5 in Rett syndrome. Nat Genet 2005;37:31–40.
[79] Samaco RC, Nagarajan RP, Braunschweig D, et al. Multiple pathways regulate MeCP2 expression in normal brain development and exhibit defects in autism spectrum disorders. Hum Mol Genet 2004;13(6):629–39.
[80] McGill BE, Bundle SF, Yayalaoglu MB, et al. Enhanced anxiety and stress induced corticosterone release are associated with increased CRH expression in a mouse model of Rett syndrome. Proc Natl Acad Sci U S A 2006;103:18267–72.
[81] Ollsen B, Rett A. Autism and RS behavioral investigations and differential diagnosis. Dev Med Child Neurol 1987;29:429–41.
[82] Gilberg C. Autistic symptoms in RS. The first two years according to mother reports. Brain Dev 1987;9:499–501.
[83] Mount R, Hastings R, Reilly P, et al. Towards a behavioral phenotype of RS. Am J Ment Retard 2003;108:1–12.
[84] Mount RH, Charman T, Hastings RP, et al. Features of autism in RS and severe mental retardation. J Autism Dev Discord 2003;33(4):435–42.
[85] Kemper TL, Bauman M. Neuropathology of infantile autism. J Neuropathol Exp Neurol 1998;57:645–52.
[86] Polleux F, Lauder JM. Towards a developmental neurobiology of autism. Ment Retard Dev Disabil Res Rev 2004;10:303–17.
[87] Schanen NC. Epigenetics of autism spectrum disorders. Hum Mol Genet 2006;15:138–50.
[88] Samaco RC, Hogart A, LaSalle J. Epigenetic overlap in autism-spectrum neurodevelopmental disorders: MECP2 deficiency causes reduced expression of UBE3A and GABRB3. Hum Mol Gen 2005;14(4):483–92.
[89] Vourch P, Bienvenue T, Beldjord C, et al. No mutations in the coding region of RS gene MECP2 in 59 autistic patients. Eur J Hum Genet 2001;9:556–8.
[90] Beyer KS, Blasi F, Bachelli E, et al. Mutation analysis of the coding sequence of the MECP2 gene in infantile autism. Hum Gen 2002;111:305–9.
[91] Carney RM, Wolpeert CM, Ravan SA, et al. Identification of MECP2 mutations in a series of females with autistic disorder. Ped Neurol 2003;28(3):205–11.
[92] Zappella M, Meloni I, Longo I, et al. Study of MECP2 gene in Rett syndrome variants and autistic girls. Am J Med Genet B Neuropsychiatr Genet 2003;119:102–7.
[93] Lobo-Menendez F, Sossey-Alaoui K, Bell JM, et al. Absence of MECP2 mutations in patients from the South Carolina autism project. Am J Med Genet B Neuropsychiatr Genet 2003;117:97–101.
[94] Shibayama A, Cook EH, Feng J, et al. MECP2 structural and 3'UTR variants in schizophrenia, autism and other psychiatric disturbances a possible association with autism. Am J Med Genet B Neuropsychiatr Genet 2004;128:50–3.
[95] Zappella M. The Rett girls with preserved speech. Brain Dev 1992;14:98–101.
[96] Zappella M, Gilberg C, Ehlers S. The preserved speech variant: a subgroup of Rett complex: a clinical report of 30 cases. J Autism Dev Discord 1998;928:519–26.
[97] Zappella M, Meloni I, Longo I, et al. Preserved speech variants of Rett syndrome. Am J Med Genet 2001;104:14–22.

[98] Kerr AM, Archer HL, Evans JC, et al. People with MECP2 mutation-positive Rett disorder who converse. J Intellect Disabil Res 2005;50(5):386–94.

[99] Villard L, Kpebe A, Cardoso C, et al. Two affected boys in Rett syndrome family: clinical and molecular findings. Neurology 2000;55:1188–93.

[100] Zeev BB, Yaron Y, Schanen C, et al. Rett syndrome: clinical manifestations in males with MECP2 mutations. J Child Neurol 2000;217:20–4.

[101] Leonard H, Silberstein J, Falk R, et al. Occurrence of Rett syndrome in boys. J Child Neurol 2001;16:333–8.

[102] Schwartzman JS, Bernardino A, Nishimura A, et al. Rett syndrome in a boy with 47 XXY karyotype confirmed by a rare mutation in the MECP2 gene. Neuropediatrics 2001;32: 162–4.

[103] Meloni I, Bruttini M, Longo I, et al. A mutation in the Rett syndrome gene, MECP2, causes X-linked mental retardation and progressive spasticity in males. Am J Hum Genet 2000;67: 982–5.

[104] Orrico A, Lam CW, Galli L, et al. MECP2 mutations in male patients with non-specific XLMR. FEBS Lett 2000;481:285–8.

[105] Gomet M, Gendrot C, Verloes A, et al. MECP2 gene mutations in non syndromic XLMR: phenotype-genotype correlations. Am J Med Genet A 2003;123:129–39.

[106] Klauck SM, Lindsay S, Beyer KS, et al. A mutation hot spot for non specific XLMR in males. Eur J Hum Genet 2005;13:523–4.

[107] Tejada MI, Penagarikano O, Rodrigues- Revenga L, et al. Screening for MECP2 mutations in Spanish patients with an unexplained mental retardation. J Med Genet 2006;70:140–4.

[108] Kammoun F, De Roux N, Boespflug Tanguy O. Screening of MECP2 coding sequence in patients with phenotypes of decreasing likelihood for Rett syndrome. A cohort of 171 cases. J Med Genet 2004;41:1–7.

[109] Lachlan KL, Collinson MN, Sanford ROC, et al. Functional disomy resulting from duplication of distal Xq in four unrelated patients. Hum Genet 2004;115:399–408.

[110] Meins M, Lehmann J, Gerresheim F. Submicroscopic duplication in Xq28 causes increased expression of MECP2 gene in a boy with severe mental retardation and feature of RS. J Med Genet 2005;42:e12–7.

[111] Ellaway C, Williams K, Leonard H, et al. Rett syndrome: randomized controlled trial of L-carnitine. J Child Neurol 1999;14:162–7.

[112] Percy AK, Glaze DG, Schultz RJ, et al. Rett syndrome: controlled trial of an oral opiate antagonist, Naltrexone. Ann Neurol 1994;35:464–70.

[113] Ramaekeres VT, Hansen SI, Holm J. Reduced folate transport to the CNS in female Rett patients. Neurology 2003;61:506–15.

[114] Neul JL, Maricich SM, Islam M. Spinal fluid 5 MTHF are normal in Rett syndrome. Neurology 2005;64:2151–2.

[115] Percy AK, Lane JB. Rett syndrome: model for neurodevelopmental disorders. J Child Neurol 2005;20(9):718–21.

[116] Tsai SJ. Lithium and antidepressant: potential agents for the treatment of Rett syndrome. Med Hypotheses 2006;67(3):626–9.

[117] Tsai SJ. Semax, an analogue of adrenocorticotropin (4–10), is a potential agent for the treatment of attention-deficit hyperactivity disorder and Rett syndrome. Med Hypotheses 2006; 68(5):1144–6.

ELSEVIER
SAUNDERS

Child Adolesc Psychiatric Clin N Am
16 (2007) 745–749

CHILD AND
ADOLESCENT
PSYCHIATRIC CLINICS
OF NORTH AMERICA

Index

Note: Page numbers of article titles are in **boldface** type.